PATHWAYS TO WELL-I DESIGN

How can we achieve and promote well-being? Drawing on examples from the arts, humanities and design, this book brings together work from a wide range of areas to reveal the unique ways in which different disciplines approach the universal goal of supporting well-being.

Pathways to Well-Being in Design recognises that the distinction between academics and practitioners often becomes blurred, where, when working together, a fusion of thoughts and ideas takes place and provides a powerful platform for dialogue.

Providing new insights into the approaches and issues associated with promoting well-being, the book's multidisciplinary coverage invites readers to consider these ideas within the framework of their own work.

The book's 12 chapters are authored by academics who are involved in practice or are working with practitioners and features real world case studies which cover a range of situations, circumstances, environments and social groups.

Pathways to Well-Being in Design responds to those wishing to enquire further about well-being, taking the reader through different circumstances to consider approaches, discussing practice and theory, real world and virtual world considerations.

This book is essential reading for anyone seeking to understand well-being, including students and professionals in architecture, landscape architecture, urban planning, design and health sciences.

Richard Coles is Emeritus Professor of Landscape in the Birmingham School of Architecture and Design, based in the Faculty of the Arts, Design and Media, Birmingham City University, UK. His research involves understanding the nature of environmental interaction and the development of environments that are supportive of the needs of users.

Sandra Costa is a Researcher and Lecturer in Landscape Architecture at the Birmingham School of Architecture and Design, Birmingham City University, UK. Her research examines the nature of person–place interactions, exploring the choreographies of the experience and how individuals negotiate well-being. She received her PhD from Birmingham City University researching immersive walking techniques involving self-narrated walking.

Sharon Watson is a Landscape Architect focusing on aspects of community engagement and research involving children. She has extensive experience of working with schools and the educational sector, where she has developed sophisticated child-centric methodologies involving the use of digital media. Her current research involves working with children in investigating their responses to the natural world and the different agencies offered by current technology, focusing on the wild places that exist in urban situations. She holds a PhD from Birmingham City University, UK.

PATHWAYS TO WELL-BEING IN DESIGN

Examples from the Arts, Humanities and the Built Environment

Edited by Richard Coles, Sandra Costa and Sharon Watson

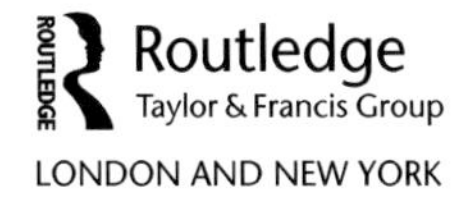

LONDON AND NEW YORK

First edition published 2019
by Routledge
2 Park Square, Milton Park, Abingdon, Oxon, OX14 4RN

and by Routledge
711 Third Avenue, New York, NY 10017

Routledge is an imprint of the Taylor & Francis Group, an informa business

British Library Cataloguing-in-Publication Data
A catalogue record for this book is available from the British Library

Library of Congress Cataloging-in-Publication Data
Names: Coles, Richard, 1949- editor.
Title: Pathways to well-being in design : examples from the arts, humanities and the built environment / edited by Richard Coles, Sandra Costa and Sharon Watson.
Description: First edition. | New York : Routledge, 2019. | Includes bibliographical references and index.
Identifiers: LCCN 2018027452| ISBN 9780815346944 (hb : alk. paper) | ISBN 9780815346951 (pb : alk. paper) | ISBN 9781351170048 (ebook)
Subjects: LCSH: Design—Human factors. | Well-being.
Classification: LCC NK1520 .P38 2019 | DDC 745.4—dc23
LC record available at https://lccn.loc.gov/2018027452

ISBN: 978-0-815-34694-4 (hbk)
ISBN: 978-0-815-34695-1 (pbk)
ISBN: 978-1-351-17004-8 (ebk)

Typeset in Bembo
by Swales & Willis Ltd, Exeter, Devon, UK

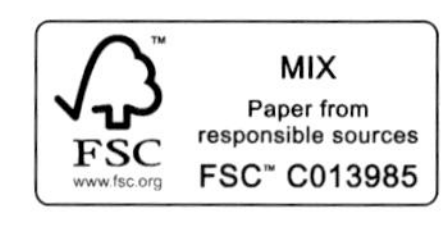

Printed in the United Kingdom
by Henry Ling Limited

CONTENTS

FIGURES

Cover image: Eastside City Park, Birmingham, UK © Sandra Costa

CONTRIBUTORS

Saamah Abdallah is a Freelance Well-Being Expert who previously worked as a Senior Researcher at the Centre for Well-being at the New Economics Foundation. He is currently focusing on well-being in local policy and in the workplace.

Darren Awang works in the Faculty of Health and Life Sciences at Coventry University. He is an Occupational Therapist teaching and undertaking research in SMART homes, assistive technology and Service Design.

Veronica Barry has over 20 years' experience in urban agriculture, community gardening and local food schemes focusing on public health, community planning, regularly speaking at conferences and public events. She is currently researching the role of food and food growing within healthy planning at the School of the Built Environment, Birmingham City University, UK.

Chris Blythe is the Director of the Federation of City Farms and Community Gardens (FCFCG), recently leading the successful merger with Care Farming UK to create a new organisation with communities and "green care" at its heart. Before joining FCFCG, Chris was Operations Leader for the Conservation Volunteers in Birmingham and the West Midlands managing the Health for Life in the Community Programme.

Elizabeth Freeman Calabrese is a Licensed Architect, Global Affiliate for the Gund Institute for Environment at the University of Vermont and is a leading educator of Biophilic Design. She encourages the holistic integration of natural systems and processes into the design process to promote both human and environmental health and well-being.

Richard Coles is Emeritus Professor of Landscape in the Birmingham School of Architecture and Design, based in the Faculty of the Arts, Design and Media, Birmingham City University, UK. His research involves understanding the nature of environmental interaction and the development of environments that are supportive of the needs of users.

Sandra Costa (PhD) is a Landscape Architect currently lecturing at the Birmingham School of Architecture and Design, Birmingham City University, UK. Her research involves user-based perceptions of the environment, examining the choreographies of interaction and innovative methodologies involving narratives and immersive walking.

Haydn Davies is Professor of Law and Head of the School of Law at Birmingham City University, currently Vice Chair of the UK Environmental Law Association and a former Co-Convenor of the Welsh Working Party. His research encompasses environmental justice, human rights, environmental protection and climate change law.

Alice Dommert is founder of Prasada: Wholebeing@Work, a Licensed Architect, Exhibit Designer, Writer and Speaker. Prasada helps HR, professional and executive teams within organisations across the United States with a holistic approach to planning and implementing policies, wellness and leadership development programmes and the design of the workplace to cohesively support employee engagement, productivity and wholebeing.

Owen Douglas is a Post-Doctoral Research Fellow in the School of Architecture, Planning and Environmental Policy at University College Dublin. He holds a BA (Mod) in Economic and Social Studies and is a Qualified Planner. His research explores spatial planning, sustainable development and population health and well-being.

Jac Fennell is a Research Assistant on the Ludic Artefacts Using Gesture and Haptics (LAUGH) Project University of Cardiff School of Art & Design. She has experience as an Interaction Designer and User Experience Consultant for multi-national companies. Her PhD focused on chance memories and supporting involuntary reminiscence by design.

Mirko Guaralda is Senior Lecturer in Architecture at Queensland University of Technology, Australia. Dr Guaralda has been working in industry and local government; he has been involved in a wide range of projects at different scales, from small dwellings and gardens, to new estates and urban strategic planning.

Nikki Holliday is a Researcher at the Centre for Innovative Research Across the Life Course, Coventry University, specialising in informing assistive technology product and Service Design through user-centred techniques. She has extensive research experience with service users and providers working on nationally funded projects.

Esther Johnson (MA, RCA) is Professor of Film and Media Arts at Sheffield Hallam University. Her documentary portraits focus on marginal worlds to reveal resonant stories that may otherwise remain hidden or ignored. Themes include personal histories, testimony, heritage, folklore, architectural vernaculars and the inhabited environment. She exhibits internationally, and broadcasts on the BBC, Channel 4, ABC Australia, Resonance FM and RTÉ radio (blanchepictures.com).

Gail Kenning is Honorary Reader in Design for Ageing and Dementia at the Centre for Applied Research in Inclusive Arts and Design (CARIAD), Cardiff Metropolitan University, a Researcher at University of Technology Sydney and Co-Investigator on the LAUGH Project. Her research is concerned with art and creativity in relation to digital media, craft, textiles, health, well-being, ageing and dementia.

Mick Lennon is a Lecturer in Planning and Environmental Policy in the School of Architecture, Planning and Environmental Policy at University College, Dublin. His research interests include the planning of salutogenic environments, green infrastructure and sustainable development.

Gill Main (PhD) is Associate Professor in the School of Education, University of Leeds. Research interests include child and youth poverty, social exclusion and well-being.

Amrit Phull is an Architectural Designer and Writer based in Toronto. Her research focuses on an ethical and culturally-aware practice of engaging with communities in the Canadian landscape, particularly in remote, subarctic Canada. She is a contributing editor of SITE Magazine.

Larissa Pople is Senior Researcher at The Children's Society, leading on well-being where she has co-authored a series of *Good Childhood Reports* and local area studies of well-being. She previously worked for UNICEF and the Independent Commission on Youth Crime and Anti-Social Behaviour.

David Prytherch is Senior Research Fellow in the Faculty of Arts & Humanities, Coventry University investigating non-pharmacological interventions for people with dementia, based on perceptual theories of intrinsic haptic reward and neuro-cognitive calming, he is Co-Investigator on the LAUGH Project.

Gwyther Rees is Associate Research Fellow in the Department of Social Policy and Social Work, University of York. He is Research Director for the Children's Worlds Project. Previously he was Research Director for The Children's Society.

Sukanlaya Sawang is an Organisational Psychologist with wide-ranging experience from Australia, the USA, the UK and Thailand, she is currently appointed as Associate Professor in Technology and Innovation at University of Leicester; Visiting Professor in Small Business Innovation and Well-being at the International Centre for Transformational Entrepreneurship, Coventry University, also Adjunct Professor at QUT Business School, Australia.

Mark Scott is Professor of Planning in the School of Architecture, Planning and Environmental Policy at University College Dublin with research interests spanning green infrastructure, ecosystem approaches in spatial planning, greenspaces and health.

John Sparrow is Professor of Occupational Psychology at Birmingham City University and Director of Visualsolve Ltd. He is a registered Practitioner Psychologist within the UK Health and Care Professional Council, a Chartered Psychologist, an Associate Fellow of the British Psychological Society and an Associate of the Institute of Reflective Practice.

Cathy Treadaway is Professor of Creative Practice at Cardiff Metropolitan University and a founder member of the CARIAD. She is Principal Investigator on the Arts and Humanities Research Council LAUGH international design for dementia research project and where she has developed the approach of Compassionate Design.

Andy Walters is Professor and Director of Research at PDR-International Centre for Design and Research located at Cardiff Metropolitan University and a founding member of the User-Centric Design Group.

Gillian Ward is Visiting Research Professor at the Faculty of Health & Life Sciences Coventry University. She is an Occupational Therapist undertaking research in assistive technology with particular focus on supporting older people and those with long-term conditions.

Sharon Watson is a Landscape Architect focusing on aspects of community engagement and research involving children. She has extensive experience of working with schools and the educational sector, where she has developed sophisticated child-centric methodologies involving the use of digital media. She holds a PhD which examined children's perceptions of nature.

INTRODUCTION

In this book we consider experiences and pathways to well-being that reveal unique accounts of the ways in which disciplines across the arts, humanities and design spectra approach the universal goal of supporting and underpinning the achievement of well-being. The work is presented through a series of chapters aiming to inform a wide audience of the initiatives being developed across these fields concerning the practice of "supporting well-being" and the scenarios surrounding their actions and responses. It recognises that, while there is a large body of work focused on well-being, both practice and research, details or the results of such are widely scattered through a range of media, not being easily accessible to scholars and practitioners. Accordingly, this volume addresses the need to bring such work together through the careful selection of material that considers the range of approaches and the underpinning knowledge essential for a fuller understanding.

Within the field of the arts, humanities and design, the distinction between the "academic" and the "practitioner" often becomes blurred; working together, a fusion of thinking takes place, with ideas explored through practitioner interventions supported by academic theory. The high value of this approach is recognised by the editors of this volume in providing a platform for cross-disciplinary dialogue which has resulted in a unique series of explorations that now form the basis of this book. These offer new insights regarding how "we", in promoting well-being, understand and approach the issues involved. We continue to be excited by the insights that these investigations offer, the new knowledge streams, including the "real world" context of the case studies, how they cross disciplines, address different circumstances and how they reference place and people's voices. In putting this book together, we hope to further encourage such dialogue.

Chapters are developed by leading academics typically involved in practice or working with practitioners. Each chapter is located within its own disciplinary/practitioner framework to present a complete niche of investigation and area of enquiry in their own right, where the impact/results are fully explored and assessed. Notwithstanding, the synergies between chapters are strong, with material applicable to a broad audience, comprehensively underpinned by theory and capable of wide application across disciplines. Accordingly, as a collaboration between academics and professionals it crosses academic divides to present a combination of diverse work which is highly relevant to a wide range of disciplines and varying circumstances. References allow the reader to follow up these aspects in the knowledge that approaches are producing effective solutions for supporting well-being and are increasing being explained by underpinning theory to which authors refer.

Many, if not all, developed countries are looking for ways to address the well-being agenda. Internationally, academics and practitioners are examining these approaches where there is growing interest in alternatives to strictly clinical models. Specifically, the book targets well-being in the context of the built environment; several authors in this book comment on issues and implications of living in urban environments and the direction that urban development is taking, typically allied to ideas of sustainable or liveable cities and growing knowledge of the problems that affect society. Accordingly, chapter authors are drawn from a range of countries, while supporting literature is drawn from international sources.

The move towards well-being

In seeking to define well-being, Huppert and So (2013, p.2) equate well-being with the concept of flourishing – "the experience of life going well . . . feeling good and functioning effectively".

Recent years have seen a substantial increase in understanding how well-being is compromised, supported, or might be supported in the planning and design of modern urban environments, with calls for the achievement of well-being to be embedded as a universal goal of society and for countries to adopt measures to support their citizens.

> Governments around the World are recognising the importance of measuring subjective well-being as a measure of progress.
>
> *(Huppert & So, 2013, p.1)*

For example, in equating happiness with well-being, a series of *World Happiness Reports* have been produced by the United Nations which ranks 155 countries by their happiness levels (Helliwell et al., 2017). These reports are critical of the ways in which we measure social progress and goals and suggest that "happiness is increasingly considered the proper measure of social progress" (Helliwell et al., 2017, p.3). This is further emphasised by the OECD who is committing itself to "redefine the growth narrative to put people's well-being at the centre of governments' effort" (OECD, 2016, p.12).

The 2017 report also quotes the head of the UN Development Program (UNDP) who at the time spoke about the "tyranny of GDP arguing that what matters is the quality of growth" (Helliwell et al., 2017, p.3). The report further explains that:

> GDP relates to the economic side of life, and to just one dimension – the output of goods and services. Subjective well-being, in contrast is a comprehensive measure of individual well-being, taking account of the variety of economic and non-economic concerns and aspirations that determine people's well-being.
>
> *(Helliwell et al., 2017, p.4).*

So well-being is increasingly promoted and understood as the proper consideration of social progress and individual governments are responding accordingly. Here in the UK, the Office for National Statistics (ONS) now collects and publishes data about well-being to stand alongside other measures of growth and has established a "National Well-Being Wheel of Measure" which is comprehensive and includes individual well-being and ratings of the quality of family life among other measures (www.ons.gov.uk/peoplepopulationandcommunity/wellbeing).

However, it would be incorrect and unfair to give the impression that well-being has been neglected by professionals and individuals, this has been far from the case, as the chapters that follow will demonstrate. There has been a groundswell of professional interest across different sectors that demonstrates how sophisticated our understanding of well-being is becoming, especially through practice and the examination of the life experience of individuals in their everyday activities, including health sectors. The range of initiatives, the disciplines involved, their remits and approaches, serve to identify and define the various dimensions of well-being in real world contexts and situations that really do make a difference. As the range of backgrounds of the chapter authors demonstrates, this is not restricted to any one profession but embraces many, especially those who are responsible for the design of the built environment and thus determine the quality of spaces and places where we work and live.

In this context, we have, in the past, used the term "multi-dimensions of well-being", by which we mean (i) the different parameters that are identified by different disciplines in its support, and (ii) the experiences or circumstances which underpin an individual's well-being, i.e. support an individual in the way that they function (function effectively) and how they feel (feel good). Accordingly, we have considered a wide range of approaches taken by professionals and academics in their investigation or application of their skills regarding this overall paradigm of supporting well-being. These dimensions are further defined by (iii) the nature of the interaction, the circumstances surrounding it, the environmental context (Costa et al., 2014), its qualities and of course life factors including life stages (Huppert & So, 2013; Coles & Millman, 2013). We feel that they must be explored by different disciplines who target or define a dimension according to their professional experience. Combining these different perspectives together thus gives us the multi-dimensions where we find substantial reinforcement of ideas, common and complementary findings and concepts which provide substantial new knowledge.

Co-creating pathways to well-being

In 2011 we initiated a series of cross-disciplinary conferences exploring these different aspects and in particular the disciplines comprising the arts, humanities and design (Coles & Millman, 2013, 2016). Our experience at these events has defined our approach to this book in presenting a range of material to demonstrate different frameworks and theory. It is specifically guided by the need to explore the development of opportunities which support the individual and thus which form a potential pathway to well-being in ways that they are meaningful to the individual; it is critical that such pathways are accessible and reflect the reality of modern life.

In considering pathways to well-being, we need to examine:

- How well-being is enacted in everyday events in un-staged encounters, exercised, devised and practised with key facilitators.
- How positive encounters are or might be embedded in our contact with the environments where we live, learn, play or work.
- How individuals are supported in ways that enables them to take control of their personal well-being.
- What constitutes a pathway or a positive encounter.
- How the impacts are expressed or captured, the techniques involved, the use of electronic media, verbalisation and narratives, through artistic endeavour, design, making and the crafts.
- What is the unique role of the practitioner and its growing relevance from a medical humanities approach.

Already referred to, is real world and real-life situations; this involves a focus on the individual in terms of the nature of an individual's experience and research approaches that respect the individual, give them voice, control, enable them to take action, inspire confidence and thus helps an individual flourish (Costa & Coles, 2018). While this does entail (and has entailed) an application of research to real-life situations, it typically involves a process of Co-Creation, an alliance between researchers and recipients of the research. More about Co-Creation is said in Chapter 2, but all chapters feature it as a component, including the circumstances which cause a negative or positive reaction, the approaches used and information on individual or group responses. Methodologies are varied and include qualitative as well as quantitative applications, case studies and design considerations, where material can be and should be considered in the context of the reader's professional and disciplinary context. The immersive methods put forward in chapters and "in the moment" data, offer unique insights into the foundations of more reflective user-led accounts.

Our own work falls under the heading of the therapeutic impact of access to greenspace where we have seen a progressive recognition of the positive impacts of access to nature as a legitimate pathway within clinical practice. This was far from so when we started; it is good to see this pathway becoming established, but it is also clear that there are conditions that need to be fulfilled before such benefits can be achieved. During a long period of research considering both urban and rural situations in Europe and the UK, we initially developed "social criteria" (Coles & Caserio, 2015) regarding access to urban greenspaces. These were based on extensive data sets and case study material, and later morphed into well-being considerations. To progress the agenda we purposely recruited researchers spanning a range of disciplines and began to more fully understand the interface between individuals, their lifestyles and how access to greenspaces helped them "flourish".

A feature of our work was taking a user-based approach. We were struck by the eloquence of the language (and other representations) used by individuals in describing their well-being experiences (Coles & Bussey, 2000; Coles et al., 2013; Costa et al., 2014) and how the approaches used actually assisted in moving the individual to a place of positivity which was then embraced and further explored with quite profound (positive) impact (Costa et al., 2014; Costa & Coles, 2018). These impacts were seen across a range of environments, blue (water-based) and green, but also in situations associated with residential streets where the presence of street trees was capable of inducing a pathway to well-being far more profound than their physical presence would suggest (Coles et al., 2013). This involved a move from what was considered relatively insignificant by one discipline to highly significant when evaluated in the context of well-being and feedback from the street community. For us it emphasises the need to consider all aspects of the built environment as a potential well-being resource, a task that we consider totally achievable if adopted by the range of built environment professions in their individual contexts allied to community ventures. Several chapters explore the remit of professions as well as Co-Creation approaches that indicate potential pathways through collaboration and that target different environments.

Accordingly, this volume invites readers to learn from those who are exploring the different dimensions of well-being, the role of the various disciplines, real-life case studies, the practices involved, the underpinning theoretical context and to consider ideas within the framework of their own disciplines, practice or responsibilities. Chapters have been carefully chosen to consider a diversity of information and present a sequence of exploration which enables the reader to progress understanding of well-being through the subject matter largely without any specialist knowledge. In the final chapter we discuss the outcomes of the individual chapters, to make observations, how ideas link together or how they are allied to the construction of pathways to well-being involving collaboration and Co-Design, but also to develop better theoretical understanding of the systems that are operating.

References

Coles, R. W. & Bussey, S. C. (2000) Urban forest landscapes in the UK, progressing the social agenda, *Landscape and Urban Planning* 52 (2–3): 181–188.

Coles, R. W. & Caserio, M. (2015) *Social Criteria for the Evaluation and Development of Urban Green Spaces, EU Report Number: D7 EVK4-CT-2000-00022*. Available at www.researchgate.net.

Coles, R. W. & Millman, Z. (2013) (eds.) *Landscape, Well-being and Environment*, Abingdon: Routledge.

Coles, R. W. & Millman, Z. (2016) (eds.) *Designs on Well-being*, Birmingham: ARTicle Press.

Coles, R. W., Millman, Z. & Flanningan, J. (2013) Everyday environmental encounters, their meaning and importance for the individual, *Urban Ecosytems* 16: 819–839.

Costa, S. & Coles, R. (2018, in press) The self-narrated walking. A user-led method to research people's experiences in urban landscapes, *Landscape Research*. Available at doi: 10.1080/01426397.2018.1467004.

Costa, S., Coles, R. & Boultwood, A. (2014) Walking narratives: interacting between urban nature and self, in Sörensen C. & Liedtke, K. (eds.), *SPECIFICS: Discussing Landscape Architecture*. Berlin: Jovis, pp.40–43.

Helliwell, J., Layard, R. & Sachs, J. (2017) *World Happiness Report 2017*, New York: Sustainable Development Solutions Network.

Huppert, F. & So, T. (2013) Flourishing across Europe: application of a new conceptual framework for defining well-being, *Social Indicators Research* 110 (3): 837–861.

OECD (2016) *Strategic Orientation of the Secretary General for 2016 and Beyond, Meeting of the OECD Council at Ministerial Level*, Paris, 1–2 June 2016. Available online at www.oecd.org/mcm/document/strategic-orientatiions-of-the-secretary-general-2016.pdf.

1

WAYS TO WELL-BEING FOR CHILDREN

Larissa Pople, Saamah Abdallah, Gwyther Rees and Gill Main

Introduction

Since 2005, The Children's Society has been engaged with the University of York in research to explore children's self-reported well-being and the factors that are associated with it. The work forms one of the most extensive national programmes of research on this topic in the world involving developing frameworks of well-being that take full account of children's own concepts of what it means (The Children's Society, 2006). This chapter presents the findings of this research with a comprehensive and detailed analysis of children's responses to questions about their subjective well-being based on nationally representative surveys (Rees et al., 2010; The Children's Society, 2017).

Over a similar timeframe, the New Economics Foundation (NEF) reviewed the evidence on determinants of well-being (as part of the Foresight Project, Aked et al., 2008) to produce messages about what individuals might do to improve their own well-being. NEF's programme of research is extensive, including evidence from neuroscience, cross-sectional surveys and longitudinal studies. *The Five Ways to Well-being* framework that was produced – Connect, Be Active, Take Notice, Keep Learning and Give – is now used in a wide range of contexts – and serves as a simple heuristic, echoing the five-a-day message around fruit and vegetable consumption.

- Connect – build social relationships, spend time with family and friends.
- Be Active – engage in regular physical activity.
- Take Notice – be mentally present focus on awareness and appreciation.
- Keep Learning – maintain curiosity about the world, try new things.
- Give – make a positive contribution to the lives of others.

(Aked et al., 2008)

Nonetheless, most of the evidence for NEF's *Five Ways to Well-being* relates to adults. Thus, The Children's Society and NEF saw a need to explore well-being-promoting activities that are pertinent to children's lives. There was a shared desire, on the one hand, to give children the opportunity to reflect on activities that they could do to improve their well-being, while on the other hand, to test out the specific relevance of the *Five Ways* framework.

The research took a mixed methods approach, comprising a combination of open, inductive enquiry through qualitative research that explored children's perspectives on activities that might enhance their feelings of well-being, as well as a deductive questioning through a survey that asked children about specific activities relating to NEF's *Five Ways to Well-being*. The methodology used and reported here emphasises the importance of a child-centric approach, giving children a voice to address wide-ranging aspects of children's well-being, the world of the child, their experiences and expectations,

The focus groups

In order to place children's voices centre stage, we start by discussing the factors that children themselves cited, unprompted, as being important for their well-being. Some of these themes fit neatly with NEF's *Five Ways*, while others are substantively different. We then report on children's responses to probing questions that were asked about the *Five Ways to Well-being*, and specifically the aspects of this framework that were not discussed unprompted.

This qualitative strand of the research involved 11 guided focus group discussions carried out in May/June 2013 in 6 schools in England. Each focus group comprised between six and eight children of the same age, including a range of ethnicities to reflect the ethnic profiles of the schools involved. Participants' ages ranged from 8 to 15 years. In these focus groups, we started by asking children open questions about the activities that they do – or could do – to contribute to making life good for them. Key probing questions included what it is about a certain activity that is good, and what might help or hinder engagement in the activities in question. After this open discussion, we introduced the *Five Ways to Well-being*, specifically those activities that had not been raised by participants themselves. So children had the opportunity to mention the *Five Ways to Well-being* unprompted, and were then led into a discussion about them.

Connect

In all of the focus groups, children asserted that being with family and friends is fundamental to a good life. Some focused on the benefits of spending time with loved ones, while for others "connecting" was part and parcel of another activity – such as playing or going on holiday.

> "I like to have people with me whatever I'úm doing."
>
> "It's like a treat when you get to see [wider family] cos you don't see them all the time."

One of the aspects of relationships that children valued most was the support that they received:

> "I think it's important to tell your parents stuff as well as your friends. Like if it were anything really serious or if it involved them I'd let them know. Like with school if anything were to happen like bullying or anything then I'd talk to my parents and they could help."

However, children also highlighted their role in *giving* as well as receiving support, illustrating the overlap that exists between different *Ways to Well-being*, in this case, Connect and Give:

> "If my mum's been working all day she'll come home and be really stressed and I'll like wash the pots to help her, like tidying up."

Friends were cherished for many reasons: for their qualities as good friends, for the activities that could be enjoyed together, and for the company that they provide:

> "You look out for each other, look after each other. Me and my friend say that we'll protect each other and stand by each other's side, like if one of us gets bullied we'll help each other cos that's what we always do."
>
> "You do things together like say, you go shopping, you play with them. They make you happy cos they keep you company. Say you're bored, you phone them up and you go and play out and you're not feeling bored anymore."

Be Active

Another strand of responses about what makes life good for children related to physical activity. This involved both organised activities, such as playing football within a club setting, as well as informal activities such as riding a bicycle in the local neighbourhood. When probed on what they enjoyed about physical activity, children often made reference to the social aspects of sports and exercise:

> "[Football] that's a good thing . . . so you can be active with your friends and you can make new friends and you can have fun."

However the well-being benefits were also felt to be important in and of themselves:

> "The park has obstacle things where you can be active and you can go on the swings, it just makes you feel happy to do it."
>
> "When I play football I get happier, either playing on the football team or playing with my mates."

As well as associating physical activity with feeling good, some children also associated it with functioning well. One girl derived a sense of vitality from exercise:

> "I used to go running in the mornings, before I hurt my knee. I would be in a better mood in the day, and feel wide awake."

Learning

Somewhat surprisingly, learning emerged unprompted in the focus group discussions as something that could engender well-being. While for some, learning was associated mainly with school, for others it encompassed learning outside of school.

> "I enjoy learning, I absolutely love learning in my favourite lessons. I also enjoy learning in other lessons cos I know they'll contribute to what I want to do when I'm older."
>
> "Well you learn every day even if you don't go to school cos there are so many things around you and you don't actually know what everything is, so you actually learn something all the time even if it isn't school or a game, just by seeing things."

Learning might be a sole pursuit or a social experience to be shared with others:

> "I really like reading my own books that are not fiction books, you can experiment with them, like I'm trying to make something at the moment with battery acid, trying to make that out of some stuff I've got around the house."
>
> "You know like grandmas and granddads? Well I really like going with them cos they've learnt all this stuff before cos they've got longer experience than your mum and dad even . . . I've learnt all about WW1 and WW2 with me grandma and granddad."

Enthusiasm for learning was also linked to the sense of achievement that it might incite, which we discuss in more detail later.

Playing, creativity and imagination

A key set of activities mentioned unprompted by children in our focus groups related to playing, doing things for fun and taking part in creative pursuits. This overarching category encompasses a broad range of activities including engaging in artistic, music-related and organised activities, playing computer games and – for younger participants in particular – simply playing.

These activities are not specifically referred to within NEF's *Five Ways to Well-being*, although they overlap with the Learning and Connect themes. It is important to highlight, however, that these activities tend to be valued by children for the pleasure that they derive from them rather than any associated learning benefits. Children described their enjoyment of playing in the park/playground or inside, alone or with friends.

> "[The adventure playground is] really fun and you get to all sorts of things there."
>
> "[Computer] games are fun. You play with other people and you can talk to your friends on it."

The benefits of listening to music, playing instruments, dancing and singing were underlined:

> "[Singing] just makes everyone happy!"
>
> "I like dancing, I go to dance classes . . . I just enjoy it, I like dancing . . . it's fun."

Pleasure was also derived from creative activities like arts, crafts and acting.

> "I like designing stuff. I like sketching things, copying things – it just makes me feel good that I can draw stuff."

Imagination was a key element of many of these activities:

> "When you're doing something where you can use your own imagination and you can do your own thing, like write a book about something, like a short fairy tale or something like that, anything can happen in there and that makes you more excited about what you're doing."

Give

Giving was not an activity that children talked about unprompted, although they often acknowledged in their comments that they liked helping others as much as they appreciated being helped. When we asked explicitly about Give activities, we framed these, in the first instance, in terms of helping at home or with siblings. These yielded mainly negative or problematic responses insofar as participants expressed clear expectations that helping out at home would be met with a reward:

> "I like helping my mum cos I get extra pocket money and I get to go on the quad bike after."

However, when the discussions were broadened out to include doing things to help others in non-specified ways, children's comments were far more positive. Giving could be achieved through everyday acts of kindness such as holding doors open for people or putting money in a charity collection tin:

> "It's like if you go to a shop and put your change in the charity box it makes you feel good cos you've helped."

When children talked freely and positively about giving, it was often linked to other activities:

> "I like making things and drawing things because I can give it to someone and make them happy . . . like my sisters and my mum."
>
> "[At dance] it's nice seeing the younger ones and how they progress and get better, it's a good feeling and makes me feel like I've helped them get there."

Take Notice

The most difficult of NEF's *Five Ways to Well-being* to explore with children was Take Notice. This is not surprising, as the principle on which it is based (mindfulness meditation) has very little precedent in UK culture and language. Thus, all of children's comments on this topic were made in response to prompting and a short, age-appropriate explanation of mindfulness. For the most part, participants had not heard of mindfulness and were not conscious of practising mindfulness, although there were a couple of exceptions to this. One was the group of older children who had the following conversation:

> "I go in the bath, like taking yourself out of everything that's busy, to calm myself down I'll just go in the bath and it makes me forget everything."
>
> "I always have candles in the bath and then I just stare at them."
>
> "Yeah, I like staring at fires."
>
> "I don't like notice a good feeling but it kind of like, what if you didn't do it? Like it's kind of, I feel like a deeper person."

One child made a connection between mindfulness and meditation, or prayer, with which she was familiar through her religious practice:

> "Like meditation you mean? Like it's part of our religion to pray, we do like praying where we focus on more important things . . . Yeah it makes you feel more calm, it makes you understand more what's going on around you and makes you improve yourself."

Finally, in one of the schools – which was chosen specifically because it practices mindfulness meditation with children – mindfulness was discussed positively:

> "I feel calm and peaceful and I feel like I want to take on the day."
>
> "It makes me feel not stressed, not like 'I need to do this, then I need to do this, then I need to do this'. It's like it gets the bad thoughts out of my head."

Cross-cutting themes: autonomy and achievement

Two cross-cutting themes also arose from children's discussions of activities that could enhance well-being – a sense of autonomy and achievement. That children recognised the importance of these concepts corroborates the self-determination theory of Psychologists Richard Ryan and Edward Deci, which highlights autonomy, competence and relatedness as universal psychological needs (Deci & Ryan, 2000).

Autonomy was a significant theme cutting across the focus group discussions. The comments of some children suggested that it could be viewed as a "way to well-being" itself, but we do not present it as such because it is arguably less amenable to being "done by" children than other activities.

Clearly, feeling independent and being able to make choices about what they do was of central importance to children:

> "Like playing with your friends, you don't want your mum holding your hand all the time, you want some independence, some time to play by yourself."
>
> "It's not the actual game playing on my PS3, it's having that time and the independence to do what I want."

Some focused on the negative aspects of having little or no say in what they did. For example, when autonomy is constrained in ways that are felt to be unreasonable, a previously enjoyed activity can cease to give pleasure:

> "I used to play the piano and my step dad made me practice every single day, like every day I had to play for an hour, and it just became horrible cos, well I really enjoyed playing the piano but the fact that he would like tell me I had to do it for an hour a day, it just really annoyed me. Now I'm trying to teach myself the guitar and I enjoy that cos no-one's telling me to do it."

Children also spoke about the sense of achievement that could be gained from different activities, the pride that they might get from developing new skills, and how these feelings made them feel good. This could be thought of as a further *Way to Well-being*:

> "I made a cake the other day and all my mum did for me was put the oven on, I did everything else."
>
> "At first I didn't know criss-cross jumping, it's so hard, but now I know and I can do it. It makes me feel proud."

The survey

The quantitative strand of the research comprised a survey administered in February/March 2013 with a socio-economically representative sample of 1,500 children aged 10 to 15 years old, and equal numbers of boys and girls in each age group. Involvement in the *Five Ways to Well-being* was assessed by asking children how much time they had spent taking part in seventeen different *Five Ways* activities. The questions were developed by considering how the *Five Ways to Well-being* have been framed for adults and the kinds of behaviours that might be appropriate for children. For example, thinking of Give, children may be unlikely to donate to charity, but they might help with chores around the house. The full question wordings and the abbreviations that we use in the report are presented in Table 1.1 below.

Figure 1.1 shows how often children reported carrying out these activities, with some activities much more common than others. For example, almost two-thirds of children (64%) reported seeing their friends outside of school most days or every day, while only 2% said that they did volunteering most days or every day.

Children's well-being was assessed using a measure of overall subjective well-being, which The Children's Society has refined from a longer version originally developed by Huebner (1991). The scale consists of the following five statements, which children were asked to respond to on a five-point scale from strongly agree to strongly disagree.

- My life is going well.
- My life is just right.
- I wish I had a different kind of life.
- I have a good life.
- I have what I want in life.

These 5 items can be combined into a single subjective well-being score from 0 to 20. We will use the shorthand "well-being" to refer to this measure of overall subjective well-being.

We conducted analysis to see whether children's well-being scores were related to their involvement in the *Five Ways to Well-being* activities that we asked about. Figure 1.2 shows the amount of variation in well-being that participation in each activity explained, once demographic variables were controlled for (age, gender, mother's education and whether the child comes from a household where no adult works). Fourteen out of the seventeen activities that children were asked about were significantly associated with well-being once demographic factors were controlled for, with the three activities with no significant association being "caring for siblings", "volunteering" and "chatting to friends".

There were differences in the amount of variation in well-being that each activity could explain. For example, just over 10% of the variation in well-being could be explained by how often children notice their surroundings – this is almost four times as much as the variation that could be explained by all of the

TABLE 1.1 Full wordings of questions about *Ways to Well-being* activities

How often do you spend time out of school . . . ?	*Abbreviation*
Be Active	
playing sports on a team (like football or netball)	Team sports
playing sports or doing exercise but not on a team (like running, swimming or dancing)	Non-team sports/exercise
walking or cycling around your local area to go to school or see friends	Walking/cycling
Keep Learning	
learning new things for fun (like music, languages, art or drama)	Learning new things
reading for fun	Reading for fun
teaching yourself new things	Teaching yourself new things
taking part in organised activities (like youth clubs or scouts/guides)	Organised activities
Give	
helping out around the house	Helping out around house
taking care of or helping out with brothers or sisters or other family members	Caring for siblings
volunteering or helping out in your community (this could include helping out a neighbour)	Volunteering
Connect	
seeing friends	Seeing friends
chatting to friends on the phone or via social websites (like Facebook, Bebo or Twitter)	Chatting to friends via social media/phone
seeing people in your family that you don't live with (like grandparents, aunts, uncles and cousins)	Seeing extended family
talking to people in your family about things that matter to you	Talking to family
Take Notice	
paying attention to how you feel physically (like feeling full of energy or tired, feeling tense or relaxed)	Attention to physical feelings
paying attention to your feelings and emotions	Attention to feelings/emotions
noticing and enjoying your surroundings (indoors and outdoors)	Noticing surroundings

demographic factors that we considered. The next strongest predictors of well-being were teaching yourself new things (almost 6%), talking to family about important matters (just over 4%) and reading for fun (4%).

Another approach is to compare the frequency of doing an activity that is associated with the lowest and highest levels of well-being (Figure 1.3). In most cases, the least optimal frequency was never or hardly ever doing the activity. The only exception is caring for siblings, where those who care for their siblings on a daily basis are less happy than those who never care for their siblings.

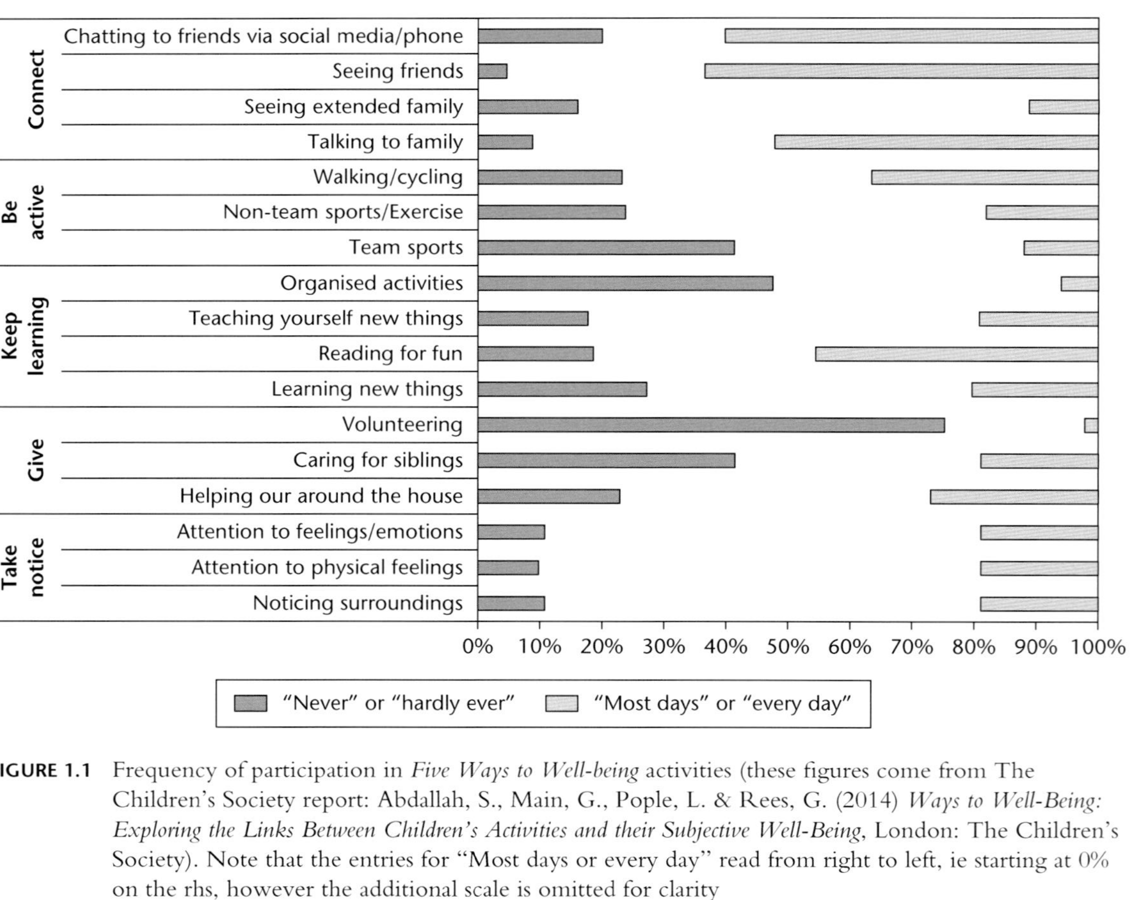

FIGURE 1.1 Frequency of participation in *Five Ways to Well-being* activities (these figures come from The Children's Society report: Abdallah, S., Main, G., Pople, L. & Rees, G. (2014) *Ways to Well-Being: Exploring the Links Between Children's Activities and their Subjective Well-Being*, London: The Children's Society). Note that the entries for "Most days or every day" read from right to left, ie starting at 0% on the rhs, however the additional scale is omitted for clarity

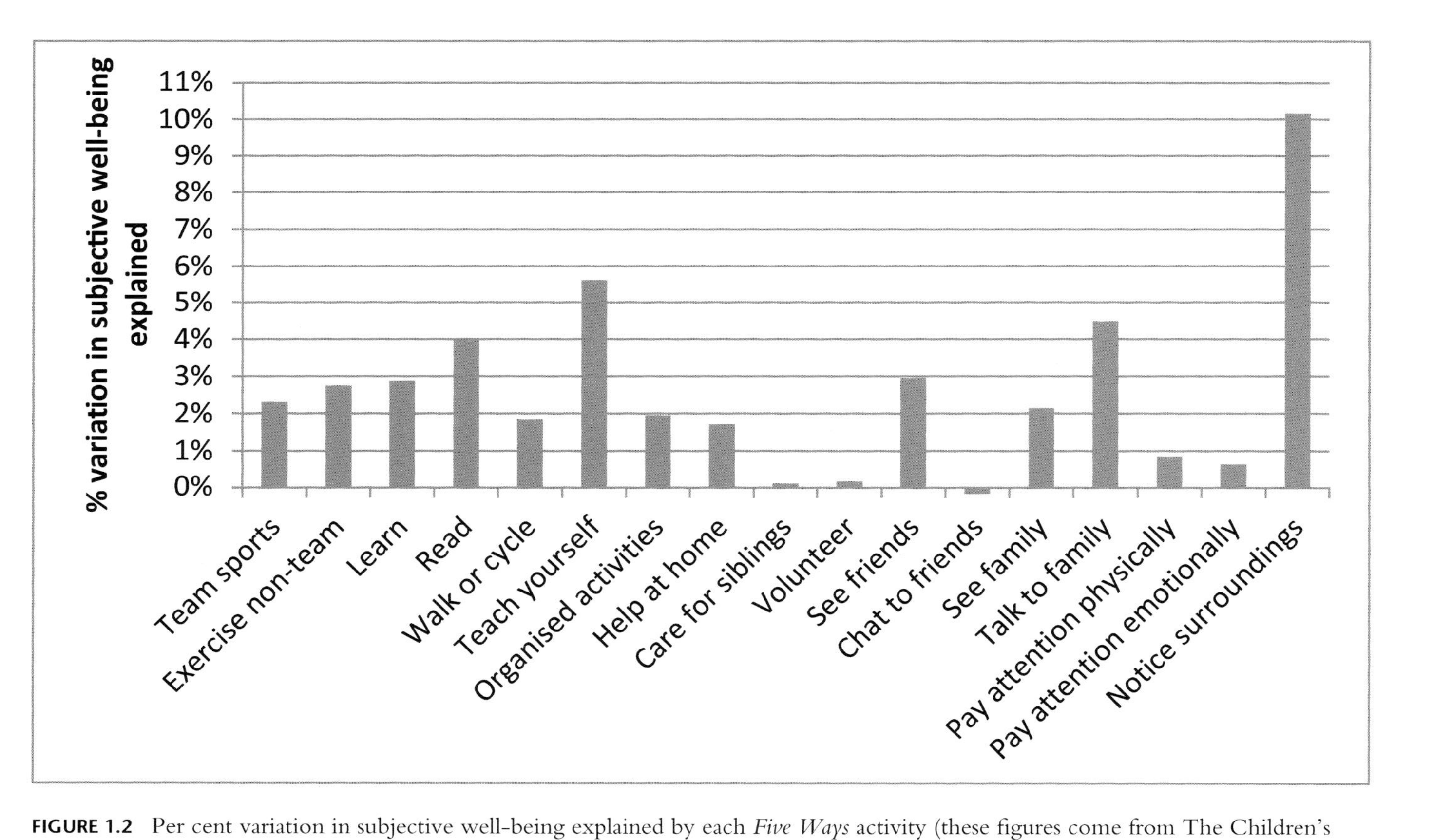

FIGURE 1.2 Per cent variation in subjective well-being explained by each *Five Ways* activity (these figures come from The Children's Society report: Abdallah, S., Main, G., Pople, L. & Rees, G. (2014) *Ways to Well-Being: Exploring the Links Between Children's Activities and their Subjective Well-Being*, London: The Children's Society)

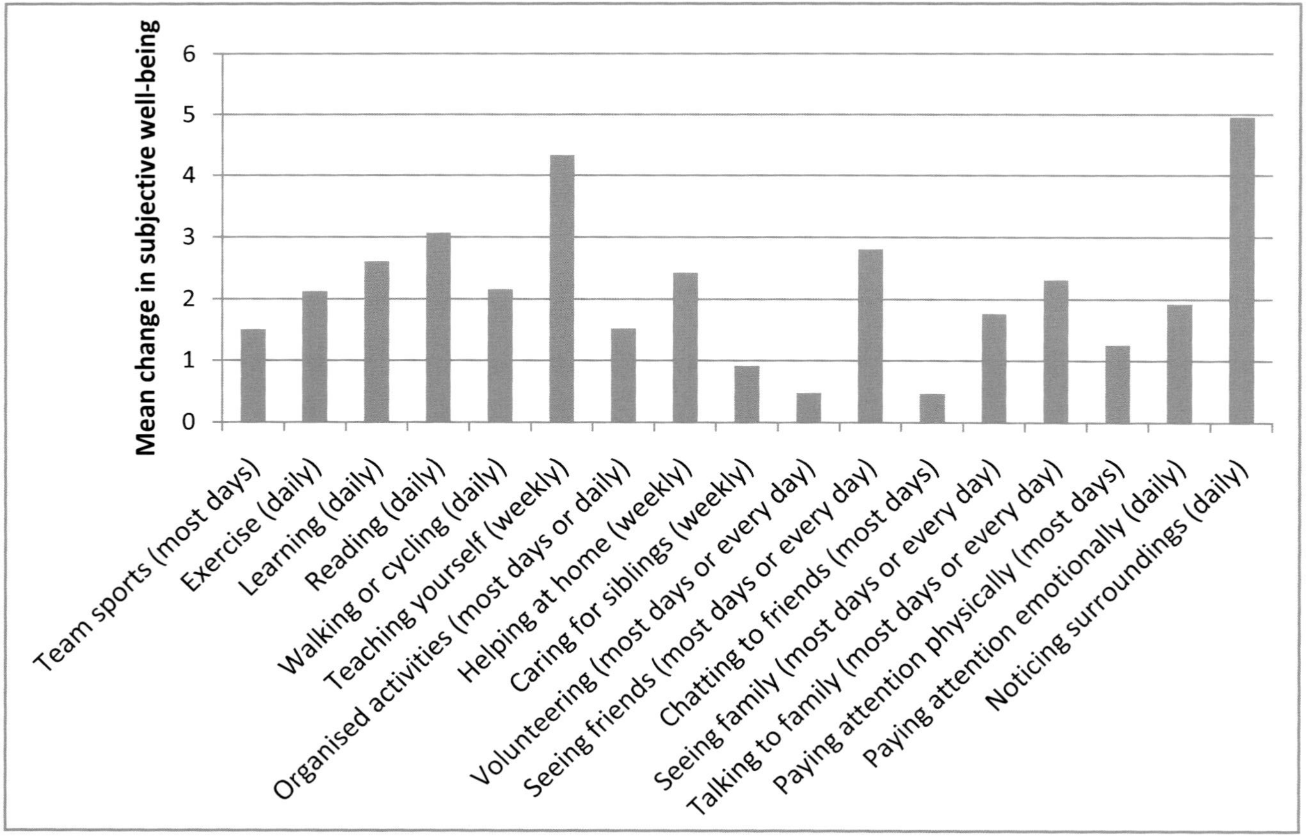

Mean change in subjective well-being

6
5
4
3
2
1
0

Team sports (most days)
Exercise (daily)
Learning (daily)
Reading (daily)
Walking or cycling (daily)
Teaching yourself (weekly)
Organised activities (most days or daily)
Helping at home (weekly)
Caring for siblings (weekly)
Volunteering (most days or every day)
Seeing friends (most days or every day)
Chatting to friends (most days)
Seeing family (most days or every day)
Talking to family (most days or every day)
Paying attention physically (most days)
Paying attention emotionally (daily)
Noticing surroundings (daily)

FIGURE 1.3 Mean difference in subjective well-being associated with optimal frequency of *Five Ways* activities

As shown in Figure 1.3 and the next section, the optimum frequency for well-being is not necessarily the maximum frequency.

The largest well-being differences were evident for children who never or hardly ever "notice and enjoy their surroundings" compared to those who do so all the time – a difference of 5.0 points on the 20-point scale after controlling for demographic factors, which is substantial. Measured this way, the next 2 most important activities were "teaching yourself new things" (a difference of 4.3 points), and "reading for fun" (a difference of 3.1 points).

Of course, due to the cross-sectional design of this study, we do not have evidence that there is a causal relationship between the *Five Ways* activities and well-being. Furthermore, there may be other unobserved factors influencing this relationship. Nonetheless, the data shows that, for most activities, frequency of participation is associated with children's well-being, even controlling for several demographic factors. Given the evidence of causal relationships for *Five Ways* activities among adults, we suggest that a plausible explanation is that the activities in some way also positively contribute to children's well-being.

Some of the *Five Ways* activities had "linear" (strictly-speaking "monotonic") relationships with well-being, but many did not.

We identified three patterns of relationship between frequency of activities and well-being: "linear", "diminishing returns" and "inverse U".

"Linear" – the more the better

For a few activities, the relationship with well-being was "linear", with every increase in frequency being associated with a similar increase in well-being. For all these activities, a multiple linear regression including frequency of the activity as a single scalar variable produced the highest adjusted r squared value, meaning that this type of regression explained more variation in subjective well-being than alternative types.

- Learning new things.
- Reading for fun.
- Organised activities.
- Talking to family.
- Attention to feelings/emotions.

"Diminishing returns"

Seeing friends was an example of "diminishing returns" – a pattern whereby the biggest increases in well-being were seen at the bottom end of the frequency scale. At the top of the scale, levels of well-being were either stable, or increases became less pronounced. We tested this by comparing the results of a multiple linear regression with the *Five Ways* activity as a linear predictor, to the results of a similar regression but with the *Five Ways* activity as categorical predictors.

Where categorical predictors produced a higher adjusted r squared value than a linear predictor, and where increases in well-being between the categories were greater towards the lower end of the frequency scale, relationships were classified as "diminishing returns". This pattern was seen in several other activities:

- Seeing friends.
- Non-team sports/exercise.
- Noticing surroundings.
- Seeing extended family.

"Inverse U" – too much is not a good thing

Some of the activities that we included in our survey had an "inverse-U" relationship with well-being, meaning that doing the activity at the maximum frequency was actually associated with significantly lower well-being than doing it at a moderate frequency. As above, we tested for this by comparing the results of a linear regression with the *Five Ways* activity as a linear predictor, to the results of the same variable as categorical predictors. Where categorical predictors resulted in a higher adjusted r squared value, and where increases in well-being could be seen towards the lower end of the frequency scale, but decreases occurred higher up, relationships were categorised as "inverse U":

- Team sports (the optimal frequency appears to be "most days").
- Attention to physical feelings (the optimal frequency appears to be "most days").
- Teaching yourself new things (the optimal frequency appears to be "weekly" or "most days").
- Helping out around house (the optimal frequency appears to be "weekly").

We then looked at each of NEF's *Five Ways to Well-being* in turn. There were not always enough children in each of the six frequency categories for us to make confident estimates, therefore, sometimes these results are grouped into three categories.

Connect

The Connect activity that explained the most variation in well-being was talking to family about things that matter to them (Figure 1.4) – 4% of variation after demographics had been controlled for. The relationship was clearly "linear", and there was a difference of 2.3 points between those who talked to their family "never or hardly ever", and those who talked to their family "most days or every day".

However, the Connect activity that was associated with the biggest difference in well-being was seeing friends (Figure 1.5). Children who "never or hardly ever" see their friends had a mean well-being score that is 2.8 points lower (on a scale of 0 to 20) than those who see their friends "most days or every day". This relationship was one of "diminishing returns" i.e. levels of well-being among children were fairly similar as long as they see their friends more than "never or hardly ever".

Seeing extended family (Figure 1.6) also showed a "diminishing returns" relationship with well-being. Well-being increased with frequency, but the differences

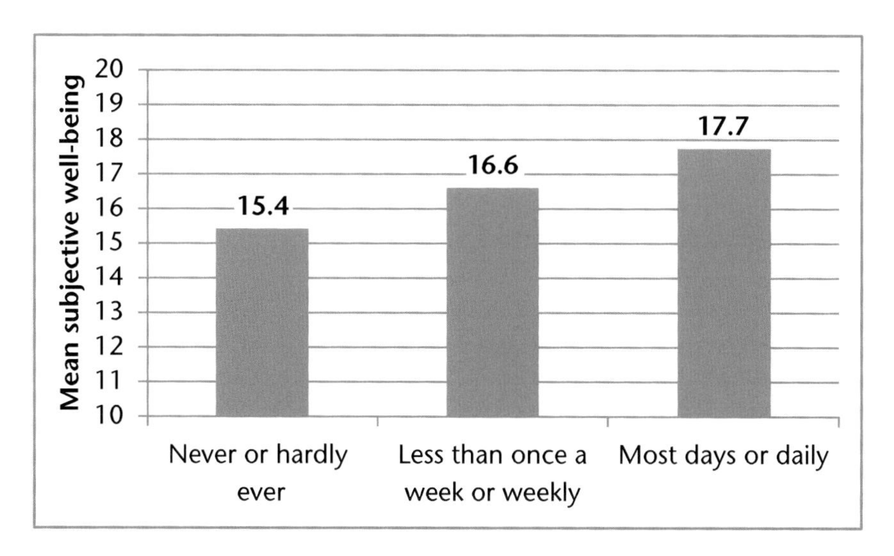

FIGURE 1.4 Children's subjective well-being according to how often they talk to their family about things that matter

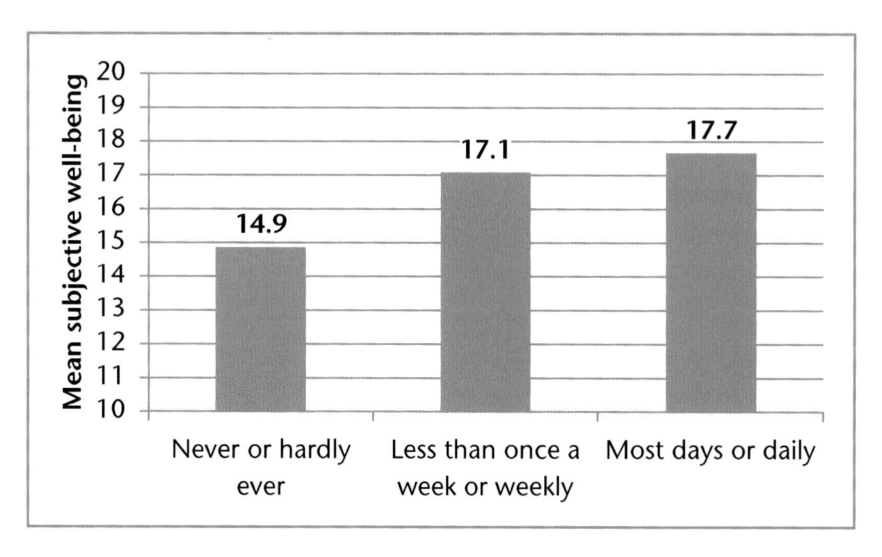

FIGURE 1.5 Children's subjective well-being according to how often they see their friends

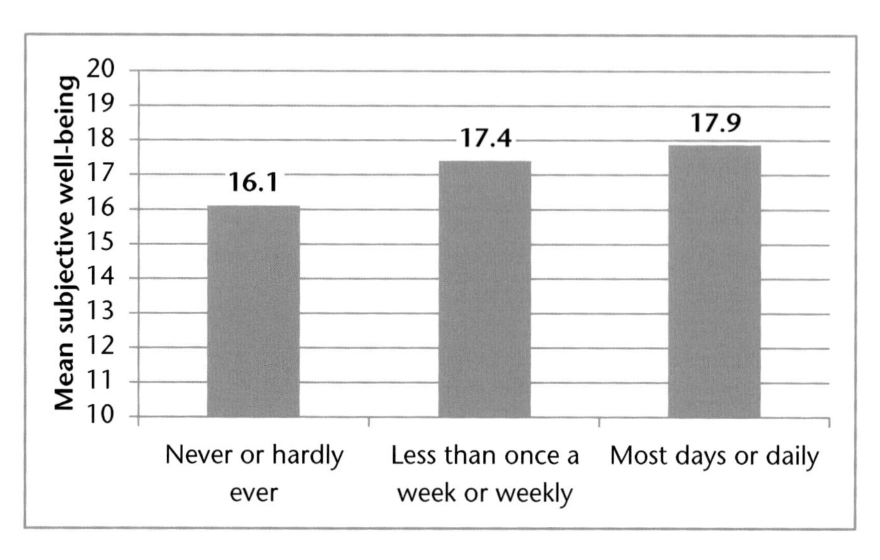

FIGURE 1.6 Children's subjective well-being according to how often they see their extended family

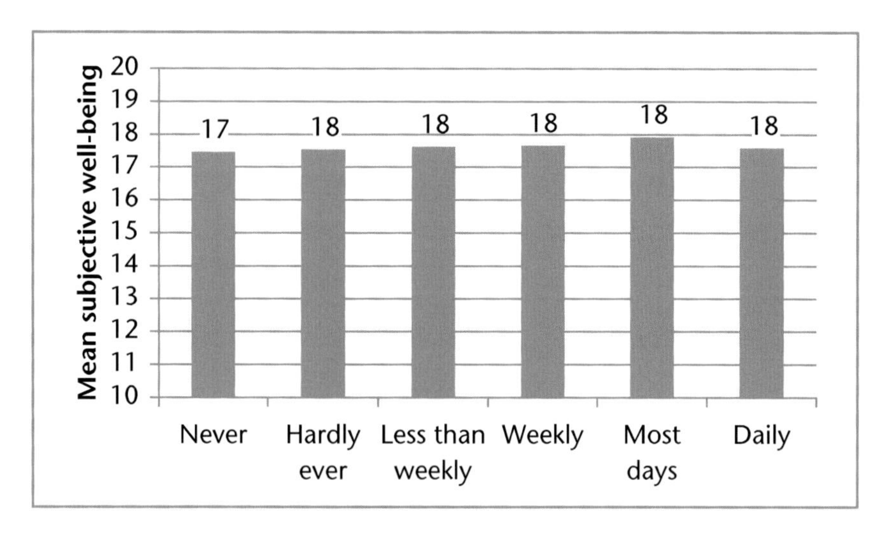

FIGURE 1.7 Children's subjective well-being according to how often they chat to their friends online

were not substantial beyond "never or hardly ever". Interestingly, chatting to friends on the phone or via social media did not have the same relationship with children's well-being as spending time with friends in person. This activity was not significantly related to well-being.

Be Active

The strongest predictor of well-being in this category was non-team sports/exercise (Figure 1.8), for which well-being increased up until a frequency of daily. However, the difference between "most days" and "daily" was smaller than the differences between lower frequencies, suggesting a "diminishing returns" relationship. For walking or cycling (Figure 1.9), the relationship is less clear, peaking once at "once or twice a week" and again at "daily". The well-being of the small proportion (8%, n=95) of children who never cycled or walked was 2.2 points below those who walked or cycled every day.

For team sports (Figure 1.10), the pattern was an inverse-U shape, with the small proportion of children who participated in team sports every day (2%, n=26) reporting significantly lower well-being. Indeed the well-being of children who took part in team sports every day was not significantly higher than the well-being of children who never did so, once demographics were controlled for.

Learning

All four of the learning activities that we asked children about in our survey – reading for fun, learning new things for fun, teaching yourself new things, and taking part in organised activities – were significantly linked with their well-being.

Teaching yourself new things (Figure 1.11) was the activity in this category that was associated with the most variation in well-being – 6% once demographics were controlled for, and children who reported doing this activity weekly had a well-being score 4.3 points higher than those who never did. However, this activity had

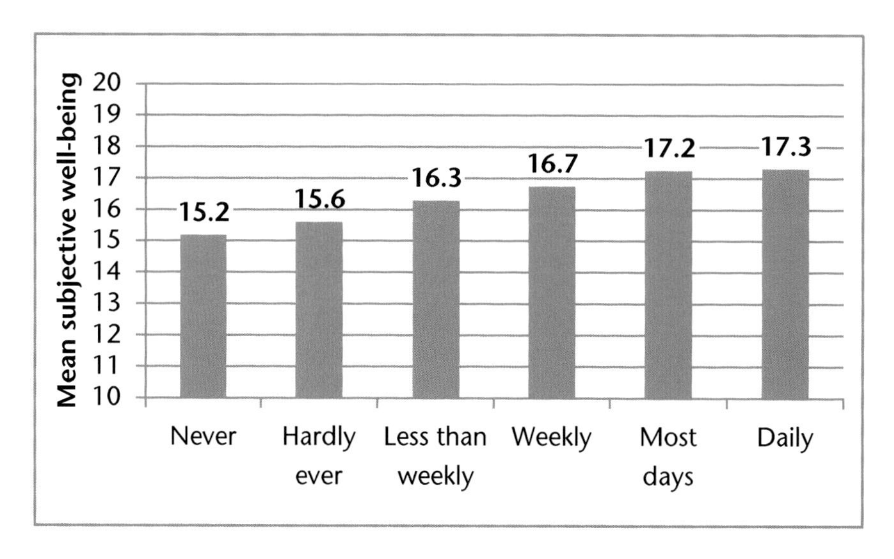

FIGURE 1.8 Children's subjective well-being according to how often they take part in non-team sports/exercise

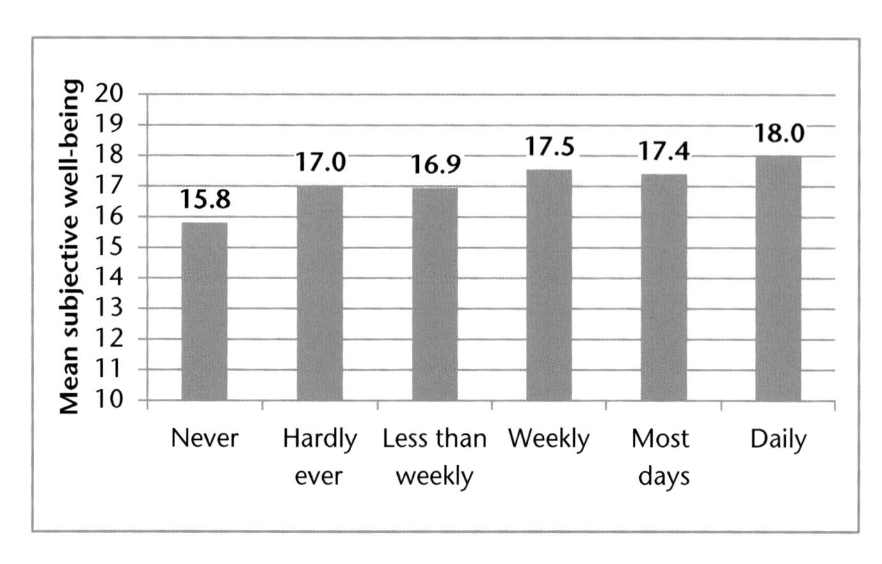

FIGURE 1.9 Children's subjective well-being according to how often they walk or cycle

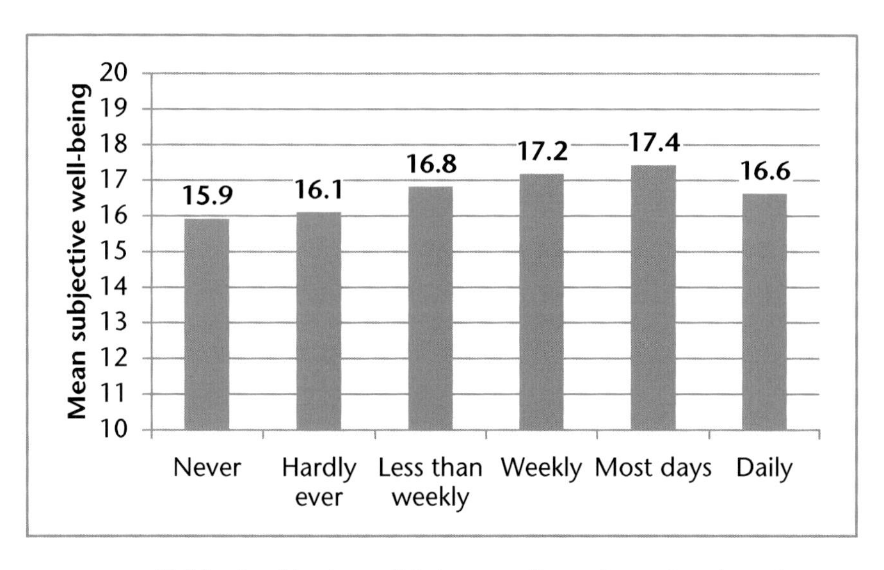

FIGURE 1.10 Children's subjective well-being according to how often they take part in team sports

an inverse-U pattern. The 3% (n=39) of children who reported teaching themselves new things "every day" had lower well-being than those who did so "most days", but their well-being was still significantly higher than those who never participated in this activity.

In contrast, reading for fun (Figure 1.12) and learning new things for fun (Figure 1.13) had a "linear" relationship with well-being and predicted 4% and 3% of variation in well-being respectively.

The fourth activity in this category – organised activities (Figure 1.14) – was the weakest predictor of well-being, explaining only 2% of variation. Nevertheless, children who carried out organised activities "most days" or more had significantly higher well-being than those who "never" did.

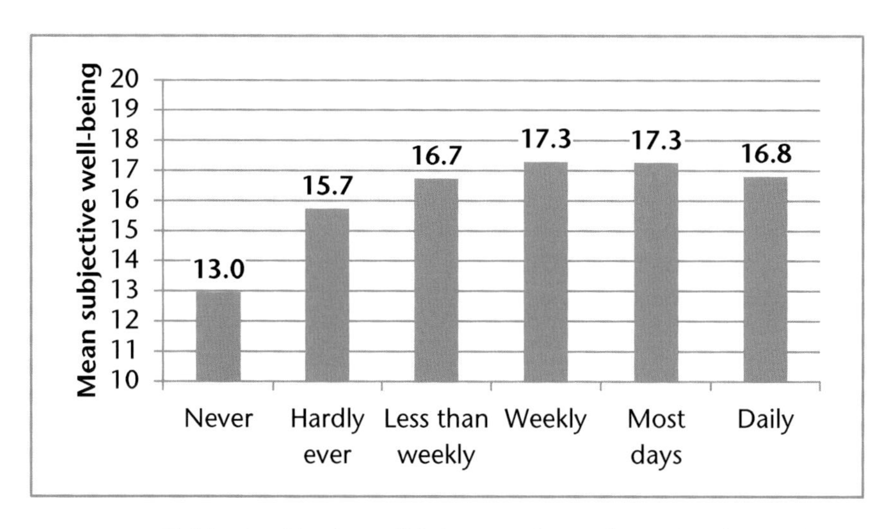

FIGURE 1.11 Children's subjective well-being according to how often they teach themselves new things

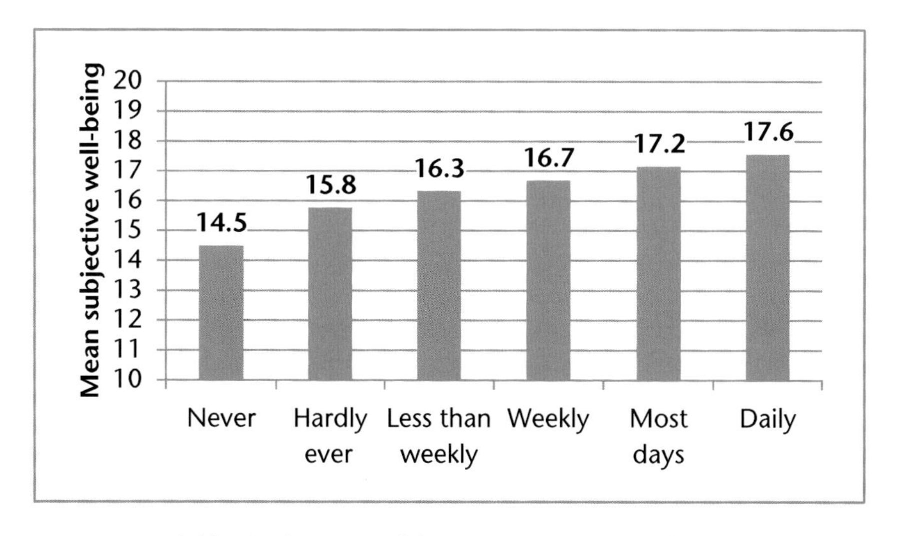

FIGURE 1.12 Children's subjective well-being according to how often they read for fun

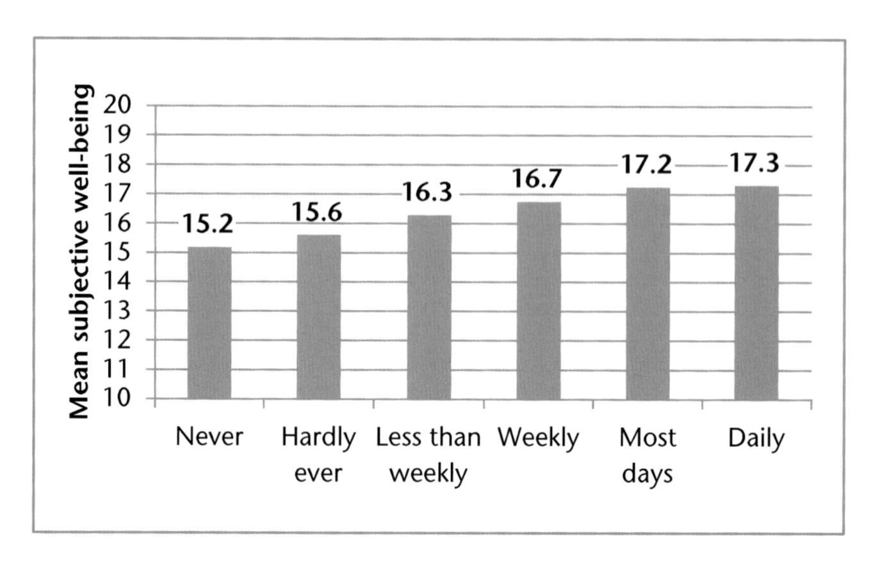

FIGURE 1.13 Children's subjective well-being according to how often they learn new things

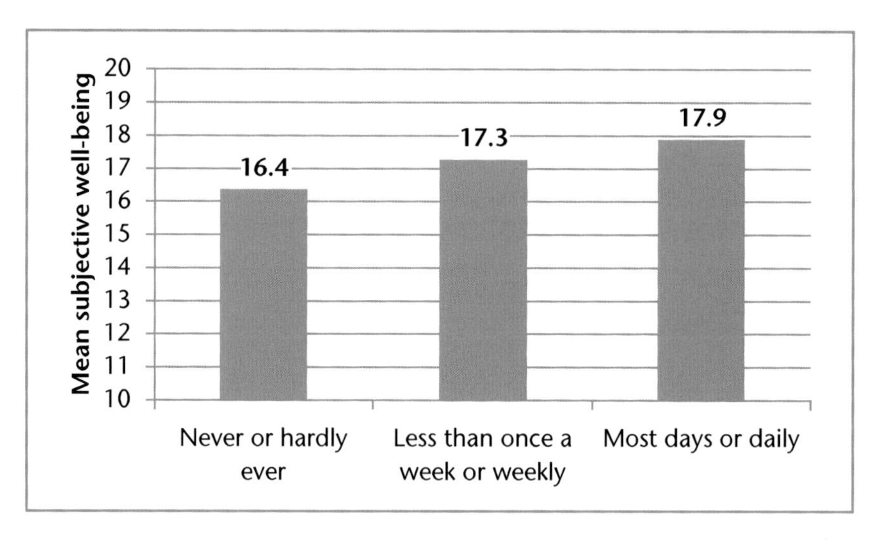

FIGURE 1.14 Children's subjective well-being according to how often they take part in organised activities

Give

The survey evidence for Give was less convincing than for the other *Five Ways to Well-being*. The strongest predictor of well-being was helping out around the house (Figure 1.15), which explained 2% of variation. Children who helped out around the house weekly had a well-being score that was 2.4 points higher than those who never helped out around the house. But this activity was also a clear example of an inverse-U pattern, with children who reported helping around the house daily having significantly lower well-being than might be expected from a "linear" relationship.

Taking care of siblings or other family members (Figure 1.16) and volunteering (Figure 1.17) were not significant predictors of subjective well-being.

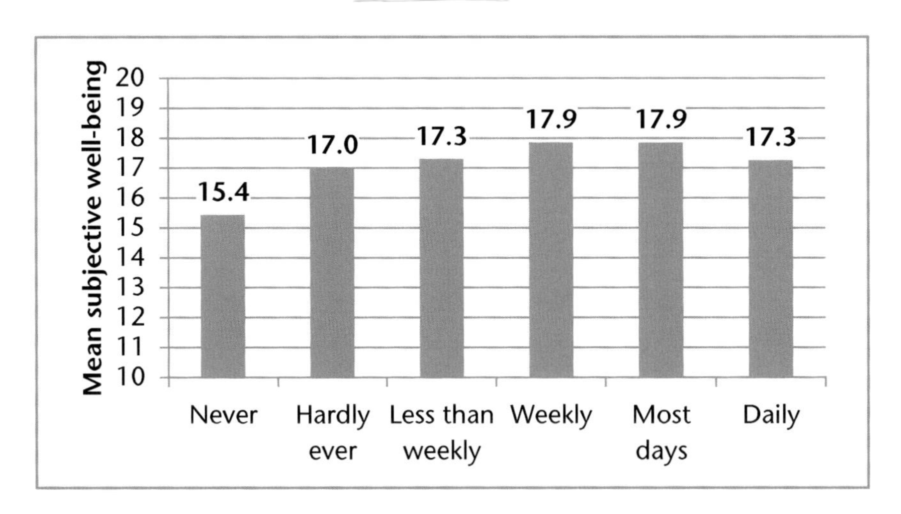

FIGURE 1.15 Children's subjective well-being according to how often they help out at home

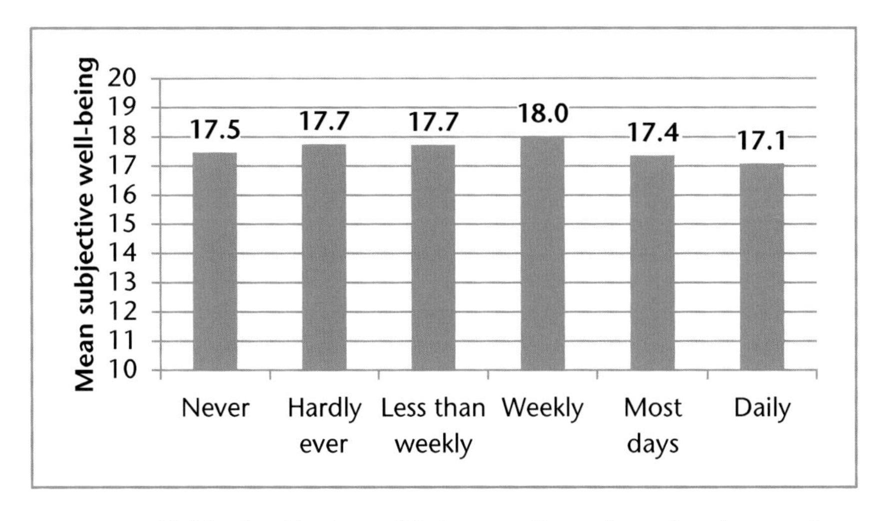

FIGURE 1.16 Children's subjective well-being according to how often they care for siblings or other family members

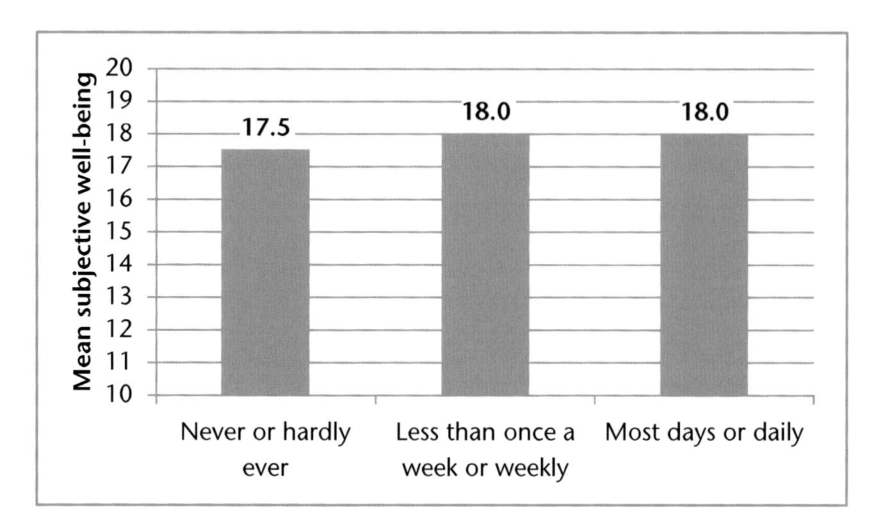

FIGURE 1.17 Children's subjective well-being according to how often they take part in volunteering

Take Notice

We found comparatively strong relationships between two of the three Take Notice activities and children's well-being. Indeed, the activity with the strongest relationship to children's well-being in our analysis was the frequency of noticing surroundings (Figure 1.18) – explaining 10% of variation in well-being, even after demographics were controlled for. The well-being of the children who reported noticing their surroundings all the time was 5 points higher than those who reported never noticing their surroundings. However, increases in well-being were more pronounced lower down the frequency scale, suggesting that the association is one of "diminishing returns".

The relationships between well-being and paying attention to "feelings and emotions" (Figure 1.19) and to "physical feelings" (Figure 1.20) were also significant, although, for the latter of these, there was some evidence that too much of this activity may be associated with lower well-being; children who reported paying attention to their physical feelings "all of the time" had lower well-being than those that reported doing so "very often".

Age and gender differences

Our analysis revealed that there are interesting age and gender differences in participation in the *Five Ways* activities that were asked about in the survey. Girls were significantly more likely than boys to "learn new things for fun", "read for fun", "chat to friends", "talk to family", "pay attention to how they feel physically" and "pay attention to how they feel emotionally". Boys were significantly more likely

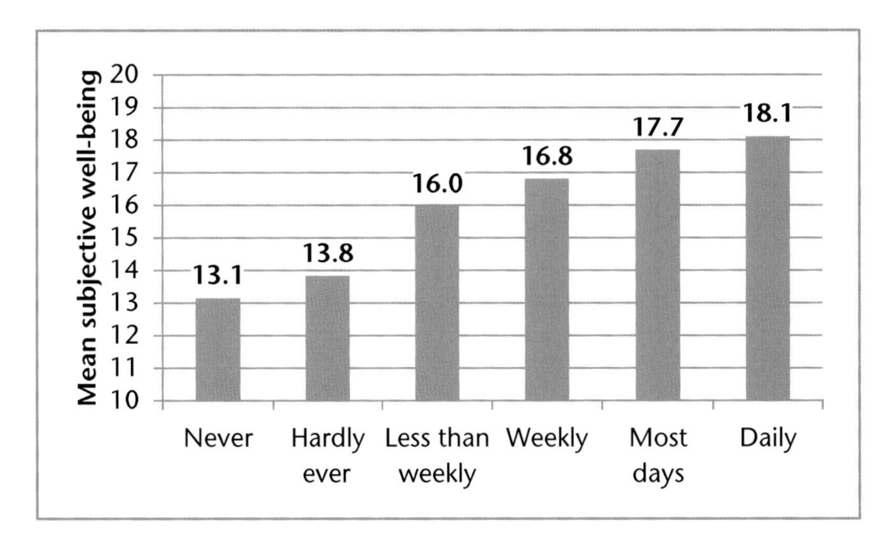

FIGURE 1.18 Children's subjective well-being according to how often they notice and enjoy surroundings

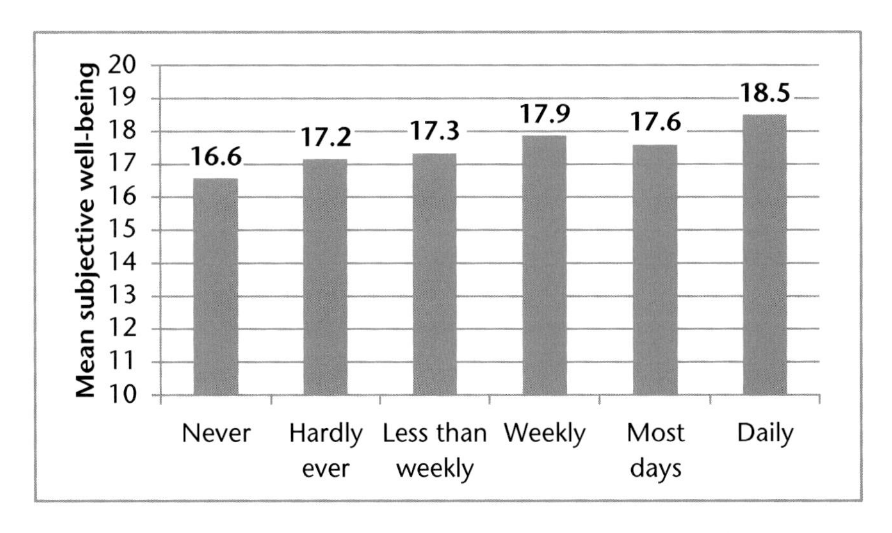

FIGURE 1.19 Children's subjective well-being according to how often they pay attention to feelings and emotions

than girls to do "team sports", "non-team sports/exercise", and "teach themselves new things". Furthermore, all bar one of the *Five Ways* activities ("teach yourself new things") were found to explain more of the variation in the subjective well-being of girls than of boys. Differences were particularly large for the Be Active activities – "'team sports", "non-team sports/exercise" and "walking or cycling".

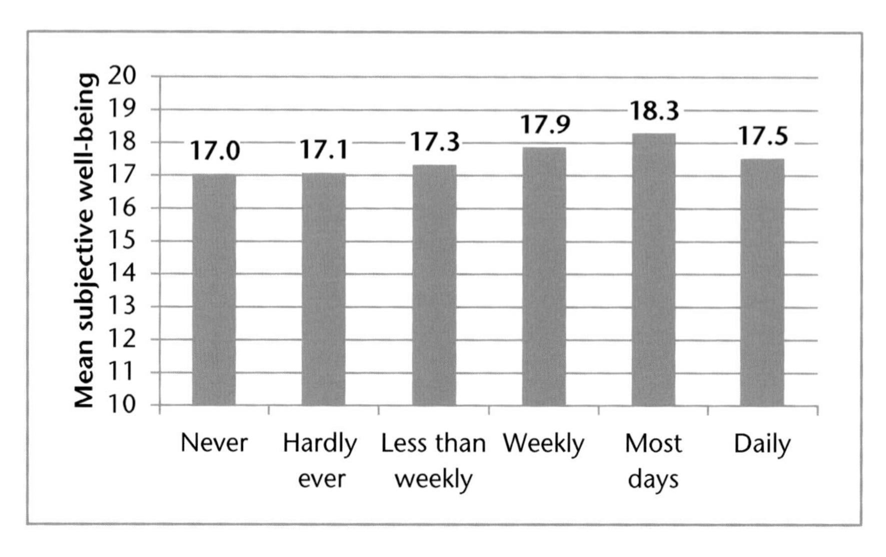

FIGURE 1.20 Children's subjective well-being according to how often they pay attention to physical feelings

Overall, participation in the *Five Ways* activities asked about in the survey declined with age, but the reverse was true of "seeing friends" and "chatting with friends online". A related finding is that well-being decreased with age. However it is not possible to conclude that the drop in well-being with age can be attributable to less frequent participation in the *Five Ways* activities, as it is also feasible that it is lower well-being that causes less frequent involvement in those activities, or that both are explained by something else. Longitudinal research would help shed light on this conundrum.

Conclusion

The focus group research that we undertook provided unprompted support among children aged 8 to 15 for the value of three of NEF's *Five Ways to Well-being* – Connect, Be Active and Keep Learning. Through prompted discussion, children also endorsed the relevance of the other two of the *Five Ways* – Take Notice and Give (in relation to acts of kindness and informal help). In addition, children drew attention to the benefits of activities related to creativity, imagination and play (which may represent an additional *Way to Well-being* for children) and the relevance of autonomy to be able to choose activities that may enhance well-being, and the sense of achievement that can be derived from carrying out activities.

The survey produced valuable evidence to support the relevance of most of the activities identified within the *Five Ways to Well-being* for children. Based on the different associations between the questions asked about each activity and well-being, the evidence for Give appears to be weakest. The survey also highlighted

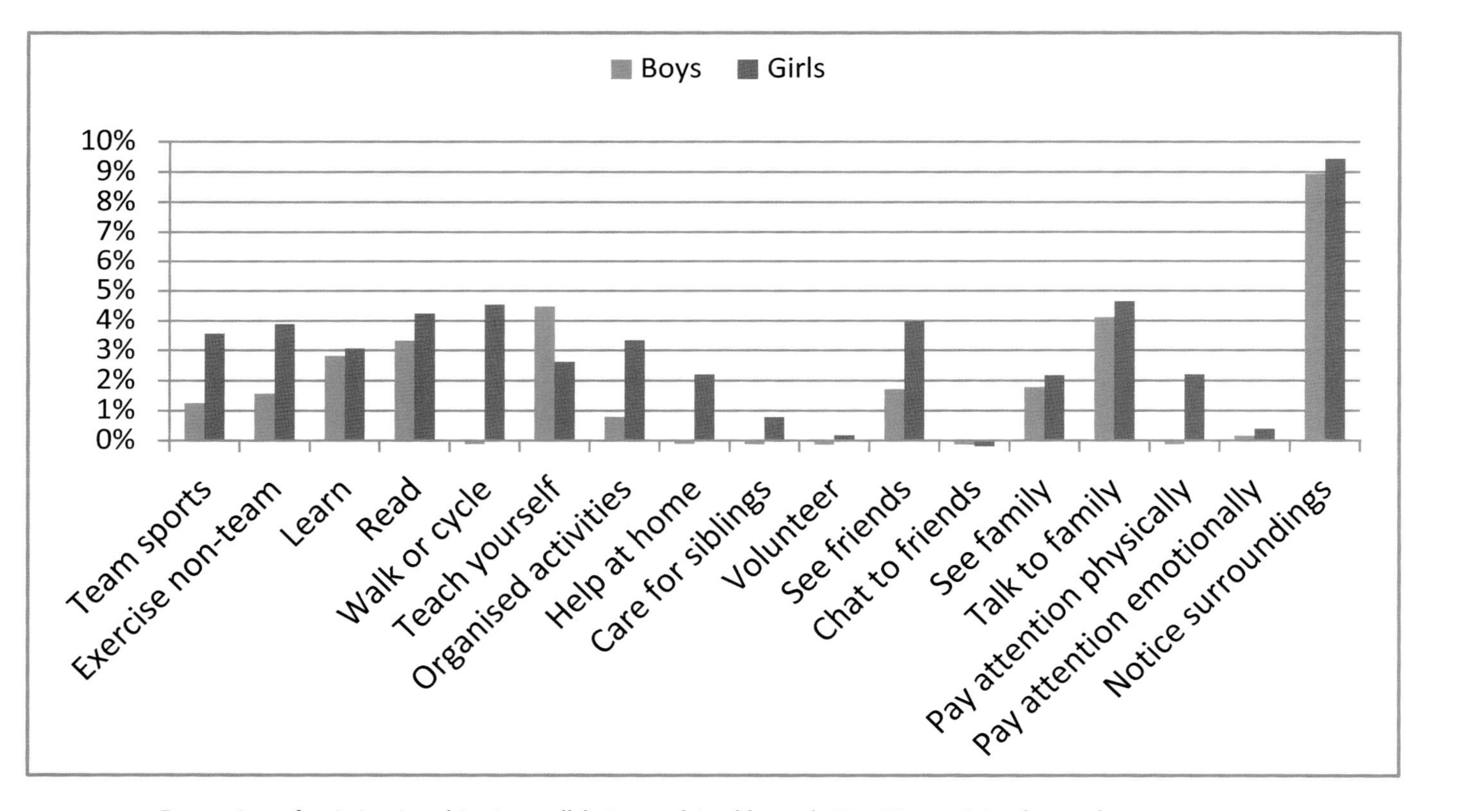

FIGURE 1.21 Proportion of variation in subjective well-being explained by each *Five Ways* activity, by gender

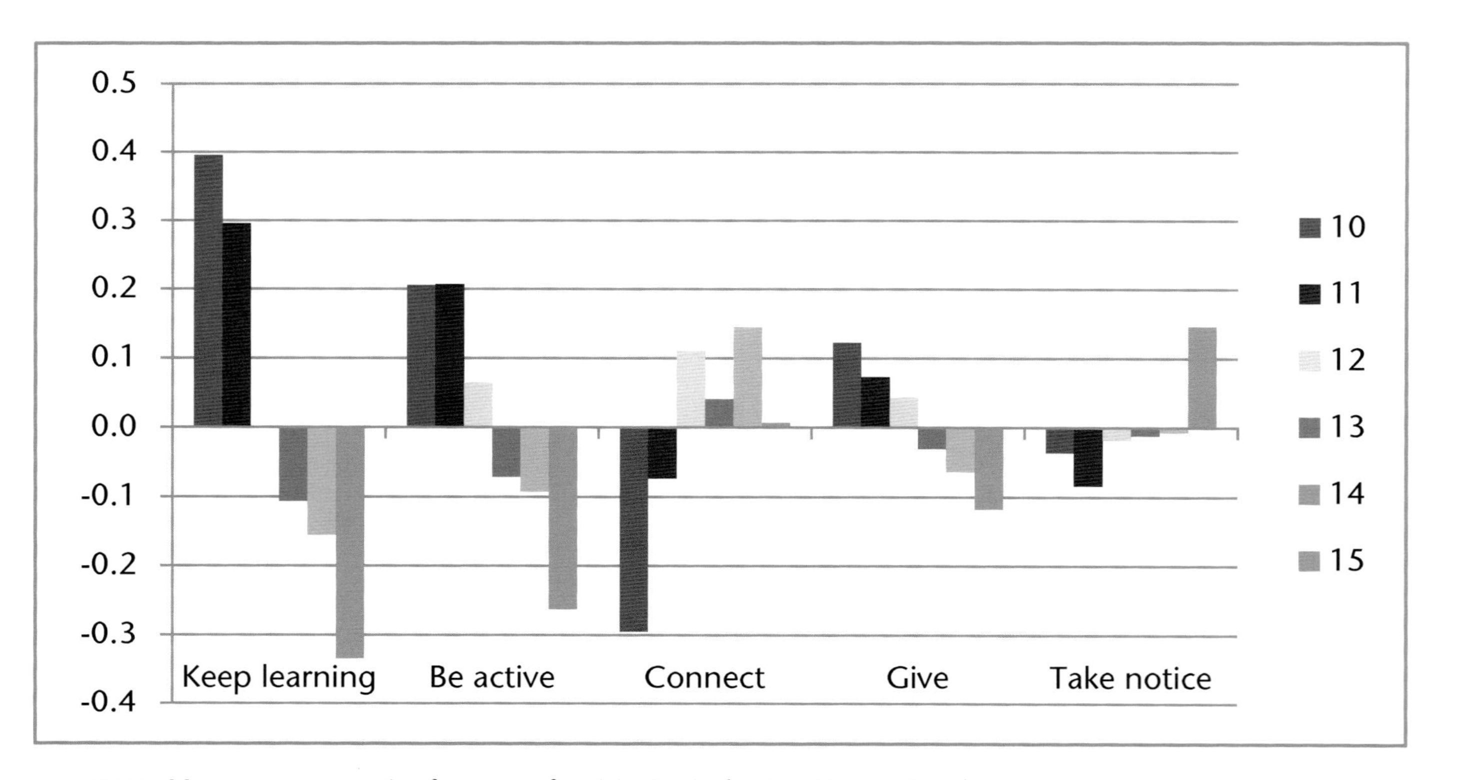

FIGURE 1.22 Mean scores representing frequency of participation in the *Five Ways* activities, by age

that some of the *Five Ways* activities were more strongly linked to well-being than others. How often children notice their surroundings (Take Notice) had the strongest association, explaining 10% of the variation in well-being. Talking to family about things that are important was the most important element of Connect, and seeing one's friends in person was more important than chatting via the phone or through social media. In the Be Active category, non-team sports/exercise was the strongest predictor of well-being, while for Keep Learning, reading for fun and other informal learning activities were more strongly associated with well-being than organised activities.

The findings of this research suggest that the *Five Ways to Well-being* framework, originally proposed on the basis of research with adults, is also useful for considering the connections between children's everyday activities and their well-being. The association between everyday activities and children's well-being does not in itself provide evidence of a causal link, although it is plausible that they do. If this is the case, then it is also possible that encouraging children to engage in these activities may lead to improvements in their well-being. There is already some evidence from research with adults of this potential. Our research therefore provides an important message for children themselves and for all those concerned with maintaining and enhancing their well-being.

References

Abdallah, S., Main G., Pople L. & Rees G. (2014) *Ways to Well-Being: Exploring the Links Between Children's Activities and Their Subjective Well-Being*, London: The Children's Society.

Aked, J., Marks, N., Cordon, C. & Thompson, S. (2008) *Five Ways to Well-being: A Report Presented to the Foresight Project on Communicating the Evidence Base for Improving People's Well-being*, London: New Economics Foundation.

Deci, E. L. & Ryan, R. M. (2000) The "what" and "why" of goal pursuits: human needs and the self-determination of behaviour, *Psychological Inquiry* 11: 227–226.

Huebner, E. S. (1991) Initial development of the Students' Life Satisfaction Scale, *School Psychology International* 12: 231–240

Rees, G., Bradshaw, J., Goswami, H. & Keung A. (2010) *Understanding Children's Well-Being: A National Survey of Young People's Well-Being*, London: The Children's Society.

The Children's Society (2006) *Good Childhood? A Question for our Times*, London: The Children's Society.

The Children's Society (2017) *The Good Childhood Report 2017*, London: The Children's Society.

2

CO-CREATING WELL-BEING EXPERIENCES WITH ASSISTIVE LIVING TECHNOLOGIES

Nikki Holliday, Darren Awang and Gillian Ward

Introduction

The use of design-influenced creative tools and methodologies, along with service blueprinting and consideration of the wider services context in which these are designed, can enable the development of effective prototype products and services that are capable of supporting the well-being of individuals. In this context, this chapter specifically explores experiences with electronic assisted living technologies (eALT) which are targeted at the needs of the elderly and vulnerable, to examine the processes involved and the experience of the design teams in meeting the needs of these target groups. As such, it considers the innovation involved, the design process and thus how this sector is responding to the agenda regarding supporting well-being specifically through eALT.

Discussion is set in the context of an increasing need by the elderly for appropriate health and well-being services, where increased age is correlated with increased likelihood of disability, long-term health conditions and poorer well-being (Steptoe, Deaton & Stone, 2015). For example, 41% of people aged over-65 years old living in England have an illness which causes some level of impairment or disability, and this figure increases to 69% of those aged over 85 years (Department for Work and Pensions, 2009), while the number of people aged 55–64 is due to increase by 18%, and those over 65 years by 39% (Cracknell, 2010; Digital, 2013; Office for National Statistics, 2015).

Further to this, fewer citizens are being offered support from their local governments (Fernández et al., 2013). Globally, annual increases in healthcare spending are beginning to slow (Deloitte, 2016). In the United Kingdom alone, healthcare spending is expected to fall from 8.2% of GDP to 6.7% by 2019.

Countries are thus beginning to recognise that, in absence of state-funded support, people should be signposted to services and products outside of statutory support (*The Care Act*, 2014; Scottish Government, 2016). This opens up an opportunity for the private sector to develop products and services to meet the needs of those who are currently not able to access statutory services (Ward et al., 2015). This is an appropriate consideration for the multi-factorial problem of ageing populations, which will require the blurring of private and public boundaries, particularly as many aspects of life which have influence over the well-being of older people are not under the remit of statutory services (PwC, 2015). Assistive Technology (AT) can address some of these aspects.

Assistive Technology

AT can be defined as "any product or service designed to enable independence for disabled and older people" (Department of Health, 2014, p.1) and spans a variety of products, both "low-tech" and "high-tech". AT can include lower-tech devices such as walking sticks, and products to help people dress, wash and eat as well as home adaptations, such as grab rails and stair lifts; such home adaptations can improve the independence safety and well-being of older people, as well as reducing care costs (Powell et al., 2017). On the higher-tech end of the scale are digital solutions which can be encapsulated by the term Electronic Assisted Living Technology (eALT), defined as "electronic technology that is developed to support the independence of community-dwelling older adults by alleviating or preventing functional or cognitive impairment, by limiting the impact of chronic disease, or by enabling social or physical activity" (Peek et al., 2014, p.237).

eALT includes digital devices, products and services which can be used to help people live independently and safely (telecare), monitor health conditions remotely (telehealth), or support health and well-being via smart device apps. There has been an exponential increase in the interest in eALT due to its purported potential to reduce healthcare costs, support care at a distance, and provide data which may be used to identify needs and treatment outcomes and predict future population health (Hostetter, Klein & McCarthy, 2014). National and international medical, financial and governmental institutions are supportive of the concept of eALT playing a role in addressing the challenges arising from ageing populations (Bhavnani, Narula & Sengupta, 2016). Further, the public are increasingly using technology in their day-to-day lives and are, or will begin to expect technology to form a part of how they manage their health and well-being on a day-to-day basis (Deloitte, 2014; PwC, 2015; Ward et al., 2017). Older people are increasingly embracing smart technologies. In 2016 (in the UK) only 28% of over-65s and 8% of over-75s owned a smartphone, however this has jumped to 39% of over-65s and 15% for over-75s (Ofcom, 2017); in the United States, 42% of over-65s and 12% of over-75s own a smartphone (Pew Research Center, 2017). In the developing economies the picture is different; Bangladesh, (where only 2% of those aged over 50 are smartphone users), Thailand and Malaysia are all seeing higher rates of smartphone use among their elder citizens (14%, 17% and 25% respectively, Telenor, 2015).

The rise of the use of fitness trackers (e.g. Fitbit, Garmin ViVosmart) and health apps (e.g. MyFitness Pal, Couch to 5k) are further testament to the notion that the public themselves are increasingly seeing a role for technology with regards to managing their own health and well-being and are willing to spend money to engage in self-management (PwC, 2015; Dinesen et al., 2016).

"Technology enabled care services"

There is an increasing evidence base supporting the role that eALT may have to play in improving health and well-being. For example, NHS England commissioned a review of eALTs (described as "technology enabled care services", or "remote assistive technologies") exploring the outcomes of eALT services from across the world (NHS England, 2017). There was some evidence for the use of SMS text messaging (e.g. in smoking cessation, adherence to antiretroviral medication), telemonitoring (diabetes, heart disease, chronic obstructive pulmonary disease), and video consultation (mental health), (NHS England, 2017). Mixed-results were found for website-based interventions, although there was evidence that some web-based interventions can reduce anxiety symptoms and improve symptoms in diabetes Type 1, although the effectiveness of web-based interventions decreases over time.

The authors of the review argued that a Participatory Design approach to developing health and well-being interventions could improve adherence rates (NHS England, 2017), and that the use of design paradigms and methodologies, including Participatory Design, Co-Production, Co-Creation and Co-Design (see Figure 2.1) are increasingly being utilised for eALT development.

Traditionally, eALT developed for use within the statutory sector has tended to be situated within the medical research paradigm, where Randomised Control Trials (RCT) are deemed the "gold standard" of evidence. However, it is argued by some that RCTs are not appropriate for the development of commercial eALT which should be aligned with commercial development and design practices (Bruseberg & McDonagh-Philp, 2002) and that RCTs are unable to keep pace with the rapid development of technology (Dinesen et al., 2016, Nicholas, Boydell & Christensen, 2016) and consumer/patient expectations (Deloitte, 2014). The largest eALT RCT to date, the Whole Systems Demonstrator (WSD) project was criticised due to its inappropriate methodology (Steventon et al., 2012).

It is argued that the heterogeneity of settings is not taken into account with RCTs such as the WSD project (Armfield et al. 2014). Indeed, a UK Department of Health working group came to the consensus that the nature of AT itself is likely to require a pragmatic approach to research, which naturally includes a variety of methodologies (Beech & Roberts, 2008). The Transatlantic Telehealth Research Network recommended the consideration of rapid cycle design evaluation and the use of innovative research methodologies to encourage the development of scalable and sustainable eALT programs (Dinesen et al., 2016) where the design research paradigm is argued to be better suited to the problems presented by the ageing population, which requires innovative solutions to improve health and well-being in this increasingly large group (Chamberlain et al., 2015; Holliday, Magee & Walker-Clarke, 2015).

The move to co-creative methods in health and well-being research

As reported above, much eALT research conducted within the health and social care sphere has traditionally been developed in a linear fashion utilising traditional social science methods (Holliday et al., 2015; Valentine et al., 2017); for example, focus groups and interviews feeding into separate design and research phases (see Figure 2.2) with designers and researchers working separately, the Researcher often being an outside observer to the design process (Fallman, 2008). This approach has been criticised for being time-consuming, and disassociating the user from the design process (Steen, Manschot & De Koning, 2011; Xie et al., 2012; Holliday et al., 2015). Increasingly, Social Scientists and Health Researchers are seeing the merit of creative and design research approaches to technology research and development (Holliday et al., 2015). Creative approaches to technology development allow embedded user involvement, research and design to occur in a simultaneous manner with the input of a variety of stakeholders (see Figure 2.3). This holistic approach enables a better understanding of "the larger context of implementation, use, location, as well as the use of real people" (Bhömer et al., 2013 p.37), allowing the development of innovative technology solutions which are embedded in user wants and needs, in a timely and feasible, and more cost-effective manner (Holliday et al., 2015). The inclusion of a wide range of stakeholders, particularly those whose well-being is at stake, allows participants to feel like "active agents"

Definitions

Participatory Design: "Defined in part by the techniques and methods used, namely strategies that allow for the direct participation of workers [stakeholders] in project definition and design specification." (Kensing & Blomberg, 1998, p.181)

Co-Creation: "Any act of collective creativity, i.e. creativity that is shared by two or more people." (Sanders & Stappers, 2008, p.6)

Co-Design: "Collective creativity as it is applied across the whole span of the design process. Thus, co-design is a specific instance of co-creation. . .the creativity of designers and people not trained in design working together in the design development process." (Sanders & Stappers, 2008, p.6)

Co-Production: "A relationship where professionals and citizens share power to plan and deliver support together, recognising that both have vital contributions to make in order to improve quality of life for people and communities." – (National Co-production Critical Friends Group, quoted in SCIE (2015))

FIGURE 2.1 Definitions used

Stakeholders
Users
Researchers
Research
Focus Groups/
Interviews
Designers
Researchers
Recommendation
to Designer
Designers
Designer
designs
something
Stakeholders
Users
Researchers
Researcher
presents design
to people
Designers
Feedback to
Designer

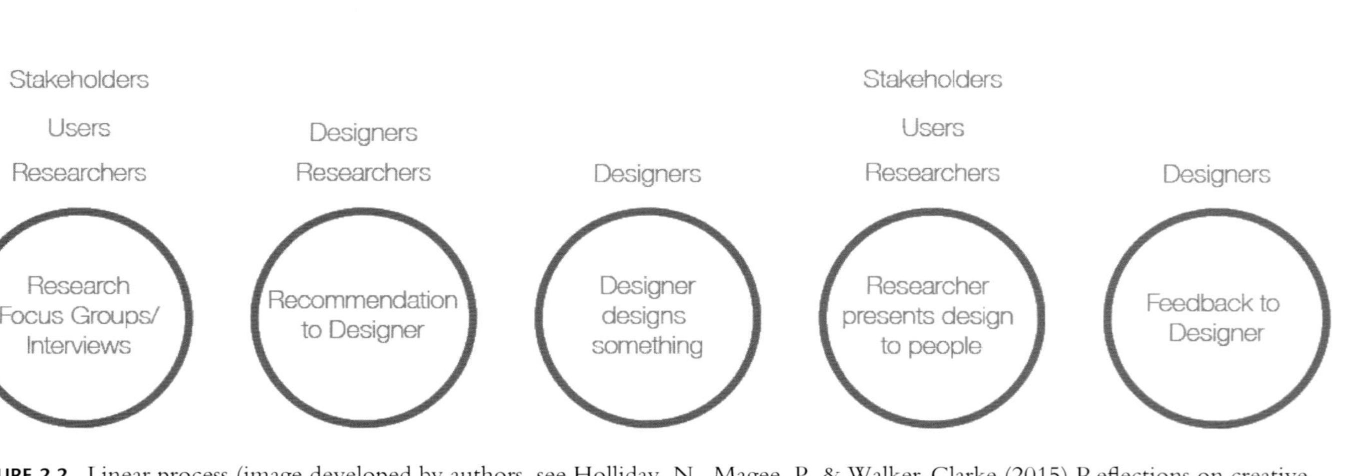

FIGURE 2.2 Linear process (image developed by authors, see Holliday, N., Magee, P. & Walker-Clarke (2015) Reflections on creative methodologies for health technology research, and the iterative process between research and design, in K. Christer (ed.), *Proceedings of the 3rd European Conference on Design4Health: 2015 European Conference*, Sheffield Hallam University. Available at http://research.shu.ac.uk/design4health/wp-content/uploads/2015/07/D4H_Holliday_et_al.pdf (July 2015)

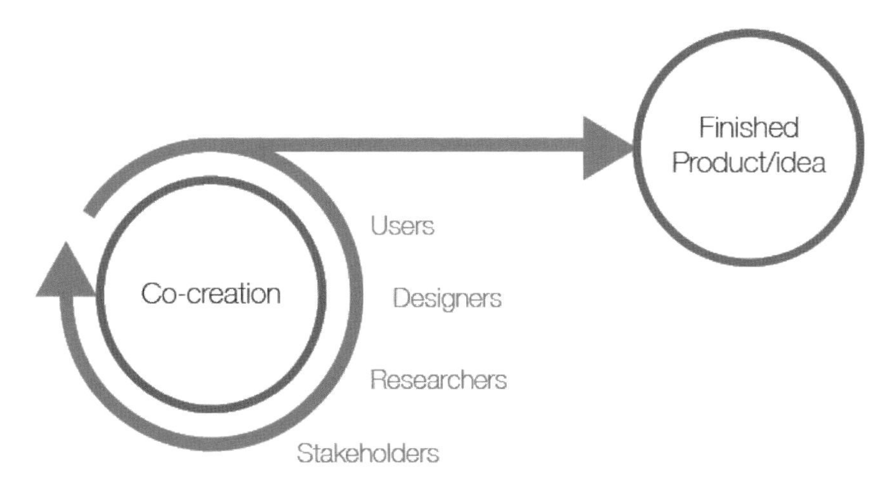

FIGURE 2.3 Multi-stakeholder approach to eALT design (image developed by authors, see Holliday, N., Magee, P. & Walker-Clarke (2015) Reflections on creative methodologies for health technology research, and the iterative process between research and design, in K. Christer (ed.), *Proceedings of the 3rd European Conference on Design4Health: 2015 European Conference*, Sheffield Hallam University. Available at http://research.shu.ac.uk/design4health/wp-content/uploads/2015/07/D4H_Holliday_et_al.pdf (July 2015)

who have control over, and a say in the development of products and services to support their well-being (Valentine et al., 2017). It is further argued that the use of creative methods can help to alleviate the effect of typical barriers to eALT adoption which include poor usability, as they have the potential to elicit rich, meaningful data from a variety of key stakeholders in a timely and cost-efficient manner and ensures user requirements are included in the design process (Holliday, Moody & Ward, 2017).

Co-Creation workshops – exploring and designing well-being with users

This chapter uses the Warm Neighbourhoods® AroundMe™ project among other examples as an example of how creative research methods, inspired by design research paradigms can address issues centred around well-being (Ward et al., 2015). The project was funded by Innovate UK's Delivering Assisted Living Lifestyles at Scalle (dallas) iFocus programme, Coventry University, on behalf of the Advanced Digital Institute. Using the Warm Neighbourhoods® AroundMe™ project, we consider the concept of Co-Creation in more detail, and how the inclusive involvement of users and key stakeholders combined with technological innovation can stimulate the development of creative and innovative ideas grounded in user need. The project occurred in four stages; Co-Creation, service blueprinting, rapid prototyping and finally a "Living Labs" trial.

The WarmNeighbouhoods® AroundMe™ service concept aimed to support older and vulnerable people to live safer at home, while enabling their friends and family to help support them. The Service Design process began with a series of Co-Creation workshops (Figure 2.4). Co-Creation was chosen as the creative approach to the Service Design, as it enabled the contribution of various stakeholder perspectives to the service, from both the "demand" (i.e. users/customers – the older/vulnerable people/their friends and family) and the "supply" side (technology, services, processes, providers) (Steen et al., 2011). The aim of the workshops was to enable the potential customers, their friends and family and industry stakeholders

Case Study: WarmNeighbourhoods® AroundMe™ Co-Creation Workshops

To design a service embedded within end-user need, potential service stakeholders (older people, friends and family, third sector representatives, technologists, eALT industry representatives, designers) were recruited to take part in two co-creation workshops.

Workshop One: The first workshop (n=12)* explored what types of technology and sensors could be used to help support an older or vulnerable person in their home, and how the service supporting the technology would work. The service designed was called AroundMe™.

Workshop Two: The second workshop (n=12)* included industry, charity, and service stakeholders, who were presented with the data generated by the end-user workshop, Their task was to develop the service further, ensuring that the ideas proposed by the first workshop were feasible for a trial and ultimately, commercialisation (Kristensson, Matthing & Johansson, 2008).

All materials generated in the workshops were preserved for analysis. Full annotations of the materials were made in situ by the researchers. Thematic Content Analysis was used to identify important themes within the data (Green & Thorogood, 2014). The older people (and their friends and family) in the first workshop were keen that the service would have a positive view of living independently, with the technology able to provide positive "I'm OK" well-being alerts, rather than just alerting when something has gone wrong. The service developed across the two workshops was rapidly prototyped ready for a small-scale trial and consisted of the following technologies: (1) Electrical appliance usage monitor; (2) Door open/close sensor; (3) Ambient temperature sensor; (4) Base unit to use co-intelligence from all sensors to determine whether or not the person is "OK" and a message of reassurance can be sent to friends and family. The base unit was programmed to send a positive well-being status message to friends and family of the main user if all sensors in the system had been triggered by a pre-agreed time, and if the ambient temperature was above 18°C.

*The Co-Creation workshops methodology is discussed in more detail elsewhere (Ward et al., 2014; Ward et al., 2015).

FIGURE 2.4 Co-Creation workshops

to engage with the concept of a commercial service to support older people to live at home longer, and to Co-Design together a prototype service. Stakeholders who attended the workshops included potential customers, informal carers, care agencies, statutory providers, industry and technology providers.

Service blueprinting

Using a persona-based approach (Service Design Tools, 2009) a fictitious scenario of a "typical" person that could be a future recipient was created to facilitate discussions within the two Co-Creation workshops. This persona was named Ada, an older person, who was struggling to remain safe and independent at home despite informal care from her daughter (Marie who lived 50 miles away) and her older friend (Alison) who lived nearby.

The creation of the persona and her situation was essential to help the workshop participants empathise with the kinds of issues that many older people in similar situations might be experiencing. The metaphor of a bus journey was used to move the focus of the discussions forward to explore what the key features of the future service might be, drawing in observations and comments from participants from the persona's viewpoint at stages of her journey. The use of the persona was an important tool to keep the participants focus on what Ada actually *needed* rather than jumping straight to conclusions about what *technology solutions* would best meet Ada's needs. This approach minimised the risk of the project re-producing a list of existing services and products (such as telecare) that are generally available thus defeating the purpose of designing a new service concept.

Having established a strong identity and context for the persona that participants could fully relate to, the research team combined the data generated within the two workshops with the Ada persona. This enabled them to begin to visualise what aspects were most important in future service possibilities. The key questions considered included:

- What the essential features were around need and how this should be expressed?
- Who were important players in the future service scenario?
- How the relevant information about needs could be communicated and to who, and
- What the realistic options were for acquiring the service and technology from the participants' perspectives?

In order to facilitate this envisioning exercise an initial Customer Journey Mapping process was created, again based on the experience and context of Ada. Customer Journey Mapping is a tool often used in business to identify critical areas of customer contact at each stage within the service journey (Pennington, 2016). Basic Customer Journey Maps include the four aspects: Aware, Join, Use, Exit. The initial map of the Ada persona and her context is shown in Figure 2.5.

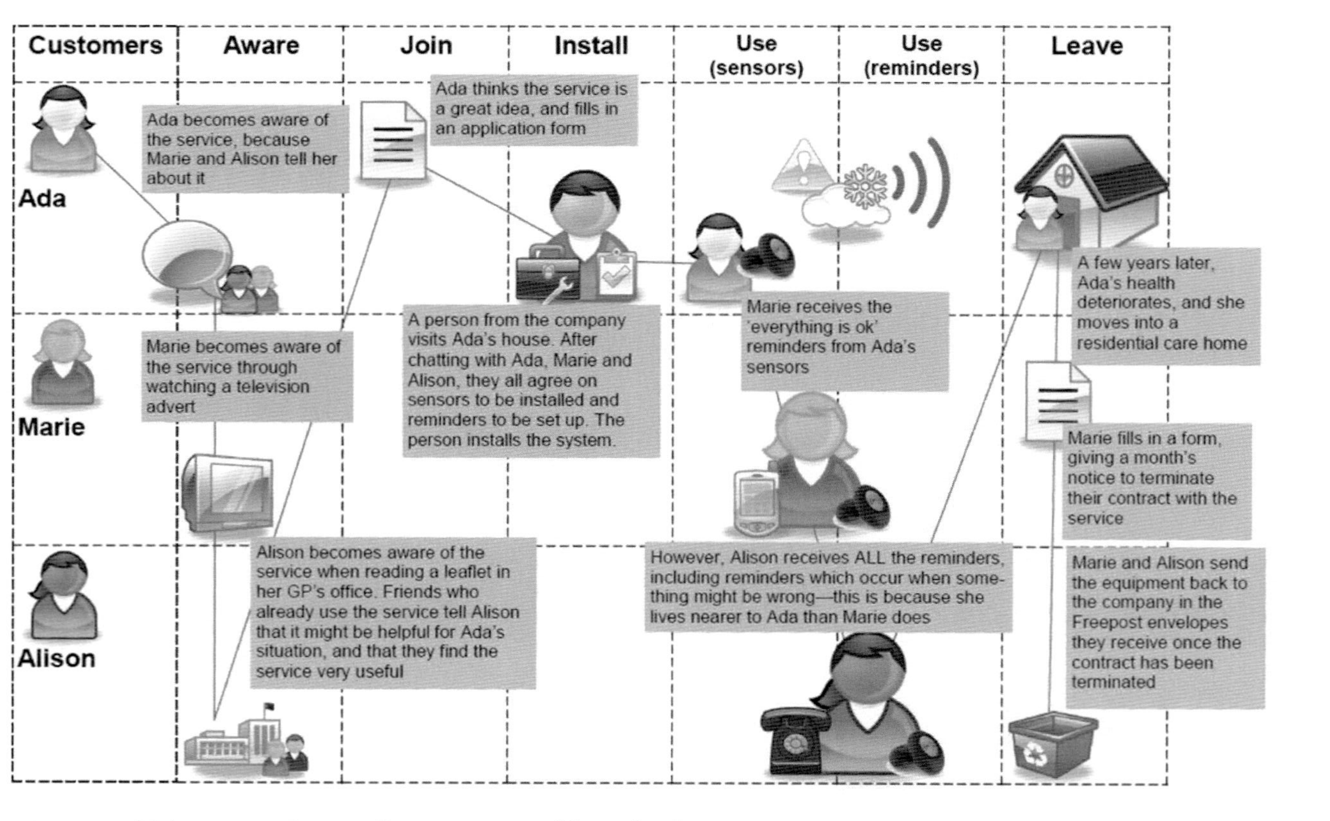

FIGURE 2.5 Ada's customer journey (image courtesy of the authors)

"Awareness" refers to the way in which the customer recognises that they have a need for a product or service and could include methods such as TV advertising, a pamphlet or brochure through the door, cold calling or an informal conversation with a friend or relative. "Joining" refers to the process of sign up or accessing the product or service. This could involve some form of application or online form, a referral from a GP to a community service or browsing for items in a shop or website to purchase. "Use" is the period when the person has accessed the product or service and the duration for which it is required. This could be quite short or an extended period, e.g. a hospital admission or 30 day holiday insurance policy for travelling abroad. "Exit" describes the process of leaving the service and/or disposing of the product after use. This is like leaving a utility provider, closing a social work case or discharge from an outpatient service.

Customer Journey Maps help to simplify what is often a much more complex process and for the purpose of designing a new service it provides an ideal starting point as it focuses primarily on the customers' perspectives as they move through a service. Additional elements can be added depending on needs. In this instance an "Install" aspect was included and "Use" aspects were broken down into two further elements to enable the team to focus in on these areas in more depth. A "Return" option could also be valuable for example if examining the journey in the context of a supermarket or restaurant experience. In the case of eALT – what would make a customer choose further supportive products from a company, or return to sign up for services to support additional family members?

Mapping the journey allows the designer to identify the possible "touchpoints" within the process where the customer encounters the service. Touchpoint analysis is a method that is used to review good practice or challenging areas of existing service provision to identify areas where lessons can be learned to enhance the customer experience (Stickdorn & Zehrer, 2009).

However, in order to design a new range of service options Customer Journey Maps in themselves are insufficient as they only provide the customer's perspective. Therefore, a Service Design Blueprint (Figure 2.6) was developed to underpin this map. Zeithaml & Bitner (2013) describe a service blueprint as an accurate and understandable map that portrays a service system. This map should be clear and accessible to a range of different people regardless of their roles or viewpoints. A key feature of blueprinting using this technique is that the "customer actions" are brought to the forefront with regards importance, and therefore guide the rest of the underpinning processes.

Service blueprinting is often attributed to (Shostack, 1982). Within a business context it is considered as a versatile technique for simultaneously depicting and visualising:

- Service process.
- Points of customer contact (touchpoints).
- Physical evidence required to support the service from the customer's point of view (Arizona State University, 2016).

Service Design Blueprints often include five elements that are overlaid beneath the Customer Journey Map (Sabine & Kleinaltenkamp, 2004).

These include:

- Physical Evidence – all tangibles that customers come in contact with and that impact customer quality perceptions.
- Customer Actions – all steps that customers take or experience as part of the service process.
- Employee On-Stage Actions (Visible) – the contact employee actions that involve face-to-face interactions with customers.
- Contact Backstage Actions (Invisible) – other contact employee actions (not involving face-to-face customer interactions) including email/phone contact with customers, preparation work, and any activities that facilitate the service process.
- Support Processes – activities that facilitate the service process and are done by individuals who are not contact employees.

Lines of interaction can be drawn across the blueprint to clarify where for example customers interact with the service or backstage employees play a role (Figure 2.6).

The research team applied this format to the customer journey and were able to redefine four different service option choices that could potentially meet the needs of the target customer. The four options were:

1. Product purchase only and self-installation.
2. Product purchase and installation by another.
3. Product rental service only and self-installation (i.e. a "plug and play" option).
4. Product rental service and installation by another.

Each option had slightly different customer touchpoints with one being the simplest service configuration. This first option is illustrated in Figure 2.6.

As part of the ongoing Co-Creation approach these Service Design Blueprints were returned to the original workshop participants for verification. Feedback requested from the participants included their views on the likely uptake of each of the different service concepts and which of the options most closely matched the ideas explored in the initial two workshops. The data collected indicated that two of the possible four options should be adopted to take the service concept forward to the development and testing phase.

The value of these powerful analysis tools and techniques should not be underestimated in the design of new service concepts. Each phase of development was carefully orchestrated and methodologies were applied that were consistent with a person-centred design approach. The tools and techniques identified in this section have subsequently been used elsewhere within undergraduate and postgraduate education at Coventry University. For example, Customer Journey Mapping was utilised as a method for Postgraduate Assistive Technology students to identify

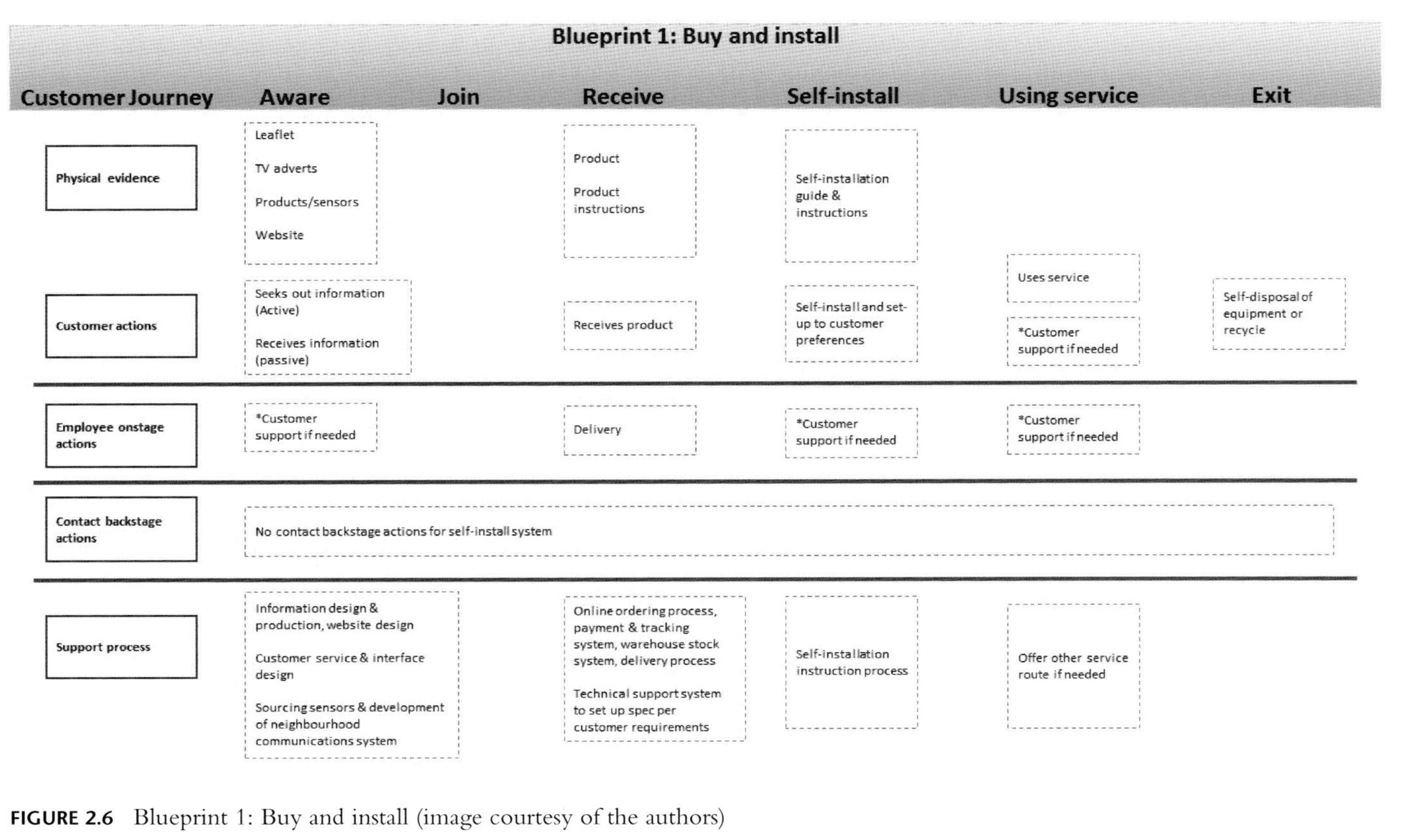

FIGURE 2.6 Blueprint 1: Buy and install (image courtesy of the authors)

challenging areas of service provision from their own employment experiences. Having identified these, students went on to address and improve the problematic touchpoints in a subsequent work based learning module. Undergraduate Occupational Therapy students have also used Customer Journey Mapping and touchpoint analysis to suggest how improvements to services could be made following their practice placement experiences in health and social care settings.

Rapid prototyping

Following the refinement of the service blueprint, the Researchers were able to match this and results of the workshops, to rapidly prototype the service using existing sensor technology, allowing a functioning prototyped service to be developed for quick, initial testing and refinement (Brown & Wyatt, 2010). Rapid prototyping with stakeholders allows development of a prototype product or service embedded in user need and societal context, which ultimately may reduce the risk of a product when entering the market, allowing researchers and older people to "[fail fast] and fail often" in the early stages of service development (Valentine et al., 2017 p.768), prior to investing in large scale trials or product/service launch.

In this project, the rapid prototype enabled the AroundMe™ service to be tested in-situ using a Living Lab methodology, which allowed the service blueprint to be tested in the context in which it would ultimately be used – the older person's home. That existing technology can be used to rapidly prototype new services from resources already available to us suggests that when considering the development of a new product or service we must avoid reinventing the wheel. Indeed, many eALT services that do find themselves with evidence of effectiveness (e.g. SMS messaging; NHS England, 2017) may often be considered "unremarkable" and "old hat" to developers and innovators who might be tempted to develop super innovative, new technologies when existing technologies and techniques may be equally (if not more effective), cheaper and more feasible to produce.

Here we can consider the case the case of the Fallcheck web-app, developed by Coventry University with Occupational Therapists, "falls" experts and older people at risk of falling. The Fallcheck web-app provides a comprehensive guide to alert to potential fall hazards that might be present in a person's home, and provides information on how to reduce or remove these hazards to prevent future falls. Initially, Fallcheck was envisaged within a 3D gaming environment, however early feedback from the steering group indicated that this was not a good fit with the intended app function of providing information to older people and their carers. Further, game programming and development can be costly and time-consuming (Kato, 2010) and would likely delay the release of Fallcheck due to the extra funding needed to fully develop a game for Android and Apple platforms. Thus, the pragmatic decision was taken to develop a web-app (see Figure 2.7), which could be rapidly prototyped in house, quickly improved with iterative feedback from professionals, carers and older people at risk of falling (Ward, Walker-Clarke & Holliday, 2017). The result of the decision to move from the cutting-edge gaming approach to the pragmatic web-app approach resulted in Fallcheck being quickly developed and is now available (free of charge) to anyone worried about falling at home (www.coventry.ac.uk/Fallcheck). Results of a recent trial of the web-app with carers and older people at risk of falling found that the web-app was acceptable and easy to use for carers and older people who may prefer the choice of using the web-app on a larger laptop or desktop screen with static interaction (Dinesen et al., 2016). Use of the web-app also increased feelings of safety at home, with 53% of trial participants making changes in their home or their relative's home to reduce home hazards based upon the advice provided (Ward & Holliday, 2016). The app has been well-received beyond the trial, with favourable independent reviews being published, and receiving the accolade of "App of the week" in *Woman's Own*, a national UK based magazine (*Woman's Own*, 2015, p.35) and further recognition by nursing and optometrists involved in falls prevention (Hayes, 2015; Harvey, 2017).

In the AroundMe™ example, the use of repurposed technology allowed us to quickly prototype the service as developed through the Co-Creation workshops and the subsequent blueprinting stage without having to endure a lengthy technological development phase. Indeed, it should be argued that it is an unethical waste

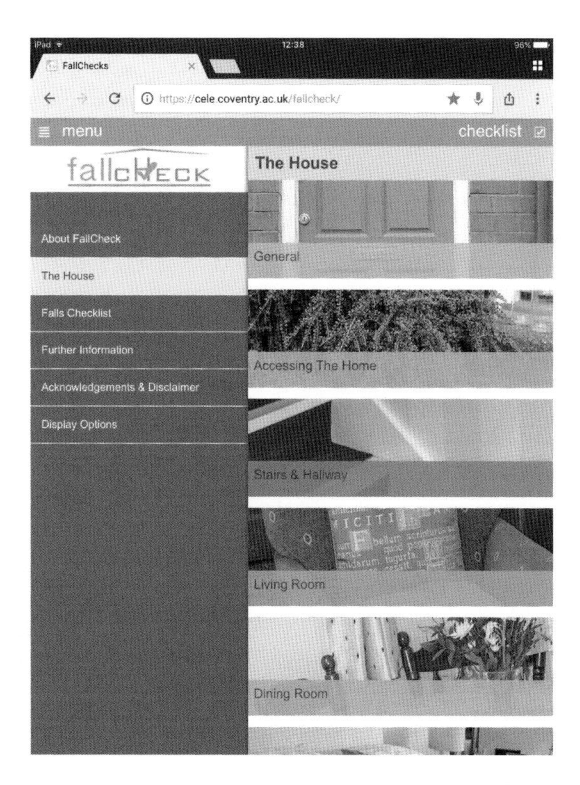

FIGURE 2.7 The Fallcheck web-app interface, a simple, non-gamified platform (© Nikki Holiday and Gillian Ward)

of Researcher time and funding to develop technologies that already exist and may be utilised. While future thinking will always be required, it is recommended that researchers and developers working in the sphere of eALT research consider how they can use creative methods to make best use of and repurpose existing technologies and focus on better application and integration of these technologies into Service Design. This can also increase the likelihood of a product achieving scalability, as the barriers of production of new parts is reduced or removed entirely and is a particularly useful approach for small or medium sized enterprises wishing to innovate new services, due to barriers removed by use of existing technologies (Yoon et al., 2015).

Trialling co-created well-being technologies

With regards to the AroundMe™ trial, we utilised a Living Lab methodology. The Living Lab method is defined as "a user-centric innovation milieu built on everyday practice and research, with an approach that facilitates user influence in open and distributed innovation processes engaging all relevant partners in *real-life contexts*, aiming to create *sustainable* values" (Bergvall-Kåreborn et al., 2009, p.3) suggesting that it is a trial methodology particularly suited to the development of eALTs (particularly commercial eALTs) which will be used within the person's own home. The Living Lab allows in-situ testing of eALT in the exact context in which it will be used, lending ecological validity to the trial – a key factor required when attempting to develop scalable solutions that will be purchased and utilised in the real world (Følstad, 2008). The Living Lab trial conducted for the WarmNeighbourhoods® AroundMe™ service is described in detail in Figure 2.8, and it allowed the researchers to discover not only whether or not the service worked within the home environment and was accepted by the participants, but also aspects of the service peculiar to its use which would not have been picked up if the technology had only been tested in a laboratory setting. For example, in one home, a participant with dementia kept

Case study: WarmNeighbourhoods® AroundMe™ Living Lab trial

The rapidly prototyped service was trialled with 12 families across the West Midlands, using a Living Lab methodology to allow in situ testing of the technology in participants' own homes (Westerlund & Leminen, 2011).* The AroundMe™ system was installed in users' homes for three months. Each system was personalised to the main user's daily routines, e.g. a person who routinely makes a cup of tea in the morning and has a bowl of cereal would have the electrical appliance usage monitor connected to their kettle, and door open/close sensor attached to a kitchen cupboard. The feedback from the trial was overwhelmingly positive. Participants found that the system promoted greater understanding, awareness, reassurance and involvement between carers of the same family. It was felt that the sensors chosen for the trial by older people and their friends and family in the co-creation workshops were appropriate to communicate wellbeing information within a "neighbourhood" of friends and family, without being too intrusive. Indeed, participants argued against the use of more intrusive sensors such as cameras:

> "Initially I didn't know whether it would bother me, but it doesn't at all. Certainly, if there was any camera work going on, that would bother me. I would feel like I would have to dress instead of lounging around in a dressing gown. . . and full make up. But no, it's perfect, absolutely perfect."
>
> *– Wendy, main user*

A criticism often levied at the use of technology to support independence and wellbeing is that it may reduce social contact (Blaschke, Freddolino & Mullen, 2009). Conversely, this trial found the opposite effect, with an increase in both quality and quantity of contact being reported. This was because the alerts acted as a reminder for friends and family to contact their loved ones, and because they were already assured regarding their wellbeing that they could then focus conversations on social topics, rather than "checking up" on the main user.

> "It works very well, because what normally happens is [I receive a message], and I pick up the phone and talk to Alice [main user] because it reminds me that it's time to talk to [her] . . . It prompts me."
>
> *– Dawn, Carer*

The service also improved the sense and awareness of their loved one's wellbeing for the friends and family of the older person. The older person themselves had an increased sense of independence and freedom, as they knew their relatives were reassured of their wellbeing.

> "I think it makes me much more aware of when [my father] is having good days and bad days."
>
> *George, Carer*

> "I don't like to feel suffocated, if you like, that they are always 'are you OK? Is everything alright?' . . . I can't stand that. But [with] this, I am doing it myself if you like, with the machine [which sends a message to George] – 'Yes everything is alright'. . . So, I think it is probably a relief for him too."
>
> *– Phyllis, main user*

*The methodology and the results of the trial are discussed in more detail elsewhere (Ward et al. 2014, Ward et al. 2015).

FIGURE 2.8 WarmNeighbourhoods® AroundMe™ Living Lab trial (see Ward, G., Holliday, N., Awang, D. & Harson, D. (2014) Technology and informal care networks: Creative approaches to user-led Service Design for the Warm Neighbourhoods® AroundMe™ service, *Interdisciplinary Studies Journal* 3 (4): 24. Also see Holliday, N., Ward, G., Awang, D. & Harson, D. (2014) Conceiving and developing a mainstream consumer service to support older or vulnerable people living independently, *ServiceDesign and Innovation 2014*, Lancaster University, April 2014)

switching off the base unit of the service as she was in the habit of switching off all electrical appliances in her home prior to going to bed.

In non-commercial, statutory settings, the Living Lab methodology may have less appeal, particularly in evidence-based medicine settings, however as described above, it is beginning to be recognised that when it comes to implementing technology in care pathways, we may have to "adapt methods to the innovative process rather than doing the opposite" (Wilson, Boaden & Harvey, 2016, p.2), or else we run the risk of real-life consumer technologies running apace those adopted in healthcare systems while we wait for "cumbersome and time-consuming" RCTs to take place (Dinesen et al., 2016). Indeed, the use of the Living Lab method allowed the researchers to test the prototyped service quickly, and allowed the researchers to adapt to the service according to participant needs (for example, the researchers had a conversation with the lady who kept switching her base unit off and it was agreed that a "Stop" sign would be placed on the plug to remind her to leave that appliance switched on).

Conclusion

The use of design-influenced creative tools and methodologies, along with service blueprinting and consideration of the wider service context in which eALT exists, can enable the development of effective prototype products and services that can support the well-being of older and vulnerable people. In the case of the AroundMe™ project, the Co-Creation workshops enabled the researchers to quickly understand the Service Design requirements from both the customer viewpoint, and those of technology industry stakeholders who were able to build upon the service co-designed by the older people and their friends and family to develop a service blueprint for a technology that not only met end-user needs but was also technologically and commercially feasible. Ultimately, this led to a service which was highly valued by the participants who took part in the Living Lab trial. This has proved to be a powerful persuader to take the service forward to commercialisation, with several national businesses interested in the commercialisation of the service. The results were reported publicly (Ward et al., 2014; Holliday et al., 2015; Ward et al., 2015) and similar services have beginning to be developed by other companies that are now available to members of the public, e.g. CanaryCare.

This chapter has outlined a specific approach to Co-Creation of eALT products and services utilised by Coventry University, however there are increasing numbers of design-influenced methodologies and tools available which are intended for those seeking to improve health and well-being, for example experience-based Co-Design and Co-Production (SCIE, 2015; Point of Care Foundation, 2017) and many researchers are adopting creative tools and methodologies for data collection and idea generation (Holliday et al., 2017). This chapter has argued that RCTs and quantitative methods may not be appropriate for the development of consumer health and well-being technologies, and the authors hope that it will provide health and well-being researchers with the inspiration to engage in co-creative methods when developing these technologies. Of course, in health and social care settings where evidence-based decision-making is crucial, evaluation must follow the innovation stage and we do not advocate missing this stage out where it is appropriate (Wilson et al., 2016). However, it is clear that creative and design methods are effective in developing eALT technologies and should be considered as a viable methodology for researchers interested in the development of health and well-being technologies which are grounded in user need and ultimately are commercially feasible and scalable.

References

Arizona State University (2016) Service blueprinting overview. Available at www.research.wpcarey.asu.edu/services-leadership/events-programs/service-blueprinting/service-blueprinting-overview.

Armfield, N. R., Edirippulige, S. K., Bradford, N. & Smith, A. C. (2014) Telemedicine – is the cart being put before the horse? *The Medical Journal of Australia* 200 (9): 530–533.

Beech, R. & Roberts, D. (2008) *Research Briefing: Assistive Technology and Older People*, London: SCIE.

Bergvall-Kåreborn, B., Ihlström Eriksson, C., Ståhlbröst, A. & Svensson, J. (2009) A milieu for innovation, in *Proceedings of ISPIM Innovation Symposium*, 6–9 December 2009.

Bhavnani, S. P., Narula, J. & Sengupta, P. P. (2016) Mobile technology and the digitization of healthcare, *European Heart Journal* 37 (18): 1428–1438.

Bhömer, T. M., Brouwer, C. E., Tomico, O. O. & Wensveen, S. S. (2013) Interactive Prototypes in the Participatory Development of Product-Service Systems, Participatory Innovation Conference, Lathi, Finland.

Bruseberg, A. & McDonagh-Philp, D. (2002) Focus groups to support the industrial/product designer: A review based on current literature and designers' feedback, *Applied Ergonomics* 33 (1): 27–38

Chamberlain, P., Wolstenholme, D., Dexter, M. & Seals, E. (2015) *The State of the Art of Design in Health: An Expert-Led Review of the Extent of the Art of Design Theory and Practice in Health and Social Care*, University of Sheffield.

Cracknell, J. (2010) *The Ageing Population*, London: House of Commons Library.

Deloitte (2014) The tail wagging the dog: how retail is changing consumer expectations of the health care patient provider relationship. Available at www2.deloitte.com/tr/en/pages/life-sciences-and-healthcare/articles/how-retail-is-changing-consumer-expectations-of-the-health-care-patient-provider-relationship.html.

Deloitte (2016) 2016 Global health care outlook - battling costs while improving care. Available at www2.deloitte.com/content/dam/Deloitte/global/Documents/Life-Sciences-Health-Care/gx-lshc-2016-health-care-outlook.pdf.

Department of Health (2014) *Research and Development Work Relating to Assistive Technology 2013-2014*, London: Department of Health.

Department for Work and Pensions (2009) *Family Resources Survey 2007/8*, London: Department for Work and Pensions.

Digital, P. A. (2013) *Living Independently: Shouldering the Burden of Chronic Disease*, Minehead: EURIM: Digital Policy Alliance.

Dinesen, B., Nonnecke, B., Lindeman, D., Toft, E., Kidholm, K., Jethwani, K., Young, H. M., Spindler, H., Oestergaard, C. U., Southard, J. A., Gutierrez, M., Anderson, N., Albert, N. M., Han, J. J. & Nesbitt, T. (2016) Personalized telehealth in the future: a global research agenda, *Journal of Medical Internet Research* 18 (3): e53.

Fallman, D. (2008) The interaction design research triangle of design practice, design studies, and design exploration, *Design Issues* 24 (3): 4–18

Fernández, J., Snell, T. & Wistow, G. (2013) *Changes in the Patterns of Social Care Provision in England: 2005/6 to 2012/13*. London: Personal Social Services Research Unit, London School of Economics and Political Science.

Følstad, A. (2008) Living Labs for innovation and development of information and communication technology: a literature review, *The Electronic Journal for Virtual Organisations and Networks* 10: 99–131.

Harvey, B. (2017) The latest in opthalmic apps, *The Optician*. Available at www.opticianonline.net/features/the-latest-in-ophthalmic-apps.

Hayes, N. (2015) App review: Fallcheck. *Nursing Standard*, 35: 27.

Holliday, N., Moody, L. & Ward, G. (2017) Electronic assisted living technology: interim systematic review results – the evidence for creative methodologies, *Studies in Health Technology and Informatics* 242: 216–223.

Holliday, N., Magee, P. & Walker-Clarke, A. (2015) Reflections on creative methodologies for health technology research, and the iterative process between research and design, in K. Christer (ed.) *Proceedings of the Third European Conference on Design4Health: 2015 European Conference*, Sheffield Hallam University.

Hostetter, M., Klein, S. & McCarthy, D. (2014) Taking digital health to the next level, Commonwealth Fund. Available at www.commonwealthfund.org/publications/fund-reports/2014/oct/taking-digital-health-next-level.

Kato, P. M. (2010) Video games in health care: Closing the gap, *Review of General Psychology* 14 (2): 113–121.

NHS England (2017) *TECS Evidence Base Review: Findings and Recommendations*, London: Health Innovation Network.

Nicholas, J., Boydell, K. & Christensen, H. (2016) mHealth in psychiatry: time for methodological change, *Evidence-Based Mental Health* 19 (2): 33–34.

Ofcom (2017) *Adults' Media use and Attitudes*, London: Ofcom.

Office for National Statistics (2015) *National Population Projections: 2014-Based Statistical Bulletin*, London: Office for National Statistics.

Peek, S. T. M., Wouters, E. J. M., van Hoof, J., Luijkx, K. G., Boeije, H. R. & Vrijhoef, H. J. M. (2014) Factors influencing acceptance of technology for aging in place: a systematic review? *International Journal of Medical Informatics* 83 (4): 235–248.

Pennington, A. (2016) *The Customer Experience Book*, Great Britain: Pearson Education MUA.

Pew Research Center (2017) Tech adoption climbs among older adults. Available at www.assets.pewresearch.org/wp-.content/uploads/sites/14/2017/05/16170850/PI_2017.05.17_Older-Americans-Tech_FINAL.pdf.

Point of Care Foundation (2017) EBCD: experience-based co-design toolkit. Available from www.pointofcarefoundation.org.uk/resource/experience-based-co-design-ebcd-toolkit.

Powell, J., Mackintosh, S., Bird, E., Ige, J., Garrett, H. & Roys, M. (2017) The role of home adaptations in improving later life, Centre for Ageing Better. Available at http://eprints.uwe.ac.uk/33945/.

PwC (2015) Connected and coordinated: personalised service delivery for the elderly. Available at www.pwc.com/gx/en/healthcare/pdf/pwc-elderly-care-report.pdf.

Sabine, F. & Kleinaltenkamp, M. (2004) Blueprinting the service company: managing service processes efficiently, *Journal of Business Research* 57 (4): 392–404.

SCIE (2015) Co-Production in social care: What it is and how to do it. Available at www.scie.org.uk/publications/guides/guide51/.

Scottish Government (2016) A national clinical strategy for Scotland. Available at www.gov.scot/Publications/2016/02/8699/4.

Service Design Tools (2009) Communication methods supporting design processes. Available at www.servicedesigntools.org/.

Shostack, G. L. (1982) How to design a service, *European Journal of Marketing* 16: 49–63.

Steen, M., Manschot, M. & De Koning, N. (2011) Benefits of co-design in service design projects, *International Journal of Design* 5 (2): 53–60.

Steptoe, A., Deaton, A. & Stone, A. (2015) Subjective wellbeing, health, and ageing, *The Lancet* 385 (9968): 640–648.

Steventon, A., Bardsley, M., Billings, J., Dixon, J., Doll, H., Hirani, S., Cartwright, M., Rixon, L., Knapp, M., Henderson, C., Rogers, A., Fitzpatrick, R., Hendy, J. & Newman, S. (2012) Effect of telehealth on use of secondary care and mortality: findings from the whole system demonstrator cluster randomised trial, *BMJ: British Medical Journal* 344 (7865): e3874.

Stickdorn, M. & Zehrer, A. (2009) (eds.) *First Nordic Conference on Service Design and Service Innovation. Service Design Tourism: Customer Experience Drive Destination Management*, Oslo, 24–26 November 2009.

Telenor (2015) The unconnected senior citizens of Asia, *M2 Presswire*. Available online at www.telenor.com/the-unconnected-senior-citizens-of-asia/.

The Care Act (2014) *The Care Act*, London: The Stationary Office.

Valentine, L., Kroll, T., Bruce, F., Lim, C. & Mountain, R. (2017) Design thinking for social innovation in health care, *The Design Journal* 20 (6): 755.

Ward, G. & Holliday, N. (2016) Usability of an app to support home hazard modification, *Gerontechnology* 15: 101.

Ward, G., Walker-Clarke, A. & Holliday, N. (2017) Evaluation of a web-based app to assist home-hazard modification in falls prevention, *British Journal of Occupational Therapy* 80 (12): 735–744.

Ward, G., Holliday, N., Awang, D. & Harson, D. (2015) Creative approaches to service design: Using co-creation to develop a consumer focused assistive technology service, *Technology & Disability* 27 (1): 5–15.

Ward, G., Holliday, N., Awang, D. & Harson, D. (2014) Technology and informal care networks: creative approaches to user led service design for the WarmNeighbourhoods® AroundMe™ service, *Interdisciplinary Studies Journal* 3 (4): 24.

Ward, G., Fielden, S., Muir, H., Holliday, N. & Urwin, G. (2017) Developing the assistive technology consumer market for people aged 50-70, *Ageing & Society* 37 (5): 1050–1067.

Wilson, P. M., Boaden, R. & Harvey, G. (2016) Plans to accelerate innovation in health systems are less than IDEAL, *BMJ Quality & Safety* 25 (8): 572–576.

Woman's Own (2015) App of the week, *Woman's Own* 2015 (25): 35.

Xie, B., Druin, A., Fails, J., Massey, S., Golub, E., Franckel, S. & Schneider, K. (2012) Connecting generations: Developing Co-design methods for older adults and children, *Behaviour & Information Technology* 31 (4): 413–423.

Yoon, J., Park, H., Seo, W., Lee, J., Coh, B. & Kim, J. (2015) Technology opportunity discovery (TOD) from existing technologies and products: A function-based TOD framework, *Technological Forecasting and Social Change* 100 (Supplement C): 153–167.

Zeithaml, V. A., Bitner, M. J. & Gremler, D. D. (2013) *Services Marketing: Integrating Customer Focus Across the Firm*, sixth edition, New York: McGraw-Hill Irwin.

3

GREENSPACE AND URBAN GREENING BENEFITS FOR HEALTH AND WELL-BEING ACROSS THE LIFE-COURSE

A pathway for the operationalisation of the green infrastructure approach

Owen Douglas, Mark Scott and Mick Lennon

Introduction

The importance of access to the natural world in supporting health and well-being is increasingly recognised, with the environment now viewed as one of the key determinants of health alongside inherited characteristics and social and economic factors (Barton, 2009). Over the past two decades, there has been a re-emergence of interest examining the impact of the environment on health in advanced economies (e.g. EEA-JRC, 2013), with a considerable expansion of theoretical and empirical studies investigating the role of contextual factors in the production and maintenance of health variations (Cummins et al., 2007). Despite the growing focus of research on the health benefits of population exposure to natural environments, urban densification, climate change and the direct negative externalities of economic growth such as air and water pollution are putting increasing pressure on natural environments worldwide (Haaland & Van den Bosch, 2015; Barton et al., 2016).

These trends are intertwined with wider social changes including shifting family and community structures and changing lifestyles characterised by inactivity (Horwitz et al., 2015) and stress (Patel et al., 2007) with the amount of time that people spend outdoors diminishing, especially in developed economies. While a substantial body of research has investigated the negative impacts on health of "environmental bads", such as poor air quality and the distribution of various forms of pollution, recent decades have seen a growing interest in the potential health creating – or *salutogenic* – effects of natural environments (Antonovsky, 1996). Attention has increasingly focused on the potential positive influence on health and well-being of "environmental goods", such as access to "nature" and the distribution of urban greenspace (Lake & Townshend, 2006). It has been argued that natural environment (including natural elements within cities), urban greenspaces and networks provide health services as part of the wider array of

Ecosystem Services (Pretty et al., 2011; Jackson et al., 2013; Lennon & Scott, 2014). In light of this, Ecosystem Services and the Green Infrastructure (GI) approach have emerged as innovative concepts to enhance population health and well-being through the promotion and maintenance of ecological integrity in both rural and urban environments.

In cities and towns, population interactions with nature generally take place in natural, semi-natural or planned greenspaces set aside for recreation (Lachowycz & Jones, 2013). Indeed, many of the nineteenth- and early twentieth-century thinkers who laid the foundations for modern planning drew intuitive links between greenspace and human health (Barton, 2010), and how it should be provided, such as Howard's Garden City movement and the US City Beautiful and urban parks movement (Howard, 1965; Ward Thompson, 2011; Arthurson et al., 2016; Scott & Lennon, 2016). Despite this well-established link, planners, urban designers and policymakers of today require clear design and management frameworks to guide its provision in the face of ever increasing development pressures and lifestyle changes (Gardsjord et al., 2014). This is particularly the case since densification processes in urban areas often lead to the loss of greenspaces.

New research techniques developed over the past two decades have provided opportunities to study and better understand the mechanisms behind associations between urban green infrastructure (comprising greenspaces, green networks and individual elements such as green roofs or urban trees) and health with increasing sophistication, thereby helping to satisfy contemporary scientific standards of evidence demanded to inform policy and practice (WHO, 2016). In order to provide the evidence in a manner which is accessible for planning and urban design professionals, this chapter adopts a life-course approach to provide a nuanced account of urban greening as a potential pathway for the operationalisation of urban green infrastructure to advance a "policy implementation framework" for enhancing the health and well-being benefits for all socio-demographic cohorts based upon greenspace integrity. In so doing, the chapter sets out a framework for the development of evidence-informed policy and cohort-specific design interventions to maximise health and well-being benefits from green infrastructure across the life-course.

Ecosystem Services, green infrastructure and well-being

Broadly conceived as "the benefits people obtain from ecosystems", Ecosystem Services are most frequently categorised according to the services advanced by the Millennium Ecosystems Assessment (Millennium Ecosystem Assessment Board, 2005). These are namely:

- Supporting Services, "necessary for the production of all other ecosystem services" (e.g. nutrient cycling, water cycling, soil formation).
- Regulating Services, "necessary for the production of all other ecosystem services" (e.g. air quality regulation, climate regulation, water purification and waste treatment).

- Provisioning Services, the provision of "products obtained from ecosystems" (e.g. food, fibre, fuel, pharmaceuticals, fresh water).
- Cultural Services, the "nonmaterial benefits people obtain from ecosystems through spiritual enrichment, cognitive development, reflection, recreation, and aesthetic experiences" (e.g. recreation and tourism, aesthetic values, sense of place, cultural heritage values) (Millennium Ecosystem Assessment Board, 2005, p.40).

In the last twenty years the Ecosystem Approach (EA) has been researched and promoted widely (FAO, 2003) as a tool to encourage "smart conservation". EA is now considered a major theoretical approach underpinning planning for complex systems (Smith & Maltby, 2003), at both the landscape scale (Potvin et al., 2011) and within urban areas (UNEP, 2008), providing a framework for looking at whole ecosystems in decision-making, and for valuing the wide-ranging Ecosystem Services they provide (DEFRA, 2005).

From a policy perspective, the ability to maximise health benefits from ecosystems and green infrastructure is undermined by fragmentation across a range of policy silos (e.g. health, natural heritage, spatial planning), suggesting the need for more holistic understandings and integrated policy implementation measures. In this context, we argue that research-led spatial planning and design supply the means by which to translate academic investigation into practical solutions when seeking to deploy an EA to enhancing human health and well-being (Barton & Tsourou, 2013) across policy domains. Specifically, GI planning provides a perspective that can help mainstream the health-related issues associated with greenspace through a focus on enhancing the mutually beneficial interactions between ecosystems and society (Tzoulas et al., 2007).

While the theory and application of GI has grown in-depth and breadth over the past decade (Dunn, 2010; Benedict & McMahon, 2012; Mell, 2013; Matthews et al., 2015), the essence of the GI perspective remains unchanged. In sum, a GI perspective can be understood as seeking to provide for "an interconnected network of natural areas and other open spaces that conserve natural ecosystem values and functions . . . and provides a wide array of benefits for people and wildlife" (Benedict & McMahon, 2006, p.1). Prominent among these "benefits" is the provision of accessible natural greenspaces for physical activity and psychological well-being for human populations.

A GI approach to spatial planning and urban design moves beyond traditional "site-based" approaches and interventions towards a more proactive approach of enhancing, restoring, creating and designing new ecological networks. Drawing on Weber et al. (2006) and Davies et al. (2006), GI networks comprise the following elements: GI hubs, representing the most ecologically important large natural areas and important sites for biological diversification (e.g. woodlands or large areas of open space, "green wedges" or "greenways"); GI parcels, or GI patches, forming smaller units than hubs and particularly important in urban areas (such as urban woodlands, amenity parks, and allotments); Individual GI elements, referring to features at a local scale which can contribute towards the wider functioning of a GI network (including planned new features incorporated into urban design such as "green roofs"); GI corridors, generally linear features which provide a networking function in linking hubs and parcels and improving ecological connectivity, particularly important in the context of habitat fragmentation; and land-use buffers, representing transition areas, providing a layer of protection between hubs/corridors and potentially damaging land-uses, such as conserved farmland providing a buffer from encroaching urban expansion, and may also include potential migration pathways for wildlife.

The literature generally endorses the view that urban green infrastructure, as part of the wider environmental context, promotes health and well-being in cities (Giles-Corti & Donovan, 2003; Giles-Corti et al., 2005; Ellaway et al., 2005; Maas et al., 2006; Kaczynski & Henderson, 2007; Tzoulas et al., 2007; Sugiyama et al., 2010; Gascon et al., 2016; WHO, 2016) and provides health services as part of a wider array of Ecosystem Services (Pretty et al., 2011; Jackson et al., 2013; Lennon & Scott, 2014). These health services are understood to range from direct positive effects on mental and physical health from increased biodiversity, to improved well-being resulting from increased exposure to nature, physical activity and social engagement in greenspaces (Sandifer et al., 2015).

In response to the identified health benefits, high-level policy frameworks and guidance documents have increasingly promoted the creation of health supporting urban environments through the increased provision of urban greenspace and re-naturing cities (for example see WHO, 2012; UN General Assembly, 2015; WHO, 2016). *Habitat III*, the United Nations' New Urban Agenda identifies the improvement of human health and well-being as a key priority urban goal (United Nations General Assembly, 2016). Signatories to the agenda have committed to the promotion of a safe, healthy, inclusive and secure environment in cities and human settlements, specifically highlighting the importance of the creation and maintenance of well-connected and well-distributed networks of greenspaces to improve physical and mental health, urban liveability and to enhance resilience to environmental risks. While such policy guidance clearly supports an emphasis on greenspace provision for population health and well-being, it does not provide detailed guidance for urban policy in terms of the specific attributes required to tackle lifestyle illnesses in multiple cohorts. Hence, this chapter addresses this knowledge deficit by employing a life-course approach to summarise the evidence for health and well-being benefits accruing from green infrastructure from prenatal development through childhood, adolescence, adulthood and old age and to propose cohort-specific planning, design and management interventions for greenspaces and GI networks. Following this, a series of cross-cutting interventions for health-promoting urban greenspace are proposed as a pathway for the operationalisation of the green infrastructure approach to development.

Green infrastructure, health and well-being across the life-course

Recognised benefits of GI elements for human health traditionally include the reduction of threats to health arising from increasing pollution, urban densification and climate change. More specifically, landscaping can act to buffer exposure to air pollution, removing ozone, particulate matter, NO_2, SO_2 and carbon monoxide from the air (Nowak et al., 2006). Increased greening has also been found to reduce perceived exposure to harmful noise and associated stress (Gidlöf-Gunnarsson & Öhrström, 2007), as well as alleviate thermal discomfort during heat stress (Lafortezza et al., 2009). Further evidence has confirmed direct biophysical effects of light, colour, bird song and scents from nature (Pretty et al., 2005; Ratcliffe et al., 2013).

In the early 1980s, the biologist E. O. Wilson developed the biophilia hypothesis, which suggests that human beings have evolved to have an affinity for nature, plants and living things (Wilson, 1984; Kellert & Wilson, 1995). Building on this, Ulrich's psycho-evolutionary theory proposes that exposure to nature may have direct restorative effect on cognition and may decrease stress (Ulrich & Addoms, 1981; Ulrich, 1984; Ulrich et al., 1991). "Green" views from the window have been shown to enhance healing and rehabilitation in hospitals and prisons (Moore, 1981; Ulrich, 1984), and views with natural elements (e.g. trees, greenspace, blue sky and water) have been found to have a positive effect on well-being while those with "unnatural" urban structures have a negative effect (Ulrich et al., 1991; Maas et al., 2006).

Similarly, research by Rachel and Stephen Kaplan – which focused on human experiences of wilderness landscapes – advanced an understanding of how exposure to nature could provide feelings of "retreat" and assist in "restoring" mental functioning (Kaplan & Kaplan, 1989). They developed the Attention Restoration Theory (ART) which suggests that people exposed to high stimulus environments which require extended periods of "direct attention" suffer mental fatigue and reduced attention span, which can in turn lead to reduced physical and mental functioning (Herzog et al., 2003). The theory suggests that nature offers "restorative settings" with specific qualities and components that can be beneficial for restoring physical and mental capabilities (Ulrich & Addoms, 1981; Kaplan, 1995). These "services" may be particularly important within an urban context where exposure to stresses may be more acutely perceived (Beyer et al., 2014; Corkery, 2015).

ART has provided a starting point for numerous investigations of urban neighbourhoods, where researchers have gauged the "restorative" effects – positive, negative or neutral – of trees and landscape elements. Studies have generally identified positive effects of green areas on the self-reported mental health of residents (Van den Berg et al., 2016). Studies have also explored the importance of greenspaces as "third places" which provide for informal and unorganised social interaction (Kent & Thompson, 2014). Higher levels of social interaction, social cohesion and the presence of strong social bonds facilitated by greenspace have been linked to multiple health outcomes (Berkman, 2004; Maller et al., 2006) and reduced crime (Kuo & Sullivan, 2001).

Building on these foundations, since the beginning of the twenty-first century century, wide-ranging studies have investigated whether there is an association between people's access to green infrastructure or nature and personal levels of activity. These studies have examined how the design of the public realm encourages people to be more physically active, if it contributes to improved health outcomes, or if it attracts people to be more active (Hillsdon et al., 2006; Kessel et al., 2009; Coombes et al., 2010). The majority of such studies have found that living in proximity to urban greenspace is generally associated with increased physical activity, positive health behaviours and improved health and well-being outcomes (Giles-Corti et al., 2005; Kaczynski & Henderson, 2007; Tzoulas et al., 2007; Sugiyama et al., 2010; Gascon et al., 2016). However, results have often varied by population cohort (see Maas et al., 2006; Gascon et al., 2016; Douglas et al., 2017) and according to perceptions of greenspace by different study groups (Ord et al., 2013; WHO, 2016).

In addition to potential variability by cohort, propensity to spend time outdoors is known to track from childhood. For example, Ward Thompson et al. (2007) identified a strong relationship between frequent childhood visits to greenspace and being prepared to visit such places alone in adulthood. Consideration of such "tracking" is important from a health standpoint since childhood inactivity has been identified as a key risk factor in many chronic diseases of later life (Marmot & Brunner, 2005; Wichstrøm et al., 2013); early socially-stimulating environments have been shown to strongly inform later emotional well-being and cognitive capacity (Danner et al., 2001; Jenkins et al., 2008).

Prenatal development

The potential benefits of GI elements to human health have been traced to the prenatal condition with positive associations between the exposure of expectant mothers to greenness and improved birth outcomes observed across the majority of studies (Dadvand et al., 2012; Agay-Shay et al., 2014; Dadvand et al., 2014; Markevych et al., 2014; Hystad et al., 2015). Where analyses have controlled for complex exposures including air pollution (Dadvand et al., 2012), neighbourhood walkability, noise (Hystad et al., 2015), race, maternal age, season of conception and child's sex, broadly consistent results have been identified (James et al., 2015).

On balance, the evidence suggests that maternal interactions with and within green environments are beneficial for prenatal development and birth outcomes. Table 3.1 summarises the key associations and suggests general planning and design interventions grounded in the GI approach.

TABLE 3.1 Planning and designing greenspaces for health and well-being in prenatal development

Associations	*Interventions and GI elements*
Positive associations between greenness and birth weight.	Maximise greenness in the urban residential environment (views of: trees, shrubbery, greenspaces, etc.).
Exposure by pregnant women to greenspace alters their levels of physical activity, reduces maternal stress, enhances social contacts among mothers, reduces maternal noise and air pollution exposure, and moderates ambient temperatures.	Provide safe and accessible walkways with regular seating areas for moderate exercise and social interaction. Greenspaces should be of sufficient size, located at a distance from noise sources and include appropriate planting regimes to supply seated 'quiet areas' for rest and relaxation.
Increased birth weights among the lowest educated and lower socio-economic status who have higher surrounding greenspace or live close to a major greenspace.	Provide well-distributed accessible green infrastructure (including GI nodes and linking elements) in areas characterised by social deprivation. Urban greenspace design should encourage use by pregnant women through the provision of attractive walkways and the frequent provision of park furniture, as well as amenities such as clean public toilets.
Stronger associations between greenness and birth outcomes for mothers of white race as compared to immigrants.	Planning and design professionals should engage with pregnant women from immigrant and minority groups to identify barriers and opportunities for urban greening.

Childhood

As a result of increased use of technology and parental and societal fears for child safety, international research has shown that children are increasingly spending less time outdoors, particularly in developed economies (Godbey, 2009; Derr et al., 2013; Mustapa et al., 2015). Studies which have investigated multiple aspects of childhood health in terms of nature and green infrastructure exposure, both physical and psychological, suggest that children increasingly suffer from a "nature-deficit disorder" (Louv, 2005).

Evidence suggests that there may be important distinctions among greenspaces that make some more health supportive than others for children (Wheeler et al., 2015). Different types of urban greenspace (e.g. "sports"/"natural") may promote physical activity to different extents among children while gender and socio-economic group also has an impact. Greenspace interventions and GI strategies must respond to these variations and attract children from all backgrounds to greenspace and away from television and computer screens (Lachowycz et al., 2012). Table 3.2 outlines key associations identified in the literature for GI-health associations in children and sets out some GI-based design interventions.

TABLE 3.2 Planning and designing greenspaces for health and well-being in childhood

Associations	*Interventions and GI elements*
Childhood inactivity and disconnection from nature leads to negative physical and mental health outcomes.	Well-equipped and well-designed greenspaces should be provided to encourage physical activity and engagement with nature among children. Evidence suggests that "designing-in" certain elements can facilitate this (e.g. paved walkways, play equipment, fields and courts).
Association between surrounding greenspace and cognitive, behavioural and social development in children. Increased neighbourhood vegetation associated with decreased risk for overweight children.	Maximise greenness in the design of the urban residential environment (e.g. incorporating trees, shrubbery and flowerbeds into the streetscape), and supply a well-distributed variety of accessible pocket parks in proximity to residential units providing local GI nodes.

Adolescence

As a specific group, adolescents are not only increasingly prone to physical inactivity, but studies have also shown that people are more likely to be physically active as adults if they were physically active in their late teens (Gardsjord et al., 2014).

In *Growing Up in an Urbanising World*, Chawla (2002) observed the neighbourhood features that teenagers valued in the 1990s compared with the 1970s remained remarkably consistent. Young adolescents reported using overgrown vacant land for exploring, creative play and hideaways and used parks for meeting friends, hanging out, active play and appreciating trees and gardens (Chawla, 2015). The characteristic most frequently reported to promote physical activity was access to greenspace (Gardsjord et al., 2014), the higher the amount and the closer the distance, the more the greenspace is used with positive effect on physical activity. The second most frequently found factor was presence of informal sports facilities and other facilities open to the public. It was found that particular types of competitive sport facilities sometimes only attract certain groups of participants, mainly dominated by boys (Limstrand & Rehrer, 2008), whereas girls might need other types of facilities such as attractive walkways, loop walks in greenspaces or within GI corridors (Cohen et al., 2006).

Another characteristic reported to be positively related to physical activity in youth is a perception of safety within greenspaces, described both as absence of crime and related to features such as lighting (Gardsjord et al., 2014). For example, greenspace maintenance and renovation were additional components frequently reported as important, a well-maintained public greenspace is likely to feel safer (Kruger & Chawla, 2002). Gender differences also feature with girls found to be more concerned with safety aspects than boys (Loukaitou-Sideris & Sideris, 2009).

Based on this growing body of research, the design of greenspaces and greenspace networks which promote physical and social well-being in teenagers emerges as a potentially important focus for policymakers in promoting life-long physical and psychological health and well-being. Where gender differences arise, sensitive design interventions can potentially address different user needs by balancing dedicated play and sporting infrastructure with safe and accessible pathways, informal sheltered seating areas and improved accessibility to GI networks. Table 3.3 identifies the key issues and GI interventions for the design of greenspaces for 'healthy adolescents' arising in the literature.

TABLE 3.3 Planning and designing greenspaces for health and well-being in adolescence

Associations	*Interventions and GI elements*
High quality neighbourhood greenspaces are highly valued by teenagers. The higher the amount and the closer the distance, the more the space is used with positive effects on physical activity and social development.	To encourage increased use, accessible greenspaces should be provided as multifunctional GI areas open for a range of different activities. Abundant paths for walking and bicycling that connect various activity zones and create opportunities for exercise should be provided. Drinking water sources, proximate to both facilities for movement and zones for relaxation/social engagement should be provided.
Informal and formal greenspaces are used by adolescents for different purposes.	Provide natural greenspaces (i.e. wildflower meadows, scrub and untended vegetated areas) for exploring, creative play, hideaways and as important zones of shelter and relaxation for teenagers. Provide more organised spaces with pathways, seated and sheltered areas for socialising. Provide sports facilities and other facilities for movement/physical activity (e.g. fields for different ball games and gymnastic bars). These zones should also include seating possibilities.
Competitive sport facilities sometimes only attract certain groups of participants, mainly dominated by boys.	While competitive sports facilities should be provided where possible, facilities such as walkways and paths should also be provided. Safe paths – lined with carefully selected planting both within and linking GI hubs and nodes to residential areas – are important for the enhancement of physical activity for adolescents by offering spaces for incidental exercise and interaction both by and between genders.
Attractive and safe greenspaces are highly valued by adolescents. Furthermore, girls have been found to be more concerned with safety aspects than boys.	In general, a well-maintained urban greenspace is likely to feel safer. As such, good maintenance and renovation regimes should be implemented. Paths should be kept clear and well-lit with passive and active surveillance encouraged to enable use outside daylight hours. While 'informal' areas should be natural looking, they should be overlooked to improve safety.

Adulthood

The association between increased greenness, re-naturing cities and improved health and well-being outcomes in adults has been investigated in numerous studies. Research broadly supports an association between increased greenness and a range of improved cardiovascular outcomes in adults (Hu et al., 2008; Mitchell & Popham, 2008; Richardson & Mitchell, 2010; Villeneuve et al., 2012; Astell-Burt et al., 2014a).

In terms of behaviour, Sugiyama et al. (2013) identified a positive association between proximity to greenspaces, in particular larger greenspaces, and a higher likelihood of walking maintenance, findings consistent with those reported in other studies examining park attributes and walking (Giles-Corti et al., 2005; Sugiyama et al., 2010). They suggest that having a park nearby or having a larger park within walking distance may help residents to maintain their walking behaviour. Furthermore, greater neighbourhood greenness or access to greenspace has been associated with reduced risk of: stress, propensity to psychiatric morbidity, psychological distress, depressive symptoms, clinical anxiety and depression prevalence, and mood disorder treatment, including the associated mediating effects of physical activity, social contact and social cohesion (Grahn & Stigsdotter, 2003; Annerstedt et al., 2012; Ward Thompson et al., 2012; Astell-Burt et al., 2013; de Vries et al., 2013; Nutsford et al., 2013; Roe et al., 2013; White et al., 2013; Astell-Burt et al., 2014b; James et al., 2015). In exploring the association between mental health and exposure to greenspace in adults' positive associations remain consistent (Sugiyama et al., 2008; Maas et al., 2009; de Vries et al., 2013).

Adults identify a preference for "serene" greenspace, followed by increased "space", "nature", "species richness", "refuge" "culture", "prospect" and "social" dimensions (Grahn & Stigsdotter, 2010). The dimensions of "refuge" and "nature" were found to be most strongly correlated, suggesting that stressed individuals may seek out the most restorative environments. Similarly, Astell-Burt et al. (2013) found that those in the greenest neighbourhoods were at a lower risk of psychological distress. This body of knowledge suggests that the greenspace-health association increases in complexity in adulthood. Since behaviours and attitudes towards physical activity and greenspace usage have been shown to develop in and track from childhood and adolescence (Danner et al., 2001; Jenkins et al., 2008), associations would seem to be characterised by complex interactions pertaining to individual-level factors, beyond gender and socio-demographics. Nevertheless, the evidence for the greenspace-health association among adults is robust. Table 3.4 below sets out the key issues identified in the literature and suggests design interventions to maximise the greenspace-health association in adults using a GI approach.

Later life

The mechanisms through which greenspace, urban greening and GI affect health and well-being may ultimately affect life-span. A range of studies record links

TABLE 3.4 Planning and designing greenspaces for health and well-being in adulthood

Associations	*Interventions and GI elements*
Higher levels of greenspace linked with lower risk of cardiovascular disease, reduced risk of ischemic heart disease, stroke mortality and Type-2 diabetes.	Maximise greenness and GI provision in the urban residential environment (trees, shrubbery, greenspaces, etc). Incorporate spaces for walking, cycling and engagement with nature (e.g. wildflower borders) in such areas.
Association between proximity to greenspaces – in particular larger greenspaces – and a higher likelihood of walking maintenance among adults.	Existing walking behaviours can be maintained by providing accessible greenspaces of a usable size proximate to urban residences. Such spaces should include a series of walking paths of different lengths that provide opportunity to traverse a variety of different environments (meadow, woodland, pond side etc.) and incorporate hills and plains to facilitate varying degrees of challenge.
Greenspace associated with reduced risk of stress, propensity to psychiatric morbidity, psychological distress, depressive symptoms, clinical anxiety and depression prevalence, and mood disorder treatment in adults.	Maximise greenspace provision and access in the urban residential environment, e.g. through GI linking and linear elements. Incorporate opportunities to engage with nature for stress relief, such as the provision of pond side benches, woodland walks and edible flowerbeds.
Those in the greenest neighbourhoods found to be at a lowest risk of psychological distress and are less sedentary, suggesting an interaction between physical activity and greenspace.	Increase proximity, exposure and access opportunities to a variety of different types of greenspaces (sizes, configurations and attributes) to supply diversity of experiences and choice. Provide allotments to facilitate engagement with nature and potential for social interaction. Incorporate communal seating areas in parks with desirable vistas to encourage use and informal social interaction among urban greenspace visitors.
The mediating effect of stress and social cohesion on green activity emphasises the potential mental and social benefits of greenspace.	
Perceived greenness associated with better physical and mental health – correlated with recreational walking and social engagement.	
Improved depression markers, greater health satisfaction, improved social relationships as well as satisfaction with a sense of community and experiences of helping among adults with disabilities and their caregivers as a result of direct exposure to greenspace.	

between greenness and mortality (James et al. 2015). In Japan, Takano et al. (2002), surveying senior citizens over a five-year period, found higher survival rates among those reporting tree-lined streets near their residence, while increased exposure to greenness proximate to place of residence has been linked with reduced overall non-accidental mortality among elderly inhabitants (Villeneuve et al., 2012). Mitchell and Popham (2008) identified a 6% lower mortality rate in UK areas characterised by high levels of greenness, while Richardson and Mitchell (2010) found that male cardiovascular and respiratory mortality rates decreased with increasing greenspace among men (but not among women) while higher rates of stroke deaths have been recorded in areas characterised by low greenness (Hu et al., 2008).

Beside mortality, Kweon et al. (1998) investigated the relationship between older adults' exposure to nearby public greenspaces and their level of social integration and attachment to local community, identifying correlations between the use of public greenspace and the strength of neighbourhood social ties and sense of community.

With increasing frailty, going outdoors independently is often the first set of activities that elderly people find difficult to perform (Shumway-Cook et al., 2003). The resulting sedentary lifestyle is considered a genuine health risk for older people (WHO, 2003). In this context, opportunities to access a high quality outdoor environments catering for the specific needs of the elderly may play an important role in maintaining and enhancing health and well-being in later life. In their study of this issue, Sugiyama and Thompson (2007) argue that the environment which makes going out easy and enjoyable likely induces more frequent and possibly habitual use of the outdoors. Hence, planning and urban design can facilitate greenspace activity and recreation among older people and their caregivers by providing proximate, accessible and safe GI networks characterised by well-maintained walking infrastructure, which is safe and wheelchair accessible. Such GI provision can act to encourage older people to observe, use and benefit from public space and nature exposure for as long as their health condition allows. Table 3.5 sets out the key issues identified in the literature and suggests GI-based design interventions facilitate older adults in accessing the outdoors.

Developing an integrated green infrastructure framework for health and well-being

In adopting the life-course approach, key variations within and between population cohorts regarding the GI attributes that promote health and well-being are clearly identified, posing challenges for the delivery of GI networks which are of benefit to multiple cohorts. This is consequent on the majority of research studies research being cohort specific and focused on a particular selection of variables. The challenge is to synthesise a multi-cohort perspective into a GI framework for health and well-being and Table 3.6 outlines four interventions which are

TABLE 3.5 Planning and designing greenspaces for health and well-being in later life

Associations	*Interventions and GI elements*
Higher survival rates from cardiovascular conditions and stroke proximate to tree-lined streets and green environments. Male cardiovascular and respiratory mortality rates decrease with increasing greenspace.	Maximise exposure to greenness in the urban residential environment by carefully incorporating planting designs into the streetscape. Provide accessible greenspace of varying sizes in close proximity to residential areas (e.g. regular spatial distribution of pocket parks).
Non-exercise specific physical activity found to reduce the risk of first time cardiovascular disease and all-cause mortality.	Incorporate opportunities for incidental and leisurely engagement with the environment into the design of greenspaces (e.g. areas for berry picking, fragrant and colourful flowerbeds).
Relationships established between the use of green outdoor common space and the strength of neighbourhood social ties and sense of community for older adult residents of inner-city neighbourhoods.	Provide accessible walkways that vary in length, degree of difficult and that traverse various environments (e.g. open grassland, riverside etc). Such walkways should be of a high-grade finish to mitigate against falls. Provide sheltered seating areas with interesting vistas that facilitate social interaction, e.g. for art classes. Provide spaces for leisurely game play appropriate to elderly abilities (e.g. a bowling greens, chess tables).

applicable across all cohorts. These are subdivided into "planning", "design" and "management" interventions to facilitate ease of reference for different disciplines involved in the delivery and maintenance of green infrastructure. The table also identifies five interventions that span the health-promoting requirements of more than one cohort. By employing this table, those engaged in greenspace provision and the development of urban greening and GI strategies can target specific interventions that maximise benefit by catering for the needs of specific and multiple user groups in any given urban context. In so doing, the framework can facilitate practitioners in the creation of inclusive health-promoting greenspaces and GI networks based on a significant bank of medical, psychological and social scientific research.

Conclusion

Urbanisation and the associated increasing rise of obesogenic environments are creating health and well-being challenges for the planning and design of urban environments (Davies, 2013). Concomitantly, enhancing, restoring and creating GI networks, hubs, corridors and smaller individual elements in urban settlements are increasingly viewed as providing "restorative" contact with nature, and locations for physical activity and social engagement, which evidence suggests positively

Interventions ▶	*Cohort cross-cutting*					*Universally cross-cutting*
Cohorts ▼	Provide formal facilities for vigorous activity, such as sports courts, all-weather pitches, outdoor gymnasiums and skate parks.	Provide facilities for less vigorous physical activity that encourages social interaction and/or engagement with nature (e.g. bowling greens, sheltered outdoor class spaces, chess tables, allotments, fragrant and colourful flowerbeds).	Provide informal GI networks for exploration and adventure (e.g. wildflower meadows, scrub and untended vegetated areas, untended woodland areas).	Incorporate opportunities for incidental and leisurely engagement with the environment into the design of greenspaces (e.g. areas for berry picking, fragrant and edible flowerbeds).	Provide GI characterised by frequent sheltered seating areas, drinking water sources and toilets.	Planning Maximise streetscape greenness and greenspace provision in the urban residential environment (exposure, proximity and accessibility) through the development of GI networks. Engage all users in GI planning, with a special focus on minority groups and those in lower socio-economic classes, ensuring equal representation from each cohort to identify barriers and opportunities for greenspace usage.
Prenatal				✓	✓	Design Provide an array of walking paths and loops of different lengths that offer opportunities to traverse a variety of different environments, and incorporate hills and plains to facilitate varying degrees of challenge.
Childhood	✓		✓	✓		Management Institutionalise good maintenance and renovation regimes. Paths and GI links should be kept clear and well-lit with passive and active surveillance encouraged to enable use outside daylight hours. While "informal" areas should be natural looking, they should be overlooked to improve safety.
Adolescence			✓			
Adulthood	✓	✓				
Later Life		✓		✓	✓	

influences well-being and triggers behavioural change towards healthier lifestyles (Beyer et al., 2014; Corkery, 2015).

While high-level "aspirational" goals advancing health-promoting environments, such as *Habitat III*, are welcome, as Barton (2010, p.97) argues:

> It is all too easy for beleaguered planners under pressure from all kinds of legitimate interests to see new objectives of "mental health" or "combating obesity", as yet more rods for their backs. Understandably, professional planners can take a jaundiced view of the exponential growth of expectations placed on them by a society desperate to find solutions to problems in the built environment.

With a view to providing improved guidance to those responsible for the design and development of the urban public realm, this chapter has sought to apply a life-course approach and an integrated greenspace planning and design framework to operationalise the green infrastructure approach for the planning and design of salutogenic and restorative environments developed from an extensive evidence base. In so doing, the variety of well-being benefits of different types of greenspace attributes for different age cohorts are demonstrated and critical decisions on the design and provision of greenspace and GI more broadly, can be enhanced through evidence-informed design.

In endeavouring to create resilient and adaptable places, the multifunctional potential of green infrastructure is increasingly recognised. The GI approach represents a holistic ecosystems approach, which includes not only the aesthetic enhancement of urban greenspaces, but also the enhancement of human health and well-being through the protection, improvement and design of green infrastructure which is suitable and appropriate for the neighbourhood, city or region (Lennon & Scott, 2014).

Funding acknowledgement

This work was undertaken as part of the Eco-Health project, funded by the Environmental Protection Agency (EPA) and the Health Service Executive under Grant, Award No. 2015-HW-MS-6, and supports the implementation of the EPA Strategic Plan 2016–2020 – Our Environment, Our Wellbeing, and Healthy Ireland, the national framework for action to improve the health and well-being of the people of Ireland.

References

Agay-Shay, K., Peled, A., Crespo, A. V., Peretz, C., Amitai, Y., Linn, S., Friger, M. & Nieuwenhuijsen, M. J. (2014) Green spaces and adverse pregnancy outcomes, *Occupational and Environmental Medicine* 71: 562–569.

Annerstedt, M., Östergren, P.-O., Björk, J., Grahn, P., Skärbäck, E. & Währborg, P. (2012) Green qualities in the neighbourhood and mental health–results from a longitudinal cohort study in Southern Sweden, *BMC Public Health* 1: 1.

Antonovsky, A. (1996) The salutogenic model as a theory to guide health promotion, *Health Promotion International* 11: 11–18.

Arthurson, K., Lawless, A. & Hammet, K. (2016) Urban planning and health: Revitalising the alliance, *Urban Policy and Research* 34: 4–16.

Astell-Burt, T., Feng, X. & Kolt, G. S. (2013) Mental health benefits of neighbourhood green space are stronger among physically active adults in middle-to-older age: evidence from 260,061 Australians, *Preventive Medicine* 57: 601–606.

Astell-Burt, T., Feng, X. & Kolt, G. S. (2014a) Is neighborhood green space associated with a lower risk of type 2 diabetes? Evidence from 267,072 Australians, *Diabetes Care* 37: 197–201.

Astell-Burt, T., Mitchell, R. & Hartig, T. (2014b) The association between green space and mental health varies across the lifecourse. A longitudinal study, *Journal of Epidemiology and Community Health* 68: 578–583.

Barton, H. (2009) Land use planning and health and well-being, *Land Use Policy* 26: S115–S123.

Barton, H. (2010) Strengthening the roots of planning, *Planning Theory & Practice* 11: 95–101.

Barton, H. & Tsourou, C. (2013) *Healthy Urban Planning*, London: Routledge.

Barton, J., Bragg, R., Wood, C. & Pretty, J. (2016) (eds.) *Green Exercise: Linking Nature, Health and Well-Being*, London: Routledge.

Benedict, M. A. & McMahon, E. T. (2006) *Green Infrastructure*, Washington, DC: Island Press.

Benedict, M. A. & McMahon, E. T. (2012) *Green Infrastructure: Linking Landscapes and Communities*, Washington, DC: Island Press.

Berkman, L. F. (2004) Social Integration, social networks, and health, in N. B. Anderson (ed.), *Encyclopedia of Health and Behavior*, Thousand Oaks, CA: Sage.

Beyer, K. M., Kaltenbach, A., Szabo, A., Bogar, S., Nieto, F. J. & Malecki, K. M. (2014) Exposure to neighborhood green space and mental health: Evidence from the survey of the health of Wisconsin, *International Journal of Environmental Research and Public Health* 11: 3453–3472.

Chawla, L. (2002) *Growing up in an Urbanizing World*, London: Earthscan.

Chawla, L. (2015) Benefits of nature contact for children, *Journal of Planning Literature*, Available at http://dx.doi.org/0885412215595441.

Cohen, D. A., Ashwood, J. S., Scott, M. M., Overton, A., Evenson, K. R., Staten, L. K., Porter, D., Mckenzie, T. L. & Catellier, D. (2006) Public parks and physical activity among adolescent girls, *Pediatrics* 118: e1381–e1389.

Coombes, E., Jones, A. P. & Hillsdon, M. (2010) The relationship of physical activity and overweight to objectively measured green space accessibility and use, *Social Science & Medicine* 70: 816–822.

Corkery, L. (2015) Beyond the park: linking urban greenspaces, human well-being and environmental health, in H. Barton, S. Thompson, S. Burgess & M. Grant (eds.) *The Routledge Handbook of Planning for Health and Well-Being: Shaping a Sustainable and Healthy Future*, London and New York: Routledge.

Cummins, S., Curtis, S., Diez-Roux, A. V. & Macintyre, S. (2007) Understanding and representing "place" in health research: a relational approach, *Social Science & Medicine* 65: 1825–1838.

Dadvand, P., Sunyer, J., Basagaña, X., Ballester, F., Lertxundi, A., Fernández-Somoano, A., Estarlich, M., García-Esteban, R., Mendez, M. A. & Nieuwenhuijsen, M. J. (2012) Surrounding greenness and pregnancy outcomes in four Spanish birth cohorts, *Environmental Health Perspectives* 120: 1481.

Dadvand, P., Wright, J., Martínez, D., Basagaña, X., Mceachan, R. R., Cirach, M., Gidlow, C. J., De Hoogh, K., Gražulevičienė, R. & Nieuwenhuijsen, M. J. (2014) Inequality,

green spaces, and pregnant women: roles of ethnicity and individual and neighbourhood socioeconomic status, *Environment International* 71: 101–108.
Danner, D. D., Snowdon, D. A. & Friesen, W. V. (2001) Positive emotions in early life and longevity: findings from the nun study, *Journal of Personality and Social Psychology* 80: 804.
Davies, C., Macfarlane, R. & Roe, M. (2006) *Green Infrastructure Planning Guide, 2 Volumes: Final Report and GI Planning*, Newcastle: University of Northumbria, North East Community Forests, University of Newcastle, Countryside Agency, English Nature, Forestry Commission, Groundwork Trusts Newcastle.
Davies, S. C. (2013) Chief Medical Officer's *Annual Report 2012: Our Children Deserve Better: Prevention Pays*, United Kingdom: Department of Health.
de Vries, S., Van Dillen, S. M., Groenewegen, P. P. & Spreeuwenberg, P. (2013) Streetscape greenery and health: stress, social cohesion and physical activity as mediators, *Social Science & Medicine* 94: 26–33.
DEFRA (2005) The Economic, Social and Ecological Value of Ecosystem Services: DEFRA Key Messages from EFTEC Report, London: Department for Environment, Food and Rural Affairs.
Derr, V., Chawla, L., Mintzer, M., Cushing, D. F. & Van Vliet, W. (2013) A city for all citizens: integrating children and youth from marginalized populations into city planning, *Buildings* 3: 482–505.
Douglas, O., Lennon, M. & Scott, M. (2017) Green space benefits for health and well-being: a life-course approach for urban planning, design and management, *Cities* 66: 53–62.
Dunn, A. D. (2010) Siting green infrastructure: legal and policy solutions to alleviate urban poverty and promote healthy communities, *Pace Law Faculty Publications* 559. Available at http://digitalcommons.pace.edu/lawfaculty/559.
EEA-JRC (2013) *Environment and Human Health*, Copenhagen: European Environment Agency.
FAO (2003) Biodiversity and the Ecosystem Approach in Agriculture, Forestry and Fisheries. Satellite event on the occasion of the Ninth Regular Session of the Commission on Genetic Resources for Food and Agriculture, Rome.
Gardsjord, H., Tveit, M. & Nordh, H. (2014) Promoting youth's physical activity through park design: linking theory and practice in a public health perspective, *Landscape Research* 39: 70–81.
Gascon, M., Triguero-Mas, M., Martínez, D., Dadvand, P., Rojas-Rueda, D., Plasència, A. & Nieuwenhuijsen, M. J. (2016) Residential green spaces and mortality: a systematic review, *Environment International* 86: 60–67.
Gidlöf-Gunnarsson, A. & Öhrström, E. (2007) Noise and well-being in urban residential environments: the potential role of perceived availability to nearby green areas, *Landscape and Urban Planning* 83: 115–126.
Giles-Corti, B., Broomhall, M. H., Knuiman, M., Collins, C., Douglas, K., Ng, K., Lange, A. & Donovan, R. J. (2005) Increasing walking: how important is distance to, attractiveness, and size of public open space? *American Journal of Preventive Medicine* 28: 169–176.
Godbey, G. (2009) *Outdoor Recreation, Health, and Wellness: Understanding and Enhancing the Relationship. RFF Discussion Paper No. 09-21*. Available at http://dx.doi.org/10.2139/ssrn.1408694.
Grahn, P. & Stigsdotter, A. U. K. (2003) Landscape planning and stress, *Urban Forestry & Urban Greening* 2: 1–18.
Grahn, P. & Stigsdotter, A. U. K. (2010) The relation between perceived sensory dimensions of urban green space and stress restoration, *Landscape and Urban Planning* 94: 264–275.

Haaland, C. & Van Den Bosch, C. K. (2015) Challenges and strategies for urban green-space planning in cities undergoing densification: A review, *Urban Forestry & Urban Greening* 14: 760–771.

Herzog, T. R., Maguire, P. & Nebel, M. B. (2003) Assessing the restorative components of environments, *Journal of Environmental Psychology* 23: 159–170.

Hillsdon, M., Panter, J., Foster, C. & Jones, A. (2006) The relationship between access and quality of urban green space with population physical activity, *Public Health* 120: 1127–1132.

Horwitz, P., Kretsch, C., Jenkins, A., Rahim Bin Abdul Hamid, A., Burls, A., Campbell, K., Carter, M., Henwood, W., Lovell, R. & Malone-Lee, L. C. (2015) Contribution of biodiversity and green spaces to mental and physical fitness, and cultural dimensions of health, in *Connecting Global Priorities: Biodiversity and Human Health- A State of Knowledge Review*, Geneva: World Health Organization and Secretariat of the Convention on Biological Diversity, pp.200–220.

Howard, E. 1965. *Garden Cities of To-Morrow*, Cambridge, MA: Mit Press.

Hu, Z., Liebens, J. & Rao, K. R. (2008) Linking stroke mortality with air pollution, income, and greenness in northwest Florida: an ecological geographical study, *International Journal of Health Geographics* 7: 1.

Hystad, P., Davies, H. W., Frank, L., Van Loon, J., Gehring, U., Tamburic, L. & Brauer, M. (2015) Residential greenness and birth outcomes: evaluating the influence of spatially correlated built-environment factors, *Environmental Health Perspectives*. Available at doi:10.1289/ehp.1308049.

Jackson, L. E., Daniel, J., Mccorkle, B., Sears, A. & Bush, K. F. (2013) Linking ecosystem services and human health: the Eco-Health Relationship Browser, *International Journal of Public Health* 58: 747–755.

James, P., Banay, R. F., Hart, J. E. & Laden, F. (2015) A review of the health benefits of greenness. *Current Epidemiology Reports* 2: 131–142.

Jenkins, R., Meltzer, H., Jones, P., Brugha, T., Bebbington, P., Farrell, M., Crepaz-Kay, D. & Knapp, M. (2008) *Mental Health: Future Challenges, Foresight, 104-08-Fo/on*, London: The Government Office for Science.

Kaczynski, A. T. & Henderson, K. A. (2007) Environmental correlates of physical activity: A review of evidence about parks and recreation, *Leisure Sciences* 29: 315–354.

Kaplan, R. & Kaplan, S. (1989) *The experience of nature: a psychological perspective*, Cambridge & New York: CUP Archive.

Kaplan, S. (1995) The restorative benefits of nature: Toward an integrative framework, *Journal of Environmental Psychology* 15: 169–182.

Kellert, S. R. & Wilson, E. O. (1995) *The Biophilia Hypothesis*, Washington, DC: Island Press.

Kent, J. L. & Thompson, S. (2014) The three domains of urban planning for health and well-being, *Journal of Planning Literature* 29: 239–256.

Kessel, A., Green, J., Pinder, R., Wilkinson, P., Grundy, C. & Lachowycz, K. (2009) Multidisciplinary research in public health: a case study of research on access to green space, *Public Health* 123: 32–38.

Kruger, J. S. & Chawla, L. (2002) "We know something someone doesn't know": children speak out on local conditions in Johannesburg, *Environment and Urbanization* 14: 85–96.

Kuo, F. E. & Sullivan, W. C. (2001) Environment and crime in the inner city does vegetation reduce crime? *Environment and Behavior* 33: 343–367.

Kweon, B., S., Sullivan, W. C. & Wiley, A. R. (1998) Green common spaces and the social integration of inner-city older adults, *Environment and Behavior* 30: 832–858.

Lachowycz, K. & Jones, A. P. (2013) Towards a better understanding of the relationship between greenspace and health: development of a theoretical framework, *Landscape and Urban Planning* 118: 62–69.

Lachowycz, K., Jones, A. P., Page, A. S., Wheeler, B. W. & Cooper, A. R. (2012) What can global positioning systems tell us about the contribution of different types of urban greenspace to children's physical activity? *Health & Place* 18: 586–594.

Lafortezza, R., Carrus, G., Sanesi, G. & Davies, C. (2009) Benefits and well-being perceived by people visiting green spaces in periods of heat stress, *Urban Forestry & Urban Greening* 8: 97–108.

Lake, A. & Townshend, T. (2006) Obesogenic environments: exploring the built and food environments, *The Journal of the Royal Society for the Promotion of Health* 126: 262–267.

Lennon, M. & Scott, M. (2014) Delivering ecosystems services via spatial planning: reviewing the possibilities and implications of a green infrastructure approach, *Town Planning Review* 85: 563–587.

Limstrand, T. & Rehrer, N. J. (2008) Young people's use of sports facilities: a Norwegian study on physical activity, *Scandinavian Journal of Public Health* 36: 452–459.

Loukaitou-Sideris, A. & Sideris, A. (2009) what brings children to the park? analysis and measurement of the variables affecting children's use of parks, *Journal of the American Planning Association* 76: 89–107.

Louv, R. (2005) Nature deficit, *Orion* July/August: 70–71.

Lovasi, G. S., Schwartz-Soicher, O., Quinn, J. W., Berger, D. K., Neckerman, K. M., Jaslow, R., Lee, K. K. & Rundle, A. (2013) Neighborhood safety and green space as predictors of obesity among preschool children from low-income families in New York City, *Preventive Medicine*, 57, 189–193.

Maas, J., Van Dillen, S. M., Verheij, R. A. & Groenewegen, P. P. (2009) Social contacts as a possible mechanism behind the relation between green space and health, *Health & Place* 15: 586–595.

Maas, J., Verheij, R. A., Groenewegen, P. P., de Vries, S. & Spreeuwenberg, P. (2006) Green space, urbanity, and health: how strong is the relation? *Journal of Epidemiology and Community Health* 60: 587–592.

Maller, C., Townsend, M., Pryor, A., Brown, P. & St Leger, L. (2006) Healthy nature healthy people: "contact with nature" as an upstream health promotion intervention for populations, *Health Promotion International* 21: 45–54.

Markevych, I., Fuertes, E., Tiesler, C. M., Birk, M., Bauer, C.-P., Koletzko, S., Von Berg, A., Berdel, D. & Heinrich, J. (2014) Surrounding greenness and birth weight: Results from the GINIplus and LISAplus birth cohorts in Munich, *Health & Place* 26: 39–46.

Marmot, M. & Brunner, E. (2005) Cohort profile: The Whitehall II study, *International Journal of Epidemiology* 34: 251–256.

Matthews, T., Lo, A. Y. & Byrne, J. A. (2015) Reconceptualizing green infrastructure for climate change adaptation: Barriers to adoption and drivers for uptake by spatial planners, *Landscape and Urban Planning* 138: 155–163.

Mell, I. C. (2013) Can you tell a green field from a cold steel rail? Examining the "green" of Green Infrastructure development, *Local Environment* 18: 152–166.

Millennium Ecosystem Assessment Board (2005) Millennium Ecosystem Assessment. Ecosystems and Human Wellbeing: A Framework for Assessment, Washington, DC: Island Press.

Mitchell, R. & Popham, F. (2008) Effect of exposure to natural environment on health inequalities: an observational population study, *The Lancet* 372: 1655–1660.

Moore, E. O. (1981) A prison environment's effect on health care service demands, *Journal of Environmental Systems* 11: 17–34.

Mustapa, N. D., Maliki, N. Z. & Hamzah, A. (2015) Repositioning children's developmental needs in space planning: a review of connection to nature, *Procedia – Social and Behavioral Sciences* 170: 330–339.

Nowak, D. J., Crane, D. E. & Stevens, J. C. (2006) Air pollution removal by urban trees and shrubs in the United States, *Urban Forestry & Urban Greening* 4: 115–123.

Nutsford, D., Pearson, A. & Kingham, S. (2013) An ecological study investigating the association between access to urban green space and mental health, *Public Health* 127: 1005–1011.

Ord, K., Mitchell, R. & Pearce, J. (2013) Is level of neighbourhood green space associated with physical activity in green space? *International Journal of Behavioral Nutrition and Physical Activity* 10: 1.

Patel, V., Flisher, A. J., Hetrick, S. & Mcgorry, P. (2007) Mental health of young people: a global public-health challenge, *The Lancet* 369: 1302–1313.

Potvin, C., Mancilla, L., Buchmann, N., Monteza, J., Moore, T., Murphy, M., Oelmann, Y., Scherer-Lorenzen, M., Turner, B. L. & Wilcke, W. (2011) An ecosystem approach to biodiversity effects: carbon pools in a tropical tree plantation, *Forest Ecology and Management* 261: 1614–1624.

Pretty, J., Barton, J., Colbeck, I., Hine, R., Mourato, S., Mackerron, G. & Wood, C. (2011) *Health Values from Ecosystems*, Cambridge: UNEP-WCMC.

Pretty, J., Peacock, J., Sellens, M. & Griffin, M. (2005) The mental and physical health outcomes of green exercise, *International Journal of Environmental Health Research* 15: 319–337.

Ratcliffe, E., Gatersleben, B. & Sowden, P. T. (2013) Bird sounds and their contributions to perceived attention restoration and stress recovery, *Journal of Environmental Psychology* 36: 221–228.

Richardson, E. A. & Mitchell, R. (2010) Gender differences in relationships between urban green space and health in the United Kingdom, *Social Science & Medicine* 71: 568–575.

Roe, J. J., Ward Thompson, C., Aspinall, P. A., Brewer, M. J., Duff, E. I., Miller, D., Mitchell, R. & Clow, A. (2013) Green space and stress: evidence from cortisol measures in deprived urban communities, *International Journal of Environmental Research and Public Health* 10: 4086–4103.

Sandifer, P. A., Sutton-Grier, A. E. & Ward, B. P. (2015) Exploring connections among nature, biodiversity, ecosystem services, and human health and well-being: Opportunities to enhance health and biodiversity conservation, *Ecosystem Services* 12: 1–15.

Scott, M. & Lennon, M. (2016) Nature-based solutions for the contemporary city, *Planning Theory & Practice* 17: 267–270.

Shumway-Cook, A., Patla, A., Stewart, A., Ferrucci, L., Ciol, M. A. & Guralnik, J. M. (2003) Environmental components of mobility disability in community-living older persons, *Journal of the American Geriatrics Society* 51: 393–398.

Smith, R. D. & Maltby, E. (2003) Using the Ecosystem Approach to Implement the Convention On Biological Diversity: Key Issues and Case Studies, Gland, Switzerland: IUCN.

Sugiyama, T. & Thompson, C. W. (2007) Outdoor environments, activity and the well-being of older people: conceptualising environmental support, *Environment and Planning A* 39: 1943–1960.

Sugiyama, T., Leslie, E., Giles-Corti, B. & Owen, N. (2008) Associations of neighbourhood greenness with physical and mental health: do walking, social coherence and local social interaction explain the relationships? *Journal of Epidemiology and Community Health* 62: e9.

Sugiyama, T., Francis, J., Middleton, N. J., Owen, N. & Giles-Corti, B. (2010) Associations between recreational walking and attractiveness, size, and proximity of neighborhood open spaces, *American Journal of Public Health* 100: 1752–1757.

Sugiyama, T., Giles-Corti, B., Summers, J., Du Toit, L., Leslie, E. & Owen, N. (2013) Initiating and maintaining recreational walking: a longitudinal study on the influence of neighborhood green space, *Preventive Medicine* 57: 178–182.

Takano, T., Nakamura, K. & Watanabe, M. (2002) Urban residential environments and senior citizens' longevity in megacity areas: the importance of walkable green spaces, *Journal of Epidemiology and Community Health* 56: 913–918.

Tzoulas, K., Korpela, K., Venn, S., Yli-Pelkonen, V., Kaźmierczak, A., Niemela, J. & James, P. (2007) Promoting ecosystem and human health in urban areas using Green Infrastructure: a literature review, *Landscape and Urban Planning* 81: 167–178.

Ulrich, R. (1984) View through a window may influence recovery, *Science* 224: 224–225.

Ulrich, R. & Addoms, D. L. (1981) Psychological and recreational benefits of a residential park, *Journal of Leisure Research* 13: 43–65.

Ulrich, R., Simons, R. F., Losito, B. D., Fiorito, E., Miles, M. A. & Zelson, M. (1991) Stress recovery during exposure to natural and urban environments, *Journal of Environmental Psychology* 11: 201–230.

UNEP (2008) Local action for biodiversity. *The United Nations Environment Programme*, Geneva: United Nations Economic Commission for Europe.

United Nations General Assembly (2015) Transforming Our World: The 2030 Agenda for Sustainable Development, New York: United Nations.

United Nations General Assembly (2016) Draft Outcome Document of The United Nations Conference on Housing and Sustainable Urban Development (Habitat III), Quito: United Nations.

Van Den Berg, M., Van Poppel, M., Van Kamp, I., Andrusaityte, S., Balseviciene, B., Cirach, M., Danileviciute, A., Ellis, N., Hurst, G. & Masterson, D. (2016) Visiting green space is associated with mental health and vitality: a cross-sectional study in four European cities, *Health & Place* 38: 8–15.

Villeneuve, P. J., Jerrett, M., Su, J. G., Burnett, R. T., Chen, H., Wheeler, A. J. & Goldberg, M. S. (2012) A cohort study relating urban green space with mortality in Ontario, Canada, *Environmental Research* 115: 51–58.

Ward Thompson, C. (2011) Linking landscape and health: The recurring theme, *Landscape and Urban Planning* 99: 187–195.

Ward Thompson, C., Aspinall, P. & Montarzino, A. (2007) The childhood factor: Adult visits to green places and the significance of childhood experience, *Environment and Behavior* 40 (1): 111–143.

Ward Thompson, C., Roe, J., Aspinall, P., Mitchell, R., Clow, A. & Miller, D. (2012) More green space is linked to less stress in deprived communities: Evidence from salivary cortisol patterns, *Landscape and Urban Planning* 105: 221–229.

Weber, T., Sloan, A. & Wolf, J. (2006) Maryland's green infrastructure assessment: Development of a comprehensive approach to land conservation, *Landscape and Urban Planning* 77: 94–110.

Wheeler B. W., Lovell R., Higgins S. L., White M. P., Alcock I., Osborne N. J., Husk K., Sabel C. E., and Depledge M. H. (2015) Beyond greenspace: an ecological study of population general health and indicators of natural environment type and quality, *International Journal of Health Geographics* 14: 17.

White, M. P., Alcock, I., Wheeler, B. W. & Depledge, M. H. (2013) Would you be happier living in a greener urban area? A fixed-effects analysis of panel data, *Psychological Science* 23 (6): 920–928. Available at https://doi.org/10.1177/0956797612464659.

WHO (2003) Health and Development Through Physical Activity and Sport, Geneva: World Health Organization.

WHO (2012) Health 2020: a European policy framework supporting action across government and society for health and well-being, *Proceedings of Regional Committee for Europe*, Geneva.
WHO (2016) *Urban Green Spaces and Health*, Copenhagen: WHO Regional Office for Europe.
Wichstrøm, L., Von Soest, T. & Kvalem, I. L. (2013) Predictors of growth and decline in leisure time physical activity from adolescence to adulthood, *Health Psychology* 32: 775.
Wilson, E. O. (1984) *Biophilia*, Cambridge, MA: Harvard University Press.

4

GROWING PATHWAYS TO WELL-BEING THROUGH COMMUNITY GARDENS AND GREENSPACE

Case studies from Birmingham and the West Midlands, UK

Veronica Barry and Chris Blythe

Introduction

Increasingly, consideration of greenspace use within cities is seen as an essential part of planning for a more healthy and sustainable future where the positive impact of green environments on longevity is well demonstrated (Mitchell & Popham, 2008; Crouse et al., 2017).

As cities expand at a rapid pace – by 2050 over 6.3 billion, or 70% of the world's population will be living in urban areas – the impacts of climate change, burden of non-communicable disease, inequalities in health and environmental degradation, call for new thinking about the way we live (WHO, 2008; United Nations, 2012). Within cities, green infrastructure is being seen as a valuable asset to human health and community resilience, and the case for consideration within city infrastructure planning is clear. This is not just about the value of greenspaces as an "add on", subjective view or lifestyle "choice", but goes to the heart of health inequalities, encompassing ways in which to support human resilience to the drivers of ill health, including tackling disparities in access to and use of greenspace (CABE Space, 2010; Marmot & Marmot Review Team, 2010; Natural England, 2010; Wolch et al., 2014; WHO, 2016).

For health agencies, the links between public health, environmental health and sustainable cities are clear. The World Health Organisation (WHO) firmly recognises the underlying environmental drivers of health inequalities and non-communicable disease. Health 2020 framework emphasises the intrinsic place of the natural and green environment to human health in supporting resilient communities (WHO, 2008; WHO, 2013). Emerging ecological, public health and planetary health perspectives frame health as a broader concept encompassing both human and ecological health and urge wider innovative "systems" thinking as the way forward (Rayner & Lang, 2012). The links between greenspace, planning and health are also referenced in policy documents, such as WHO Healthy Cities and through legislation such as England's *National Planning Policy Framework* (WHO, 1998; DCLG, 2012).

Benefits of greenspace to health

Set within these wider debates, the contribution of greenspace to health and well-being is being increasingly understood. As contact with the natural environment becomes less of an everyday experience, particularly in urban areas, a genre of literature has developed concepts to explain nature's intrinsic value, linking its loss with discordant effects on human well-being. Some attribute humans with a deep and innate drive to affiliate with nature. E. O. Wilson explored the term "biophilia", a principle now inspiring the International Biophilic, Cities Movement to embrace the natural environment to the heart of city planning (Wilson, 1984; Beatley, 2011). Others argue contact with greenery supports "attention restoration" and recovery from stress (Kaplan & Kaplan, 1989). Richard Louv's *The Last Child in the Woods* (Louv, 2008) powerfully explores the rise of "nature-deficit disorder" among children, seen as stemming from cumulative effects of loss of contact with the natural world, while Moss (2012) tracked the increasingly restricted opportunities for contact with the natural environment among children in England, highlighting concerns for their development, health and well-being.

Health and well-being benefits from greenspace can be manifested through numerous pathways, including ambient, "passive" or immersive exposure, by living or being in areas of natural greenery, or through "active" interaction such as walks in parks, gardening, or conservation activities (Shanahan et al., 2015). Environmental challenges to human health in cities, through air and noise pollution, heat stress, flood risk, exacerbated by climate change, can be buffered by presence of greenspaces and vegetation (Nowak & Crane, 2006; Gidlöf-Gunnarsson & Öhrström, 2007; Lafortezza et al., 2009; James et al., 2015). As new methods emerge to measure physiological and emotional changes – for example, using measurement of salivary cortisol levels, EEGs to track brain waves, and use of interactive "apps" – evidence of the impact of exposure to natural greenspace is becoming clearer. These indicate both physical changes and subjective experiences of well-being, capturing a sense of "flow" or "awe" stimulated by immersion in greenspace, contrasted to emotions generated from exposure to built-up environments (MacKerron & Mourato, 2013; Roe et al., 2013; Aspinall et al., 2015).

The body of evidence that human relationship with greenspaces is beneficial to health is expanding (de Vries et al., 2003; Lee & Maheswaran, 2011; Pretty et al., 2011; James et al., 2015). Immersion in accessible greenspace for leisure and recreation can drive healthier behaviours, including increased physical activity, social interaction and support "prosocial" attitudes (Tanako et al., 2002; Sugiyama et al., 2008; Maas et al., 2009). Contact with greenspace, both active and passive, has been seen to improve recovery, reduce and mitigate stress, lower blood pressure and support mental well-being (Ulrich, 1984; Kaplan & Kaplan, 1989; Kaplan, 2001; Hartig et al., 2003; Wells & Evans, 2003; Barton & Pretty, 2010; Pretty et al., 2011; Bragg et al., 2013; Gascon et al., 2015). Contact with soil, and soil-based micro-organisms is also understood to hold benefits to physical and mental health (Ege et al., 2011).

Urban agriculture and gardening as part of greenspaces for health

Urban agriculture, allotments and community gardens feature as a particular cultural and physical use of land in the literature on greenspaces and health. These multifunctional spaces, varied in the way they are established and organised and sometimes set apart from debates about management and governance of the wider "natural" and "wild" green environment, are increasingly being seen to hold potential for planning multifunctional greenspace use (Lovell, 2010; Viljoen & Wiskerke, 2012; Lohrberg et al., 2016). These garden spaces arise from development of land, often derelict, brownfield or "temporary", and range from grassroots projects to those more formalised in structure. They present opportunities to support human interaction with greenspace and gardening, bringing social, educational, therapeutic, health and well-being benefits for individuals and communities (Fieldhouse, 2003; Hawkins, 2011, 2015; Leng, 2016; Lohrberg et al., 2016; Federation of City Farms and Community Gardens, 2017).

Davies et al. (2014) and Buck, (2016), reviewing international literature, outline the evidence for health benefits of gardening and food growing within the wider greenspace literature. Studies are variable, but, overall they demonstrate multiple benefits of gardening and food growing across a range of health conditions and groups, increased physical activity, improved fruit and vegetable consumption and weight outcomes (Alaimo et al., 2008; Zick et al., 2013). Other benefits show enhanced recovery from illness, improved functioning among those with dementia, and physical and mental health benefits for the elderly (Hawkins et al., 2011; Adevi & Lieberg, 2012; Hewitt et al., 2013). Van den Berg et al. (2010), showed improved health outcomes and stress restoration among allotment gardeners compared to non- gardeners. Others have focused on demonstrating the potential "upstream" cost benefits to the economy through improved health outcomes and associated health care savings (Pank & Gorgie City Farm, 2011).

Formalising the pathways between health and greenspace

At policy context and evidence levels, attempts have been made to formalise some of the pathways to well-being and to make the case for greenspaces use to be incorporated into planning and implementation of *health service pathways* (FPH & Natural England, 2010). For example, "forest bathing" (Shinrin Yoku) as a public health intervention in Japan, the establishment of Horticulture Therapy as a professional association in the US, and wide use of "care" and "social farming" across Italy, Norway and Belgium (Hassinck & Van Dijk, 2006; Lee et al., 2011).

Different concepts and terms have arisen to describe the interaction between an individual and the environment for health benefits. Terms, including "eco-therapy", "green care", and "nature-based care" describe the more formalised pathways, interventions supported and facilitated using nature and natural settings. Bragg and Atkins et al. (2016), following collaborative discussion with a range of UK providers, proposed a distinction between three levels of engagement with nature through green projects; contact with nature in everyday life, nature as health promotion, and "green care" where nature is used as a deliberate therapeutic *intervention*, although they acknowledge that these distinctions in real-life are often less clear. Community gardens can offer all three pathways both spatially and temporally, in a range of activities to multiple users (Lund et al., 2015).

In the UK, dialogue between health and "green" organisations is developing fast (Davies et al., 2014; Green Care Coalition, 2017). This in part driven by the search for new solutions to the burgeoning burden of disease, demographic and health pressures bringing increasing costs (in the UK) to the National Health Service (NHS). So-called "lifestyle" related illnesses, such as obesity, diabetes, CHD, some cancers, along with mental health treatment, costs the NHS billions of pounds a year; obesity alone cost £6.1 billion in 2015 (Public Health England, 2017). The "NHS five year forward view" calls for innovative thinking to tackle some of the wider drivers of illness, with a strong focus on prevention and working with patients on self-care and lifestyle change (NHS England, 2014). There is also a recognition of the need for health service "estate" to maximise its influence and greenspace use to model more sustainable and environmentally friendly ways of working (NHS Scotland, 2017).

For example, Merseyside and Croydon (2017) have pioneered concepts of a "Natural Health Service", forming coalitions to offer a range of formal and informal ways for people to access natural environments for health, working closely with GPs and Health Commissioners to develop referral pathways (Mersey Forest, 2017; Wild in the City, 2017). Other areas are piloting the use of "social prescribing" to stimulate reduction of the demand on GP and Acute Services, to link patients with non-clinical need with wider voluntary and community support, for example through joining a Green Gym®, park walking groups or community gardening programmes (Bragg & Leck, 2017).

Birmingham and the West Midlands; consideration of greenspace and health

Birmingham as England's second largest city with over one million residents, and proud industrial heritage, sits at the heart of the West Midlands region, as one of seven metropolitan authorities. Recent devolution of powers from central government, has led to the establishment of a West Midlands Combined Authority (WMCA) in 2016, embracing the seven authorities at its core as constituent members. Although early days, this has been seen by some as a potential platform for more collaborative and strategic consideration of greenspace and health. A coalition of local nature-based organisations used the opportunity of the WMCA mayoral elections in 2017 to launch a vision for a "25 year natural capital plan" for the region, arguing that natural capital should be at the heart of economic and strategic planning (Birmingham and Black Country Wildlife Trust, 2017).

Pledged in 2014 to become UK's first Biophilic City, Birmingham has worked for some time to integrate heath and the natural environment into strategic planning (Banzourkov, 2017). With over 570 parks and 73,000 hectares of greenspace, the city has potential to maximise the health benefits to its residents. Birmingham Council's Green Living Spaces Plan (Birmingham City Council, 2013; Franchina et al., 2017) has pioneered an innovative mapping-based approach at a landscape and neighbourhood scale. It lays the pathway for putting greenspaces at the forefront of planning decisions, underpinned by considerations of inequalities in health, environmental hazard exposure, climate change and access to greenspace. Natural Health Improvement Zones (NHIZ) have been identified, building on data in multi-layered maps indicating areas of high air pollution, poor environmental quality and poor health. This evidence has supported focused action through collaborative multi-agency work to intensify provision of greenspaces and greenery in these areas, with the aim of improving health, with input from Public Health in monitoring improvements. Similarly, "Multiple Challenge Maps" combine all aspects to give an overview of how the city's Ecosystem Services are performing. The development of a BUCCANEER (Birmingham Urban Climate Change Adaptation with Neighbourhood Estimates of Environmental Risk) tool supports climate adaptation planning, mapping heat island and flood risk against wider environmental features (Birmingham City Council, 2013; Tomlinson et al., 2013). Birmingham has also pioneered an innovative Natural Capital Planning Tool (NCPT) to provide developers with a tool to assess impact of new developments at the planning stage, on a range of ecosystems services and environmental features and to make subsequent changes to developments in favour of greenspace enhancement (Hölzinger, Laughlin & Grayson, 2015).

Diverse voluntary, community and statutory sector collaborations across the region have sought to raise the profile and value of greenspaces to health and well-being. This has included strategic work by the Birmingham Green Commission, Sustainability West Midlands, the Wildlife Trusts' development of a network of Nature Improvement Areas (NIA), the Green Gym® and conservation work by the Trust for Conservation Volunteers (TCV). Parks in Birmingham and the West Midlands borough of Dudley, have been enhanced to provide opportunities for health and well-being activities, supported by Birmingham Open Spaces Forum (BOSF) and the West Midlands parks forum plus partnerships with councils and public health. Other groups support development of and collaborative work between the diverse community gardens and allotments across the city and include formal and informal growing spaces, such as Martineau Gardens, Thrive's Kings Heath Park Project, and gardens showcased by the Growing Birmingham umbrella group (Growing Birmingham, 2017). Not all activity is strategically planned or coordinated but has arisen in response to specific local and community-based initiatives often faced with challenges of competing land use and limited funding.

In the wider region, Sandwell Public Health's strategic establishment of a ground-breaking community and urban agriculture initiative offer Ideal for All Growing Opportunities, garden sites offering preventive public health and therapeutic opportunities, led by deprived communities involving gardening and food growing (Davis & Middleton, 2012; Barry, 2017). Sandwell Public Health also pioneered in-depth monitoring and mapping of the links between health, planning, environment and inequality, including assessment of environmental hazards into Joint Strategic Needs Assessments, and experimentation with "green walls" to reduce air pollution (Middleton, 2010; Sandwell Primary Care Trust, 2013). Similarly, through Healthy Towns funding, Dudley MBC and Public Health pioneered work in healthy planning, incorporating development of infrastructure in parks and interconnected greenspace for health to encourage physical activity.

Case study: Queen Elizabeth Hospital, Birmingham

The grounds of one of Europe's biggest hospitals might be an unlikely place to come across groups of enthusiastic children and adults picking heritage apples, making and tasting juice and celebrating a new harvest. Yet this is just one of the developments within the greenspaces surrounding Birmingham's Queen Elizabeth Hospital, situated in the heart of the city and part of a wider linkage between the hospital's land assets with preventive health (UHB, 2017).

The new Queen Elizabeth Hospital Birmingham (QEH), Edgbaston, Birmingham has over 8,000 staff and throughput of 80,000 patients a year (UHB, 2017; NHS Forest, n.d.). The hospital sits on a scheduled ancient monument, Metchley Roman Fort (AD 48), which requires careful preservation and as such has presented opportunities to innovatively develop the land (University of Birmingham, 2000). The land (over 1,600m^2) surrounding the hospital now includes wildflower and hay meadows, woodland, orchards and food growing spaces created through partnerships of residents, patients and voluntary groups, supported by corporate and public funding (NHS Forest, n.d.). Greenspaces and trees provide peaceful, therapeutic spaces for staff and visitors away from the stresses of the busy hospital (UHB, 2017). Links are developing between the greenspaces and the hospital's health professionals, giving them support to make use of the grounds as a resource for rehabilitation and dementia programmes. The contrast

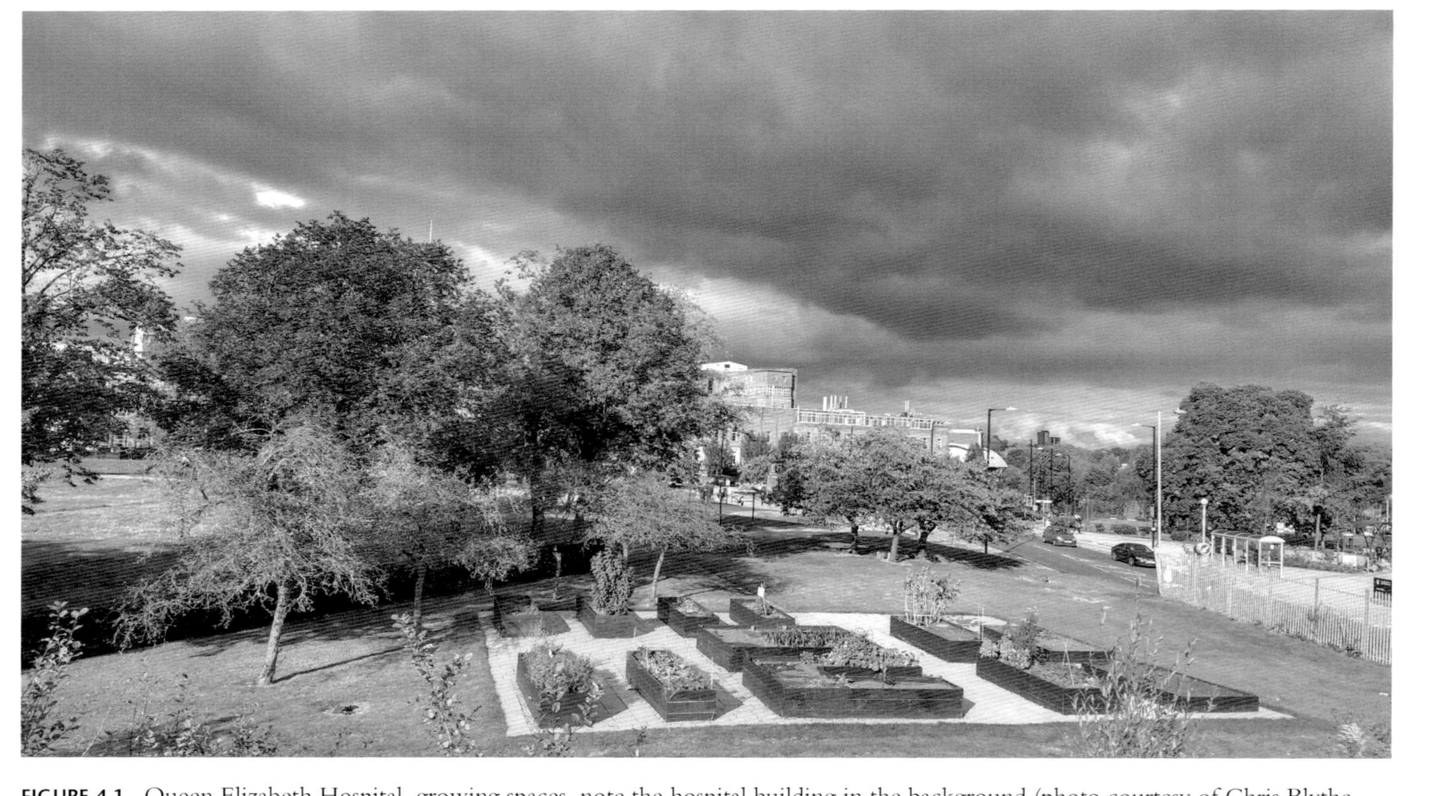

FIGURE 4.1 Queen Elizabeth Hospital, growing spaces, note the hospital building in the background (photo courtesy of Chris Blythe Federation of City Farms and Community Gardens)

between the hospital building, and its linked greenspace presents a more holistic view of health and well-being, demonstrating preventive approaches as well as acute care (Figure 4.1).

Creating the community growing food space within the hospital grounds was made possible through the input of the Trust for Conservations Volunteers' (TCV) Health for Life in the Community programme funded by Mondelēz International. TCV has created fifteen Health for Life garden and growing "hubs" across south Birmingham, supporting the programme's aim to increase physical activity, improve understanding of healthy diets and provide opportunities for people to grow their own food, responding to health issues in the city, including obesity, diet-related illness and physical inactivity.

Working with residents, hospital staff, corporate volunteers and schools, TCV created a garden "hub" at QEH, growing fresh vegetables in raised beds. Weekly Green Gym® sessions, run by TCV staff combine physical activity and outdoor work, gardening, cooking and eating (TCV Health for Life, 2016). Volunteers from all ages and backgrounds, including those with mental health issues, poor health and long-term unemployed, use the gardens. Activities embrace the wider site with maintenance of the woodland, orchard and hay meadows with plans to extend food growing areas in order to supply the hospital canteen, modelling sustainable production

Participants in activities of the broader Health for Life programme complete health questionnaires covering physical activity levels, healthy eating and gardening skills. Ongoing use of the questionnaire has enabled baseline comparisons – the programme found 84% of participants said they had become physically more active, with numbers exercising 5 days a week up from 9% to 17%, 91% of people grew their own food as a result of involvement, and 68% consumed more fruit and vegetables, 87% participants increased social activity (made new friends) and 86% spent more time outdoors (TCV Health for Life, 2016).

In contrast to more informal community gardens, interaction with the hospital garden, orchard and conservation activities are supported by a member of staff. Comments from garden volunteers demonstrate the importance of the immersion in and active engagement with the greenspace. Some spoke of the activity giving them a greater of sense connection to the processes of the natural world:

> "As a child I was always outside . . . coming to the city was the biggest change, you miss it initially, then you adjust . . . I find these gems in the city, it's more relaxing standing, looking out, seeing something green, it's much more energising for me . . . another level of connection and empathy."
>
> "I think you've more connection . . . [when gardening] . . . you start off, with seeds, nurture them, it's something that changes, and stays with you and you get something at the end, whereas if you're just visiting a garden, you appreciate it but its momentary. This is more lasting."

Participants speak of well-being benefits from working outside, including stress reduction, feelings of being "present", improved fitness and more understanding of healthier eating:

> "When it's like a sunny day, normally, you wouldn't have a reason to be outside, but when you come here you know you are going to be outside . . . I like being outside, you are more in the moment, not thinking about the other stresses you have, just thinking about what you are doing, especially when you are like learning about gardening."

Others spoke of the pleasure of seeing the site transforming, creating a place others can enjoy:

> "I remember this was a roundabout, and this is definitely preferable, to walking through the cars, queued down the road, this is much more tranquil."

Social interaction and reduced isolation motivates many of the volunteers and gaining confidence and meeting others was also a key part of activity:

> "There's no better way of keeping fit, having a banter, contributing to community . . . it's nice to see, people from the hospital taking a stroll . . . seeing it enjoyed by other people."
>
> "I like the social side, I was unemployed . . . its rubbish . . . when you are not working, you just want to speak to someone, that's one of the reasons I like coming here . . . well-being."

Staff involved expressed satisfaction in seeing people change over time:

> "For me it's watching the volunteers, there is a social focus . . . it's watching volunteers develop and seeing the transformation in confidence, building up trust, as well, it's a stimulating enough environment for them to come back week after week . . . a fantastic process, it's not a short-term thing, when you are there planting, you don't know if you will be there to harvest."

Jasmine Road Community Gardens

In contrast to the gardens at Queen Elizabeth Hospital, Jasmine Road Community Garden sits hidden from view once derelict, piece of council works land, at the back of Kate's Hill, one of the West Midland Borough of Dudley's most deprived housing estates. Many residents in the area face long-term, generational, unemployment following the collapse of Dudley's industrial base during the 1980s. The impact of economic downturn is manifested in persistent poor health outcomes, with higher than average obesity, CHD, and long-term conditions (Jasmine Road Community Garden, 2015; Public Health England, 2015). Jasmine Road is seen by Public Health as a "local health asset", being a resource that "enhances the ability

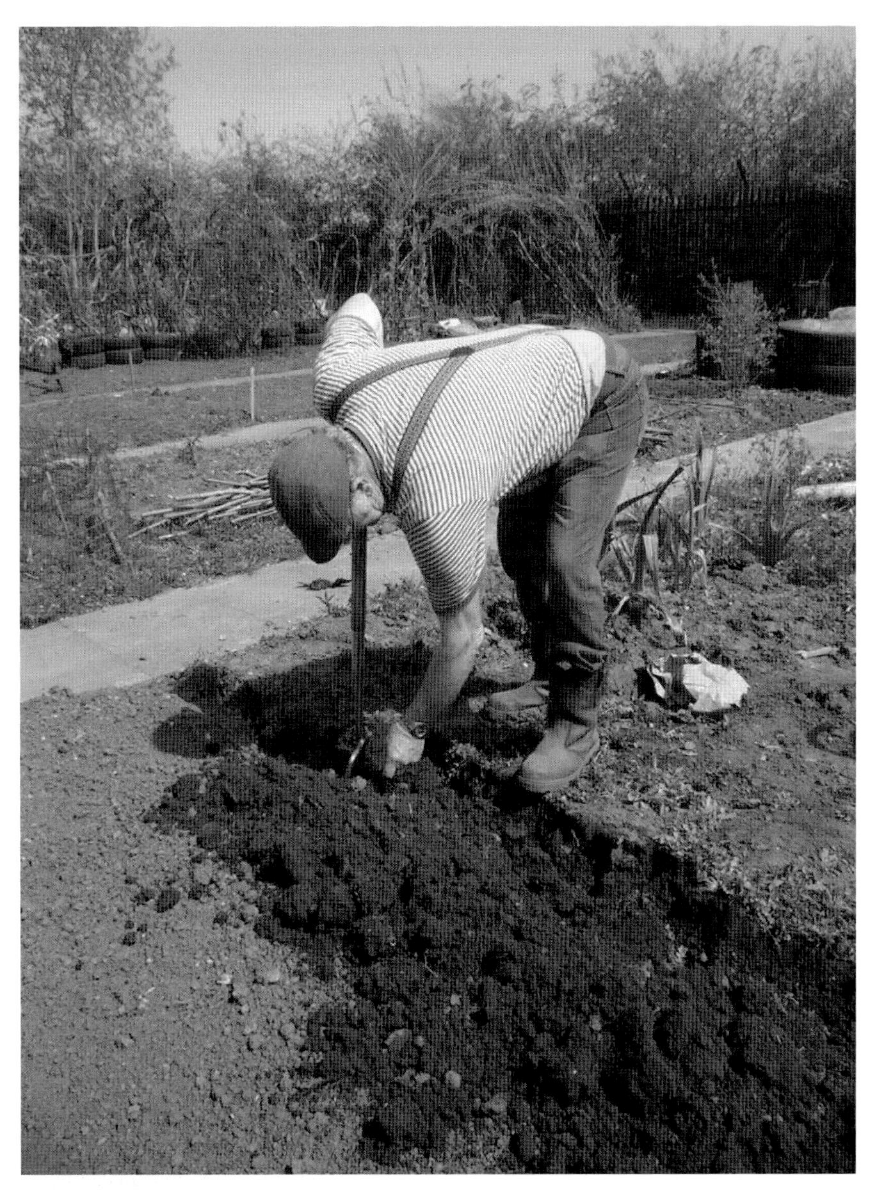

FIGURE 4.2 Growing spaces identified as a "local health asset" (photo courtesy Jasmine Road Community Gardens)

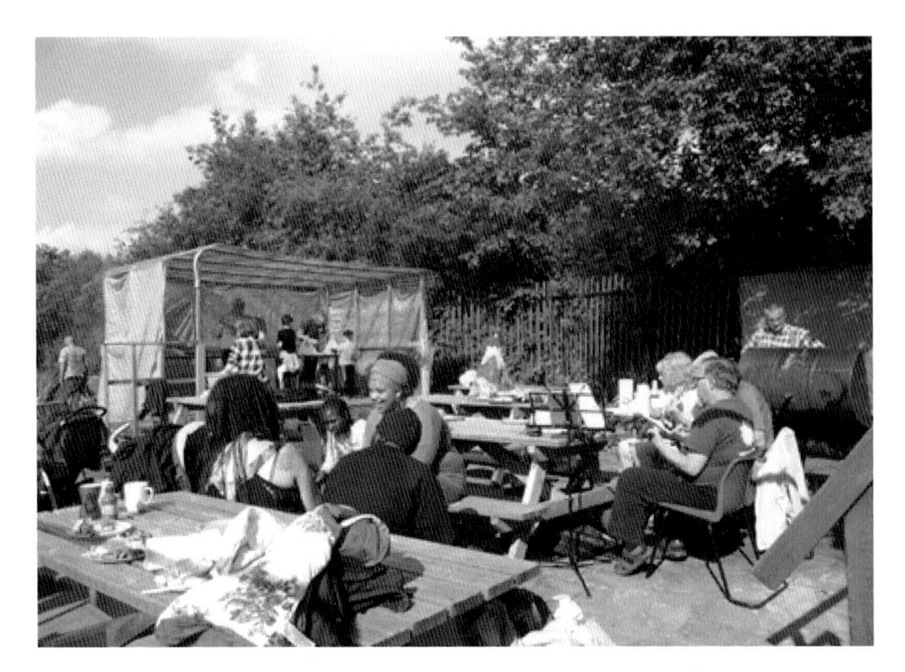

FIGURE 4.3 Jasmine Road Community Gardens encourages a flexible approach to activities underpinning community and well-being (photo courtesy Jasmine Road Community Gardens)

of individuals and community . . . to maintain and sustain health and wellbeing" and has attracted attention (capacity building support and occasional funding) as a way of working to improve health outcomes spanning out from the garden to the wider neighbourhood (Morgan & Ziglio, 2007, 18). It is an example of MBC's "asset based" approach to health and local governance, working closely with communities to build resilience, recognising that links between people, place, and health outcomes are underpinned by a range of "social determinants" embedded in local history and experience (Dudley MBC, 2014).

Pathways for engagement in the garden are flexible and fluid, ranging from someone dropping in to enjoy the sights and smells, sit on a bench, tending a vegetable or flower bed, feeding the chickens, harvesting fresh produce, or through more formal visits by local schools, events and workshops. Run by a committee of local volunteers, the community gardens are "a catalyst to support people . . . within their own communities . . . break down barriers . . . providing a safe haven to support the health and wellbeing of all" (Jasmine Road, 2015, p.5).

The informality of engagement leads to a more collective approach, with participants managing, planning and creating the garden, through individual and communal plots, through crafts, cooking and shared community events. Volunteers use the gardens for individual and collective work, with a strong ethos of creativity, change, and self-determination, where the very act of creating and maintaining the garden space, or "place-making" contributes to experiences of personal and community well-being, reflected in comments from gardeners themselves:

> "We're about an active life rather than a passive one, real rather than virtual, fresh air rather than indoor . . . a contrast between the way life is moving at the moment."
>
> "We build temporary structures that work for a bit and are replaceable, we recreate them or build new things. We build with recycled materials . . . these introduce people to a different way of life, hands on, dealing with things instead of sweeping them away."

This sense of active participation and ability to shape the surroundings seemed to have an impact on how individuals perceive themselves, giving a sense of self-efficacy, personal satisfaction and space for recovery from life's stresses:

> "I had panic attacks . . . this site has allowed me to do things, it's a real 'can do' place, everybody can do the things they want to do . . . my anxiety is much lower, I'm doing more . . . things . . . this is one of the most successful thinks I have done."
>
> "The garden gives people's lives meaning, everything changes from grey to technicolour when they have a project. People can use this space in their own way."

The relationships between the garden and participants was mediated directly, through their own individual experiences and needs, giving a sense of personal story:

> "People can use this space in their own way, I mean 'x' has built in her raised bed, a memorial garden for her sister, there is a little path down the middle of it, and every bit of it has a symbolic meaning, and there are layers of meaning as well . . . this has given her a real interest."
>
> "The boys who have a raised bed, they come up every day and see things grow . . . it's a healthy relationship between them and the space."

Garden users showed a sense of pride in the activity of creation, expressing strong emotional links with both people and place:

> "You certainly get really good quality food from it, but you also get a fantastic amount of friendship, that's really good, and better than the kind of relationships sometimes within my own family, these men and women here mean a lot to me . . . that is about healthy living."

One volunteer emphasised that the garden was *'non-medical'* despite being ultimately about building health and well-being in the widest sense:

> "There is nobody here who has a clean bill of health, and most people are here for their own reasons, and it's a lifeline for them."
>
> "I've been coming here since I finished work, when I was 63, so about 8 years up here, I thought I would do something up here as it will keep me fit, really it keeps me going . . . coming up to the garden . . . while I am doing it I feel better, so I have to keep going."

Discussion

The two case studies, set within the wider context in the West Midlands, illustrate well-rehearsed individual stories, found within the myriad of often hidden and unnoticed greenspaces and community gardens across England and beyond. At their heart is ability of participants, beyond medical settings and through immersion in natural spaces, to build their own sense of empowered health improvement and enhanced well-being. Few of these schemes work within formalised "green care" or medical pathways but happen alongside or in spite of these. This activity embodies what Shah and Marks observe as the wider aspects of well-being beyond the narrow definition of health, "as well as a feeling of being satisfied and happy, well-being means developing as a person, being fulfilled and making a contribution to the community", certainly provided through engagement in these greenspaces (Shah & Marks, 2004, p.2).

The challenge ahead, is how the dialogue between the medical profession and those working to support wider integration of greenspace and well-being will proceed. On one level, many argue greenspaces can provide solutions for new ways of working and preventive agenda, espoused within the NHS Forward View, and Sustainability Transformation Plans (STPs). On another level, it calls for recognition of the spectrum of approaches to bring out the benefits of greenspaces for health. This includes highlighting both formal "green care" pathways, with clear links to health care delivery and valuing the *embedded public health benefits* found within everyday interactions taking place across the smaller, diverse and often unnoticed network of greenspaces and community gardens (Bragg & Atkins, 2016). This will require collaboration and creative responses to health needs at a local level.

Buck (2016) indicates that, despite the growing evidence of the diverse benefits of gardening and greenspace, gardens remain "the elephants outside the room, providing multiple pathways to health gain" but challenging to policy makers (Buck, 2016, p.42). Medical professionals need, in order to understand the value of nature-based health and well-being activity, commissioners and clarity of scale, quality, and process, along with a demonstration of potential long-term savings. The challenge to Commissioners and practitioners alike, is that there is a huge variety of greenspace activity and projects, some more formalised than others, with varied pathways and routes. Care farms and Therapeutic Horticulture projects for example, have developed clear pathways for referral, engagement, and follow up for the medical profession to navigate. Small scale community-based gardens, like Jasmine Road, in contrast, often do not offer medical pathways in a formal sense, yet achieve significant impact on social inclusion, reduced isolation, and community well-being. Models for delivery, need to recognise the spectrum of approaches, and avoid creating a sense of a "two tier" system, whereby those with formal pathways and quality standards end up being seen as the more valid or valuable. In a world of increasing competition for funds faced by the voluntary sector, this could be potentially divisive.

Where and with whom the governance of this sits is another matter. The NHS, as Naylor et al. (2013) envisages, urgently needs new approaches to health commissioning, recognising the economic burden of disease, while embracing preventive public health agenda, wider determinants and lifestyle factors (Naylor et al., 2013). While Buck acknowledges that the system within health presents a myriad of complex and ever-changing structures, difficult for those on the outside to penetrate, he also argues that enough evidence is "out there" and that health services and others need to take the plunge in embracing the opportunity presented by greenspaces for health (Buck, 2016). Will the way forward be through absorption of greenspace activity into existing medical pathways and procedures, for instance, embracing "green care" into social prescribing and community referral schemes via GPs, integration into recovery and rehabilitation pathways working with physiotherapists, occupational therapists, and others? Or will it be through a recognition that it is possible to "let go", and widen the understanding that health and well-being is created beyond medical realms with a move towards a new and integrated model? This could involve a shift towards recognition of the value and cost saving elements of greenspace across the life-course, supporting "co-production" of healthy activity in greenspaces, and creation of place-based population health systems.

Much needs to be considered and worked through by multiple stakeholders, including issues such as land use, ownership, risk, cost, funding sustainability, accountability and use of public money, evaluation and demonstration of social return on investment. This is set against a backdrop of an ongoing debate about austerity, NHS demand and the balance of immediate demands of critical versus longer term preventive care. For greenspace stakeholders, the challenge is how to act collaboratively, recognising the diversity of approaches and aims across varied projects, and without valuing one approach above another, or losing recognition of the incidental well-being provided through greenspaces. There is a need to develop consistent opportunities to Commissioners, presenting clear pathways and frameworks tailored to diverse needs; something that initiatives like The Natural Health Service and Green Care Coalition are trying to develop, through offering a "palette" of greenspace opportunities and entry points across a region, and clearer conceptual frameworks (Green Care Coalition, 2017).

The medical and urban planning world needs to shift as well for these opportunities to become more mainstream and move beyond small project focus to a joined-up approach. For change to happen it requires creative, brave, systems-based thinking, where health planning, and sustainability considerations combine with spatial planning and begin to work together. This is slowly beginning to happen in the West Midlands, with examples like Queen Elizabeth Hospital, and soon to be built Midland Metropolitan Hospital sites, demonstrating how creative and responsible use of health "estate" and surrounding greenspace can play its part in contributing to health, well-being and sustainable development. Birmingham's use of innovative environmental risk mapping and the Natural Capital Planning Tool, highlights a way in which greenspaces can be valued for health, giving developers a strong economic case for consideration. Ross and Chang (2014) and Barton et al.'s (2015) explorations of healthy planning, highlight the possibilities of connected greenspace for health and well-being, with potential to realise this in emerging models like NHS Healthy New Towns and Garden Villages, how to fund, support and make best use of parks as public multifunctional space, along with frameworks for joined-up thinking. Fears that greenspaces will be "over medicalised" through links with health system infrastructure can be allayed if spatial planning were to embrace greenspace and health. Birmingham's endorsement of the of Biophilic Cities, approach could see a future where nature, greenspace and health are embraced as integral to daily experience and signifying a blue print for future urban expansion across the region (Biophilic Cities, 2017).

Acknowledgements

Antony Cobley, Head of Inclusion, Engagement and Wellbeing, and staff and volunteers at QEHB University Hospitals Birmingham NHS Foundation Trusts.

Neil Rimmington, Assistant Inspector of Ancient Monuments, English Heritage,

The Mondelēz International Foundation and staff and volunteers from TCV.

The many corporate volunteers who supported the development QEH grounds, including Mondelēz International, PriceWaterhouse Coopers, and Royal Bank of Scotland, Helping Britain Blossom Project, Bulmers Foundation and Jasmine Road Community Garden, Dudley.

References

Adevi, A. A. & Lieberg, M. (2012) Stress rehabilitation through garden therapy: A caregiver perspective on factors considered most essential to the recovery process, *Urban Forestry & Urban Greening* 11 (1): 51–58.

Alaimo, K., Packnett, E., Miles, R. A. & Kruger, D. J. (2008) Fruit and vegetable intake among urban community gardeners, *Journal of Nutrition Education and Behavior* 40 (2): 94–101.

Aspinall, P., Mavros, P., Coyne, R. & Roe, J. (2015) The urban brain: analysing outdoor physical activity with mobile EEG, *Br J Sports Med* 49 (4): 272–276.

Banzourkov, I. (2017) Director. *Nature in the City. A Biophilic Birmingham.* (Documentary short). Available at http://biophiliccities.org/partner-cities/birmingham-uk/.

Barry, V. (2017) Growing health: Community agriculture in Sandwell, in R. Roggema (ed.) *Agriculture in an Urbanizing Society. Volume Two: Proceedings of the Sixth AESOP Conference on Sustainable Food Planning*, Newcastle on Tyne: Cambridge Scholars Publishing, pp.905–923.

Barton, H., Thompson, S., Burgess, S. & Grant, M. (2015) (eds.) *The Routledge Handbook of Planning for Health and Well-Being: Shaping a Sustainable and Healthy Future*, London: Routledge.

Barton, J. & Pretty, J. (2010) What is the best dose of nature and green exercise for improving mental health? A multi-study analysis, *Environmental Science & Technology* 44 (10): 3947–3955.

Beatley, T. (2011) Biophilic Cities: Integrating Nature into Urban Design and Planning, Washington, DC: Island Press.

Biophilic Cities (2017) http://biophiliccities.org/, last accessed 1 December 2017.

Birmingham and Black Country Wildlife Trusts (2017) A 25 year natural capital vision for the West Midlands combined authority. Available at www.bbcwildlife.org.uk/what-we-do/voice-nature/west-midlands-combined-authority.

Birmingham City Council (2013) *Green Living Spaces Plan 2013*, Birmingham: Birmingham City Council.

Bragg, R. & Atkins, G. (2016) *A Review of Nature-Based Interventions for Mental Health Care – Natural England Commissioned Report 2014.* London: Natural England. Available at http://publications.naturalengland.org.uk/publication/4513819616346112, last accessed on 1 December 2017.

Bragg, R. & Leck, C. (2017) *Good Practice in Social Prescribing for Mental Health: The Role of Nature-Based Interventions*, Natural England Commissioned Reports, Number 228, York: Natural England Publications.

Bragg, R., Wood, C. & Barton, J. (2013) *Ecominds Effects on Mental Wellbeing: An Evaluation for Mind*, London: Mind. Available at www.mind.org.uk/media/354166/Ecominds-effects-on-mentalwellbeing-evaluation-report.pdf.

Buck, D. (2016) *Gardens and Health: Implications for Policy and Practice, Report Commissioned by the National Gardens Scheme*, London: The King's Fund. Available at www.kingsfund.org.uk/publications/ gardens-and-health, last accessed 1 December 2017.

CABE Space (2010) *Urban Green Nation: Building the Evidence Base*, London: Commissioner for Architecture and the Built Environment. Available at http://webarchive.nationalarchives.gov.uk/20110118095356/http:/www.cabe.org.uk/publications/urban-green-nation.

Crouse, D., Pinault, L., Balram, A., Hystad, P., Peters, P., Chen, H., Van Donkelaar, A., Martin, R., Ménard, R., Robichaud, A. & Villeneuve, P. (2017) Urban greenness and mortality in Canada's largest cities: a national cohort study, *Lancet Planetary Health* 1: e289–e297.

Davies, G., Devereaux, M., Lennartsson, M., Schmutz, U. & Williams, S. (2014) *The Benefits of Gardening and Food Growing for Health and Wellbeing*, London: Garden Organic; Sustain.

Available at www.farmtocafeteriacanada.ca/wcontent/uploads/2014/06/GrowingHealth_BenefitsReport.pdf, last accessed 13 July 2016.

Davis, L. & Middleton, J. (2012) The perilous road from community activism to public policy: fifteen years of community agriculture in Sandwell, in A. Viljoen & J. S. C. Wiskerke (eds.), *Sustainable Food Planning: Evolving Theory and Practice*, Wageningen: Wageningen Academic Publishers.

DCLG (2012) *National Planning Policy Framework*, London: Department for Communities and Local Government.

de Vries, S., Verheij, R. A., Groenewegen, P. P. & Spreeuwenberg, P. (2003) Natural environments – healthy environments? An exploratory analysis of the relationship between greenspace and health, *Environ. Plan. A* 35: 1717–1731.

Dudley Metropolitan Borough Council (2014) *All About Dudley Borough. Joint Strategic Needs Assessment 2014*, Dudley: Dudley MBC. Available at www.allaboutdudley.info/AODB/publications/2014%20JSNA%20synthesis%20docuement.pdf, last accessed 11 November 2017.

Ege, M. J., Mayer, M., Normand, A. C., Genuneit, J., Cookson, W.O., Braun-Fahrländer, C., Heederik, D., Piarroux, R. & von Mutius, E. (2011) Exposure to environmental microorganisms and childhood asthma, *New England Journal of Medicine* 364 (8): 701–709.

European Commission (2013) Communication from the Commission to the European Parliament, The Council, the European Economic and Social Committee and the Committee of the Regions. Green Infrastructure (GI) - Enhancing Europe's Natural Capital. COM(2013) 249 final.

European Commission (2015) Towards and EU Research and Innovation Policy agenda for Nature-Based Solutions and Re-Naturing Cities. Final Report of the Horizon 2020 Expert Group on "Nature-Based Solutions and Re-Naturing Cities", Luxembourg: EU Commission.

Faculty of Public Health and Natural England (2010) (eds.) *Great Outdoors: How Our Natural Health Service Uses Green Space to Improve Wellbeing: An Action Report*, London: Faculty of Public Health.

Federation of City Farms and Community Gardens (2017) Available at www.farmgarden.org.uk/, last accessed 20 November 2017.

Fieldhouse, J. (2003) The Impact of an allotment group on mental health clients' health, wellbeing and social networking, *British Journal of Occupational Therapy* 66: 286–296.

Franchina, A., Scott, A. J. & Carter, C. E. (2017) *The Green Living Spaces Plan: Evaluation and Future Prospects*. Report Submitted to Birmingham City Council, Birmingham: Birmingham City University.

Gascon, M., Triguero-Mas, M., Martínez, D., Dadvand, P., Forns, J., Plasència, A. & Nieuwenhuijsen, M. J. (2015) Mental health benefits of long-term exposure to residential green and blue spaces: a systematic review, *International Journal of Environmental Research and Public Health* 12 (4): 4354–4379.

Gidlöf-Gunnarsson, A. & Öhrström, E. (2007) Noise and well-being in urban residential environments: the potential role of perceived availability to nearby green areas, *Landscape and Urban Planning* 83 (2): 115–126.

Green Care Coalition (2017) Available at https://greencarecoalition.org.uk/, last accessed 1 December 2017.

Growing Birmingham (2017) Available at www.growingbirmingham.org/, last accessed 1 December 2017.

Hartig, T., Evans, G. W., Jamner, L. D., Davies, D. S. & Gärling, T. (2003) Tracking restoration in natural and urban field settings, *Journal of Environmental Psychology* 23: 109–112.

Hassink, J. & Van Dijk, M. (2006) (eds.) Farming for Health: Green-Care Farming Across Europe and the United States of America (Vol. 13), Berlin: Springer Science & Business Media.

Hawkins, J. L., Smith, A., Backx, K. & Clayton, D. A. (2015) Exercise intensities of gardening tasks within older adult allotment gardeners in Wales, *Journal of Aging and Physical Activity* 23: 161–168.

Hawkins, J. L., Thirlaway, K. J., Backx, K. & Clayton, D. A. (2011) Allotment gardening and other leisure activities for stress reduction and healthy aging. *Hort Technology* 21: 577–585.

Hewitt, P., Watts, C., Hussey, J., Power, K. & Williams, T. (2013) Does a structured gardening programme improve well-being in young-onset dementia? A preliminary study, *British Journal of Occupational Therapy* 76: 355–361.

Hölzinger, O., Laughlin, P. & Grayson, N. (2015) Planning for Sustainable Land-Use: The Natural Capital Planning Tool (NCPT) Project, London: RICS.

James, P., Banay, R., Hart, J. & Laden, F. (2015) A review of the health benefits of greenness, *Current Epidemiology Reports* 2 (2): 131–142.

Jasmine Road Community Garden (2015) *Jasmine Road Community Gardens. Business Plan 2015*. Dudley: Jasmine Road Community Gardens.

Kaplan, R. (2001) The nature of the view from home: psychological benefits, *Environment and Behavior* 33 (4): 507–542.

Kaplan, R. & Kaplan, S. (1989) *The Experience of Nature: A Psychological Perspective*, Cambridge: Cambridge University Press.

Lafortezza, R., Carrus, G., Sanesi, G. & Davies, C. (2009) Benefits and well-being perceived by people visiting green spaces in periods of heat stress, *Urban Forestry & Urban Greening* 8 (2): 97–108.

Lee, A. C. & Maheswaran, R. (2011) The health benefits of urban green spaces: a review of the evidence, *Journal of Public Health* 33 (2): 212–222.

Lee, J., Park, B. J., Tsunetsugu, Y., Ohira, T., Kagawa, T. & Miyazaki, Y. (2011) Effect of forest bathing on physiological and psychological responses in young Japanese male subjects, *Public Health* 125: 93–100.

Leng, C. H. & Wang, J. D. (2016) Daily home gardening improved survival for older people with mobility limitations: an 11-year follow-up study in Taiwan, *Clinical Interventions in Aging* 11: 947–959.

Lohrberg, F., Lička, L., Scazzosi, L. & Timpe, A. (2016) (eds.) *Urban agriculture Europe*, Berlin: Jovis.

Louv, R. (2008) *Last Child in the Woods: Saving our Children from Nature-Deficit Disorder*, New York: Algonquin Books.

Lovell, S. T. (2010) Multifunctional urban agriculture for sustainable land use planning in the United States, *Sustainability* 2 (8): 2499–2522.

Lund, I. E., Granerud A., Eriksson B. G. (2015) Green care from the provider's perspective, *Sage Open* 5 (1). Available at https://doi.org/10.1177/2158244014568422.

Maas, J., van Dillen, S. M. E., Verheij, R. A. & Groenewegen, P. P. (2009) Social contacts as a possible mechanism behind the relation between green space and health, *Health Place* 15: 586–595.

MacKerron, G. & Mourato, S. (2013) Happiness is greater in natural environments, *Global Environmental Change* 23 (5): 992–1000.

Marmot, M. & Marmot Review Team (2010) *Fair Society, Healthy Lives. The Marmot Review, Strategic Review of Health Inequalities in England Post-2010*, London: Marmot Review. Available at www.instituteofhealthequity.org/Content/FileManager/pdf/fairsocietyhealthylives.pdf.

Mersey Forest (2017) Natural choices for health and wellbeing. Available at www.merseyforest.org.uk/our-work/natural-choices-for-health-and-wellbeing/.

Middleton, J. (2010) The Three Greens for Health. Director of Public Health Annual Report for Sandwell. *2009–10*, Sandwell: Sandwell Partnership.

Millennium Ecosystem Assessment (2005) *Ecosystems and Human Well-being: Synthesis*, Washington, DC: Island Press.

Mitchell R. & Popham F. (2008) Effect of exposure to natural environment on health inequalities: an observational population study, *The Lancet* 372: 1655–1660.

Morgan, A. & Ziglio E. (2007) Revitalising the evidence base for public health: an assets model, *Global Health Promotion* 14 (supplement 2): 17–22.

Moss, S. (2012) *Natural Childhood*, London: The National Trust.

Natural England (2010) Nature nearby – accessible natural greenspace guidance, *NE 265*. Available at www.naturalengland.org.uk/regions/east_of_england/ourwork/gi/accessiblenaturalgreenspacestandardangst.aspx.

Naylor, C., Imison C., Addicott, R., Buck, D., Goodwin, N., Harrison, T., Ross, S., Sonola, L., Tian, Y. & Curry, N. (2013) *Transforming our Health Care System: Ten Priorities for Commissioners*, London: The King's Fund. Available at www.kingsfund.org.uk/sites/files/kf/field/field_publication_file/10PrioritiesFinal2.pdf, last accessed 1 December 2017.

NHS England (2014) NHS Five year forward view. Available at www.england.nhs.uk>five-year-forward-view.

NHS Forest and Centre for Sustainable Healthcare (n.d.) University Hospitals Birmingham. Case study by the centre for sustainable healthcare. Available at http://nhsforest.org/sites/default/files/Birmingham_University_Hospitals_case_study_web_final.pdf, last accessed 1 December 2017.

NHS Scotland (2017) NHS greenspace demonstration project. Available at www.healthscotland.com/topics/settings/nhsgreenspace/index.aspx.

Nowak, D., Crane, D. & Stevens, J. (2006) Air pollution removal by urban trees and shrubs in the United States, *Urban for Urban Green* 4: 115–123.

Pank H. (2011) *Gorgie City Farm Community Gardening Project: Social Returns on Investment (SROI) Report*, Edinburgh: Federation of City Farms & Community Gardens Gardening Project.

Pretty, J., Barton, J., Colbeck. I., Hine, R., Mourato, S., MacKerron. G. & Wood, C. (2011) Health values from ecosystems. *Chapter 23, in UK National Ecosystem Assessment. Technical Report*, Cambridge: UNEP-WCMC, pp.1153–1182.

Public Health England (2015) *Dudley Health Profile 2015*, London: Public Health England. Available at file:///c:/users/id916420/downloads/healthprofile2015dudley00cr%20(1).pdf, last accessed 1 December 2017.

Public Health England (2017) Guidance. health matters: Obesity and the food environment. Available at www.gov.uk/government/publications/health-matters-obesity-and-the-food-environment/health-matters-obesity-and-the-food-environment--2.

Rayner, G. & Lang, T. (2012) *Ecological Public Health: Reshaping the Conditions for Good Health*, Abingdon: Routledge.

Roe, J. J., Thompson, C. W., Aspinall, P. A., Brewer, M. J., Duff, E. I., Miller, D., Mitchell, R. & Clow, A. (2013) Green space and stress: evidence from cortisol measures in deprived urban communities, *International Journal of Environmental Research and Public Health* 10 (9): 4086–4103.

Ross, A. & Chang, M. (2014) *Planning Healthy Weight Environments*, London: Town and Country Planning Association. Available at www.tcpa.org.uk/pages/planning-out-obesity-2014.html, last accessed 1 December 2017.

Sandwell PCT & Sandwell MBC (2013) Environment and Health in Sandwell. *Joint Strategic Needs Assessment*, Sandwell: Sandwell PCT.

Shah, H. & Marks, N. (2004) *A Well-Being Manifesto for A Flourishing Society*, London: The New Economics Foundation.

Shanahan, D., Lin, B., Bush, R., Gaston, K., Dean, J., Barber, E. & Fuller, R. (2015) Toward improved public health outcomes from urban nature, *American Journal of Public Health* 105: 470–477.

Sugiyama, T., Leslie, E., Giles-Corti, B. & Owen, N. (2008) Associations of neighbourhood greenness with physical and mental health: do walking, social coherence and local social interaction explain the relationships? *Journal of Epidemiology and Community Health* 62: e9.

Tanako, T., Nakamura, K. & Watanabar, M. (2002) Urban residential environments and senior citizens longevity in megacity areas: the importance of walkable green spaces, *Journal of Epidemiology and Community Health* 56: 913–918.

Tomlinson, C. J., Prieto-Lopez, T., Bassett, R., Chapman, L., Cai, X. M., Thornes, J. E. & Baker, C. J. (2013) Showcasing urban heat island work in Birmingham –measuring, monitoring, modelling and more, *Weather* 68 (2): 44–49.

Trust for Conservation Volunteers (2016) *Health for Life Report to Modelez International Foundation. Year 4, June 2015–November 2015.* Available at www.tcv.org.uk/sites/default/files/health-for-life-report-year4.pdf, last accessed 29 November 2017.

Ulrich, R. (1984) View through a window may influence recovery from surgery, *Science* 224 (4647): 420–421.

United Nations (2012) *World Urbanization Prospectus, the 2011 Revision: Highlights*, New York: United Nations, Department of Economic and Social Affairs, Population Division.

University of Birmingham (2000) *The Romans in Britain. Metchley Roman Fort*, Birmingham: University of Birmingham. Available at www.birmingham.gov.uk, last accessed 1 December 2017.

Van den Berg, A. E., van Winsum-Westra, M., de Vries, S. & van Dillen, S. M. (2010) Allotment gardening and health: a comparative survey among allotment gardeners and their neighbors without an allotment, *Environmental Health* 9 (1): 74.

Viljoen, A. & Wiskerke, J. S. (2012) (eds.) *Sustainable Food Planning: Evolving Theory and Practice*, Wageningen: Wageningen Academic Publishers.

Wells, N. M. & Evans, G. W. (2003) Nearby nature: a buffer of life stress among rural children, *Environment and Behavior* 35 (3): 311–330.

Whear, R., Coon, J. T., Bethel, A., Abbott, R., Stein, K. & Garside, R. (2014) What is the impact of using outdoor spaces such as gardens on the physical and mental well-being of those with dementia? A systematic review of quantitative and qualitative evidence, *Journal of the American Medical Directors Association* 15 (10): 697–705.

Wild in the City (2017) The natural health service. Available at http://wildinthecity.org.uk/programmes-2/the-natural-health-service/.

Wilson, E. O. (1984) *Biophilia*, Cambridge, MA: Harvard University Press.

Wolch, J. R., Byrne, J. & Newell, J. P. (2014) Urban green space, public health, and environmental justice: the challenge of making cities "just green enough", *Landscape and Urban Planning* 125: 234–244.

World Health Organization (1998) *The World Health Report 1998 – Life in the 21st Century: A Vision for All*, Geneva: World Health Organization.

World Health Organization (2008) *Commission on the Social Determinants of Health*, Geneva: World Health Organization.

World Health Organisation (2016) *Urban Green Spaces and Health*, Copenhagen: WHO Regional Office for Europe.

World Health Organization Europe (2013) *Health 2020. A European Policy Framework and Strategy for the 21st Century*, Copenhagen: Regional Offices for WHO Europe.

Zick, C. D., Smith, K. R., Kowaleski-Jones, L., Uno, C. & Merrill, B. J. (2013) Harvesting more than vegetables: the potential weight control benefits of community gardening, *American Journal of Public Health* 103 (6): 1110–1115.

5

BIOPHILIA AND THE PRACTICE OF BIOPHILIC DESIGN

Elizabeth Freeman Calabrese and Alice Dommert

Introduction

The places and spaces that we love as humans tell much about the origins of our species and what we innately need not only to survive but to flourish. Close your eyes and take a moment and think about where you like to go on vacation or celebrate a special occasion. What are your favourite childhood memories and what were the smells, sounds and emotions involved? When and where do you feel the most creative, calm and balanced?

This chapter provides a framework for the understanding and application of Biophilic Design, exploring the concept of biophilia as an inherent inclination to affiliate with nature, the nonhuman environment, as essential to human health, fitness and well-being (Wilson, 1984; Kellert & Wilson, 1993; Kellert, 2005, 2012; Kellert et al., 2008; Kellert & Calabrese, 2015). The prevailing paradigm regarding the design of the modern built environment has encouraged environmental degradation and separation from nature. Biophilic Design offers an ecological and ethical remedial response to the stressful impacts of city life, addressing the breach of modern society from the natural world. It is this conscious process of Biophilic Design that forms the subject of this chapter.

> Biophilia, if it exists, and I believe it exists, is the innately emotional affiliation of human beings to other living organisms. Innate means hereditary and hence part of ultimate human nature.
>
> *(Wilson, 1984)*

Increasingly, research shows the state of human disease and the environmental degradation we see continuing to grow is reflective of our waning direct and indirect connections with nature (Kellert & Wilson, 1993; Kellert, 2005; Kellert et al., 2008).

In this context, two key questions need addressing:

- What impact does the built environment where we work and live have on our health, well-being and our ability to thrive?
- How can we balance the need and desire for our comforts and conveniences, our evolving technologies and our inherent need for the elements of nature?

Biophilia reflects our biocentric connections and leads to the consideration of Biophilic Design which seeks to restore this connection in ways that reflect the reality of a modern world. René Dubos (1980), in *The Wooing of the Earth*, speaks of the possibilities of mutual adaptation:

> The relationship between humankind and nature can be one of respect and love rather than domination . . . The outcome can be rich and lastingly successful only if both partners are modified by their association so as to become better adapted to each other . . . With our knowledge and sense of responsibility for the welfare of humankind and the Earth, we can create new environments that are ecologically sound, aesthetically satisfying, economically rewarding, and favorable to the continued growth of civilization.

Biocentric connections

> It is assumed that humans are a product of evolution and that they reflect that heritage in their information-handling patterns, in their biases, in their very nature.
>
> *(Kaplan & Kaplan, 1983)*

Humans have evolutionary anchored behaviour systems (Wilson, 1984; Öhman, 1986) and as a species our behaviour systems have been characterised by a biocentric existence (Figure 5.1). Despite the prevalence and scope of modern technology, we retain this innate need for connection with nature.

The earliest modern Homo sapiens lived approximately 200,000 years ago and as a species we have spent the majority of our evolution in Africa migrating to other reaches of the earth 60,000–70,000 years ago. Hunting and gathering were the primary means of sustenance until 10,000 years ago when humans began to raise food on a larger scale through agriculture resulting in significant population growth. The first cities formed roughly 6,000 years ago and the mass production of goods and services began with the industrial revolution about 400 years ago (Harari, 2015). Electricity and modern technology have only influenced the human-built environment for a mere 200 years (Figure 5.1).

Homo sapiens evolved in the context of the natural world, not a technologically dominated environment; we were a foraging culture for the majority of our species' existence (Wilson, 1984; Kellert & Wilson, 1993). We relied on physical

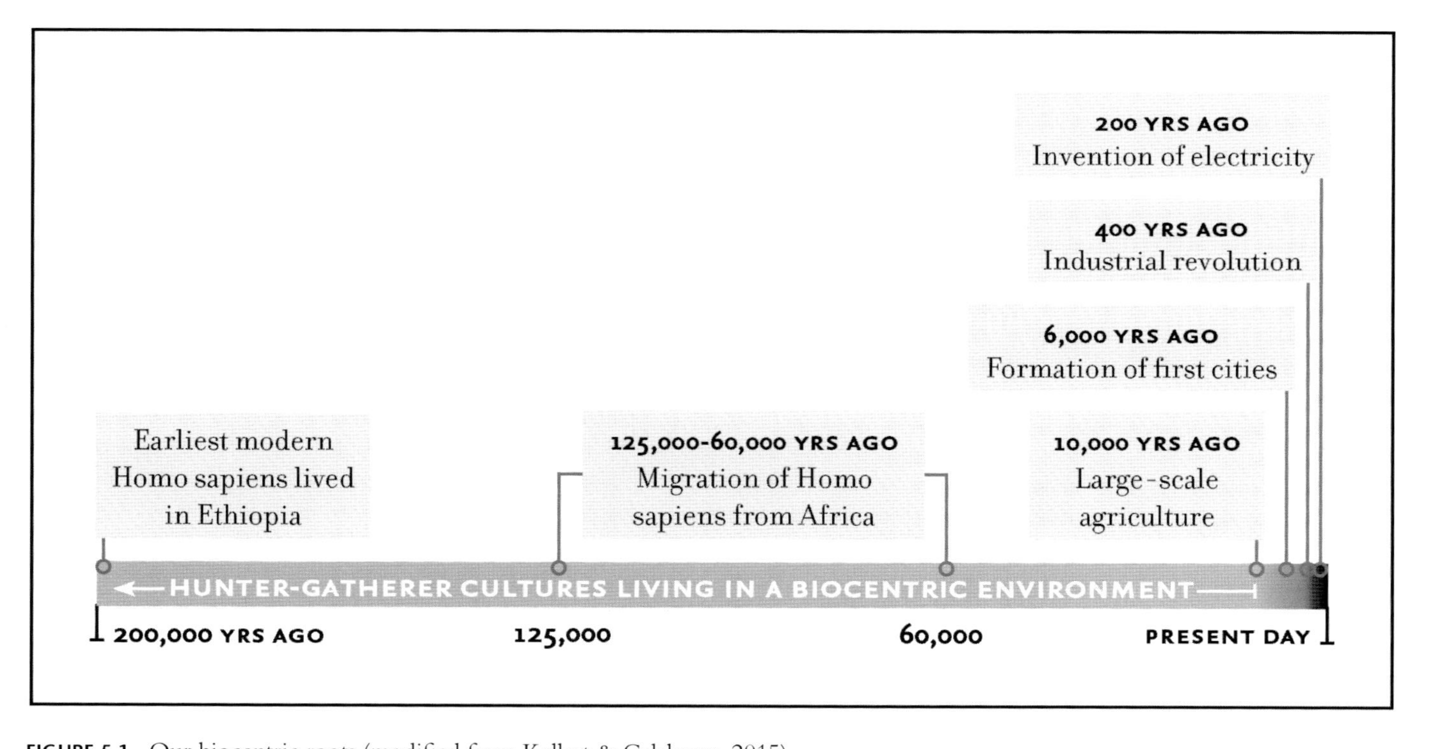

FIGURE 5.1 Our biocentric roots (modified from Kellert & Calabrese, 2015)

stamina, agility and diverse strategies to navigate the terrain in which we lived, to hunt and trap animals and collect wild food. A keen understanding of the seasons, weather patterns and animal migration were vital to our survival as a species. We had to "know nature" in order to survive. However, by the early twenty-first century, hunting and gathering was no longer a way of life for the majority of human beings (Heerwagen & Orians, 1986, 1993; Harari, 2015).

Advancements in agriculture and technology have eliminated our need to "know nature" as our ancestors did in order to survive. Furthermore, we now have the ability to hermetically seal ourselves inside of structures created of chemically derived materials with artificial lighting and mechanically controlled air in the name of energy efficiency, value engineering and progress, thus disconnecting us even more so from the natural world – in schools, hospitals, eldercare facilities, affordable housing, prisons and high-rise office buildings. But towards the end of the twentieth century, research began to substantiate the deleterious effects of this isolation and re-establish the inherent need to connect with the natural world and natural systems and processes (Heerwagen & Orians, 1993; Ulrich, 1993; Todd & Todd, 1993; Kellert, 1997, 2005).

In 1984, Roger Ulrich, PhD, was involved with ground-breaking research and the resulting paper, "View through a window may influence recovery from surgery", analysed the medical records of patients recovering from a common gallbladder surgery. Two recovery rooms were used in the study, one with a window view of trees with leaves and the other with a view of a brown brick wall. Patients who had a view of the trees complained less, required less pain medication and healed faster than the patients with the view of the brick wall (Figure 5.2). This study was one of the first to conclude "hospital design and siting decisions should take into account the quality of patient window views" (Ulrich, 1984).

Since Ulrich's work, research supporting our need to connect with nature for health and well-being is mounting across fields and disciplines. In a recent publication of *Environmental Health Perspectives*, "Nature contact and human health: A research agenda", a multidisciplinary team "recognized the need to balance linear, reductionist approaches to research with complex, systems-based approaches". The authors concluded,

> According to the best available evidence, nature contact offers considerable promise in addressing a range of health challenges, including many, such as obesity, cardiovascular disease, depression, and anxiety that are public health priorities. Nature contact offers promise both as prevention and as treatment across the life-course. Potential advantages include low costs relative to conventional medical interventions, safety, practicality, not requiring dispensing by highly trained professionals, and multiple co-benefits. Few medications can boast these attributes.
>
> *(Frumkin et al., 2017)*

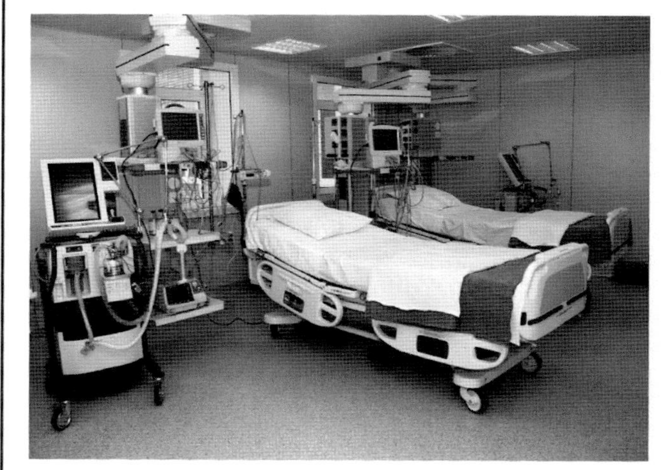

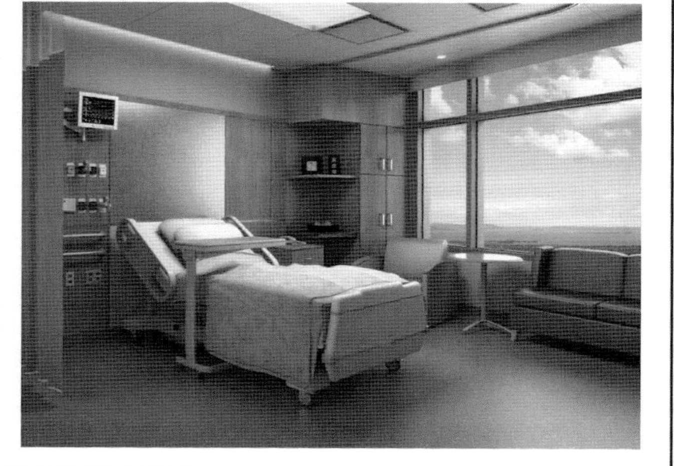

FIGURE 5.2 "View through a window may influence recovery from surgery", note typical hospital rooms similar to the room on the left often have no natural daylight as compared to the room on the right that includes natural daylight, nature-inspired materials and colours in the interior finishes. Patients heal faster, take less pain medication and complain less when they have a view of nature (Ulrich, 1984) (source: left – Calabrese/Shutterstock and right – permission of William McDonough + Partners)

Evidence-Based Design (EBD), a process of using research to guide decisions about the built environment to achieve the best possible outcomes, is being used in the healthcare field and acknowledges the mental and physical benefits of exposure to nature (Cama, 2009; Marcus & Sachs, 2014; Shepley & Samira, 2017). Being around, in, or near nature can lower blood pressure, reduce stress and anxiety, aid in recovery and healing, improve patient and staff morale, reduce conflicts and help to create a healthier sense of being (Ulrich, 1993, 2008; Frumkin, 2001, 2008; Kellert & Heerwagen, 2007; Bowler et al., 2010; Kou, 2010; Townsend & Weerasuriya, 2010; Annerstedt & Währbor, 2011; Louv, 2012; Wells & Rollings, 2012).

In 2005, Richard Louv introduced the term "nature-deficit disorder" in his 2005 book, *Last Child in the Woods*, attributing the continued increase of children's behavioural problems is due, in part, to limited time outdoors in the natural environment (Taylor et al., 2001; Louv, 2005). Natural play offers children multisensory experiences, including movement, balance, sights, smells, touch and sounds.

The evidence for biophilia as a human condition for children and adults, and the penalties of disconnection with the natural world are strong; as Dr William Bird, MBE, Founder of Intelligent Health, UK, states:

> Our bodies are meant to be active and we're designed to be connected to nature. We're hunter-gatherers and our bodies currently exist in an alien environment of being indoors all the time and living under artificial lights and so on. Owing to this, our bodies respond with chronic inflammation which leads to cancer and long-term illness.
>
> *(www.intelligenthealth.co.uk, p. 1)*

Interface and HermanMiller are demonstrating that work environments based on biophilia have numerous business benefits in the workplace including improved employee retention, enhanced cognitive performance, decreased absenteeism, higher employee satisfaction and increased profitability (Browning et al., 2012, 2014; HermanMiller, 2018; Human Spaces, 2018). Google and Amazon are examples of major corporations now utilising biophilic elements in the planning and design of their campuses. Furthermore, three major building certification programs include biophilia and Biophilic Design: The Living Building Challenge (ILFI, 2018), WELL Building Standard (IWBI, 2018) and Fitwel (Fitwel, 2018).

Biophilic Design

Biophilic Design was pioneered by Dr Stephen Kellert and is based on the concept of biophilia with the intent of creating healthy habitats for humans as biological organisms (Kellert, 1997; Kellert et al., 2008). Most people in developed countries now spend on average 90% of their time inside human-built environments. With the invention of televisions, computers, tablets and smartphones, our lives have become increasingly interconnected and reliant on technology (Kellert et al., 2008).

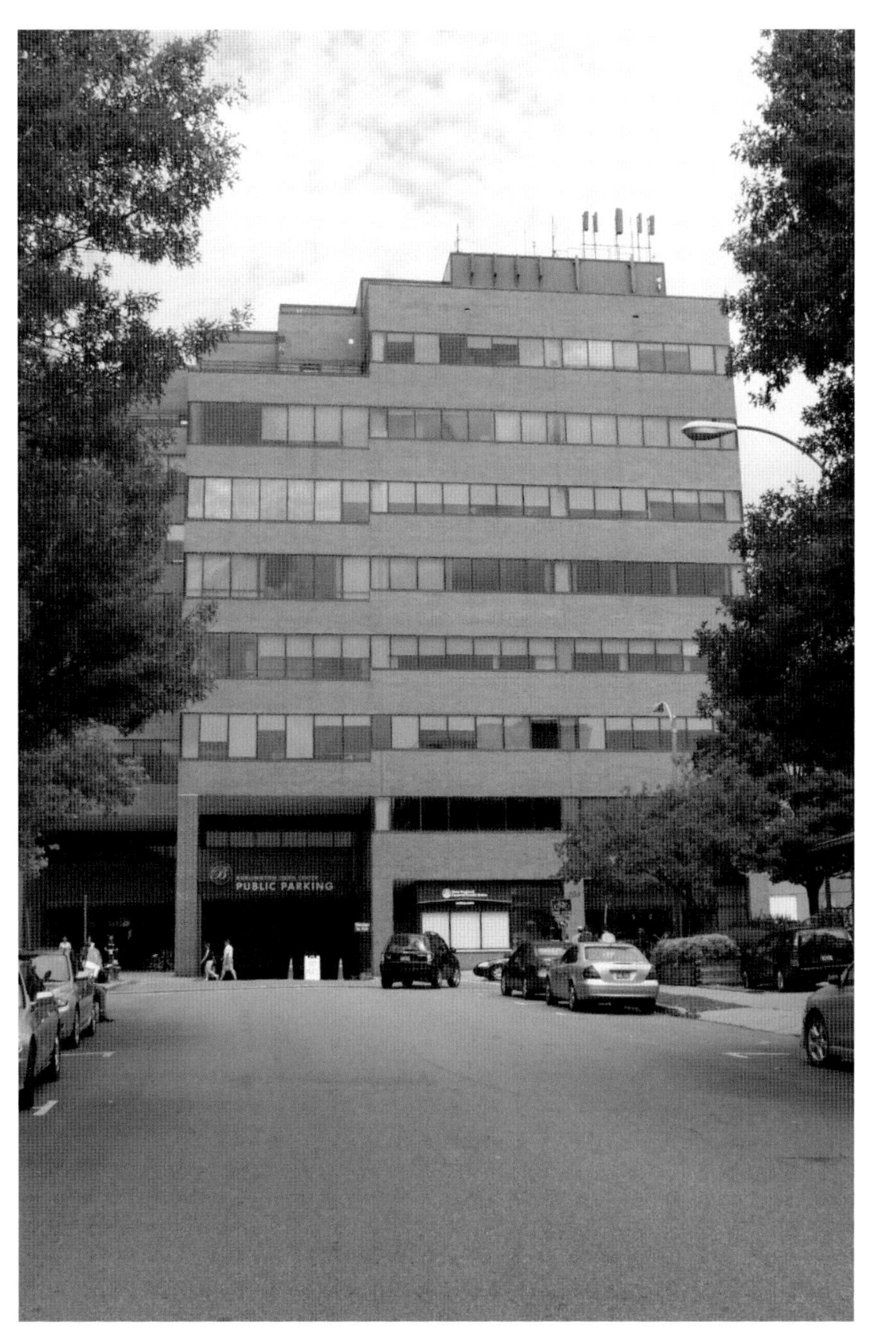

FIGURE 5.3 Modern building can create a barrier to the natural world. Many structures built with mechanical air conditioning have fixed glass facades that create a barrier to the natural world. Typically, the glass in these windows is tinted for energy efficiency, however the tint can negatively affect the natural colour spectrum of light for the occupants inside. Such facades can lack a sense of place within the streetscape (Calabrese)

Biophilic Design re-establishes our connections with the natural world by providing pathways that bring nature into the modern built environment by directly and indirectly integrating nature and natural systems and processes. Many of our most beloved places that offer the best examples of Biophilic Design demonstrate a strong genius loci – sense of place. They embody a natural integration with the local geography, climate, culture and ecology and are designed with nature as a priority (Figure 5.4). The essence and powerful allure of a truly biophilic space have a strong natural resonance (Alexander et al., 1977; Alexander, 1979; Salingaros, 2015).

> There is one timeless way of building. It is thousands of years old, and the same today as it has always been. The great traditional buildings of the past, the villages and tents and temples in which man feels at home, have always been made by people who are very close to the center of this way. And as you will see, this way will lead anyone who looks for it to buildings which are themselves as ancient in their form as the trees and hills, and as our faces are.
>
> *(Alexander, 1979)*

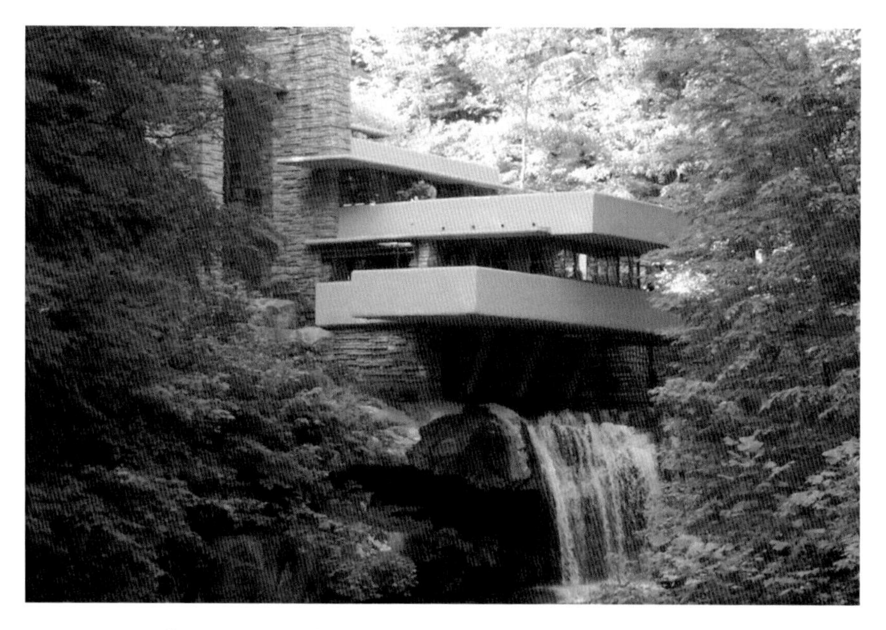

FIGURE 5.4 Falling water. Built in 1939 by Frank Lloyd Wright, this is a classic example of a structure designed to connect occupants to the surrounding natural landscape and ecology (Hildebrand, 1991) (Somach (Own work) [CC BY-SA 3.0 (https://creativecommons.org/licenses/by-sa/3.0)], via Wikimedia Commons)

PRINCIPLES OF BIOPHILIC DESIGN (KELLERT & CALABRESE 2015)

1. **Biophilic design fosters a repeated and sustained engagement with nature.**
2. **Biophilic design focuses on human adaptations to the natural world that over evolutionary time have advanced people's health, fitness and wellbeing.**
3. **Biophilic design encourages an emotional attachment to particular settings and places.**
4. **Biophilic design promotes positive interactions between people and nature that encourage an expanded sense of responsibility and stewardship for the human and natural communities.**
5. **Biophilic design encourages ecologically connected, mutually reinforced and integrated design solutions.**

FIGURE 5.5 The Five Principles of Biophilic Design (modified from Kellert & Callabrese, 2015)

The Biophilic Design Framework

Biophilic Design is a conscious process of design for a built environment that supports our ability to flourish, individually, as communities and as a greater humanity. Biophilic Design helps to identify why certain places resonate and inspire us and provides design Principles to guide architects and designers, engineers and landscape architects, urban planners and community members.

The practice of Biophilic Design developed by Dr Stephen Kellert and Elizabeth Calabrese offers a simplified Biophilic Design Framework. The Framework consists of five key Biophilic Design Principles (Figure 5.5). These Principles provide the intentions of the Biophilic Design approach to foster cohesive, holistic, ecological design solutions that reconnect us to nature and to each other. Although the term Biophilic Design is relatively new, this design approach is as ancient as our species and is based on our intuitive and innate wisdom.

Biophilic Design offers three experiential ways to integrate nature into the design process – Direct Experience of Nature, Indirect Experience of Nature and Experience of Space and Place and each Experience has associated Attributes (Figure 5.6). Together the Principles, Experiences and Attributes provide a design ecology of varied strategies where different elements of natural biophilic orientation can be integrated into the design process, hence the Biophilic Design Framework (Kellert & Calabrese, 2015).

Biophilic Design, in seeking to restore contact with nature, is underpinned by ancient connections with the natural world that reflect a biocentric existence. As discussed, biophilia indicates that we still require these connections to function effectively and that they are rooted in our direct contact with nature and survival strategies; it is these which are considered first.

Direct Experience of Nature

The Direct Experience Of Nature can be accomplished by opening spaces up to the surrounding natural environment, by bringing nature into the built

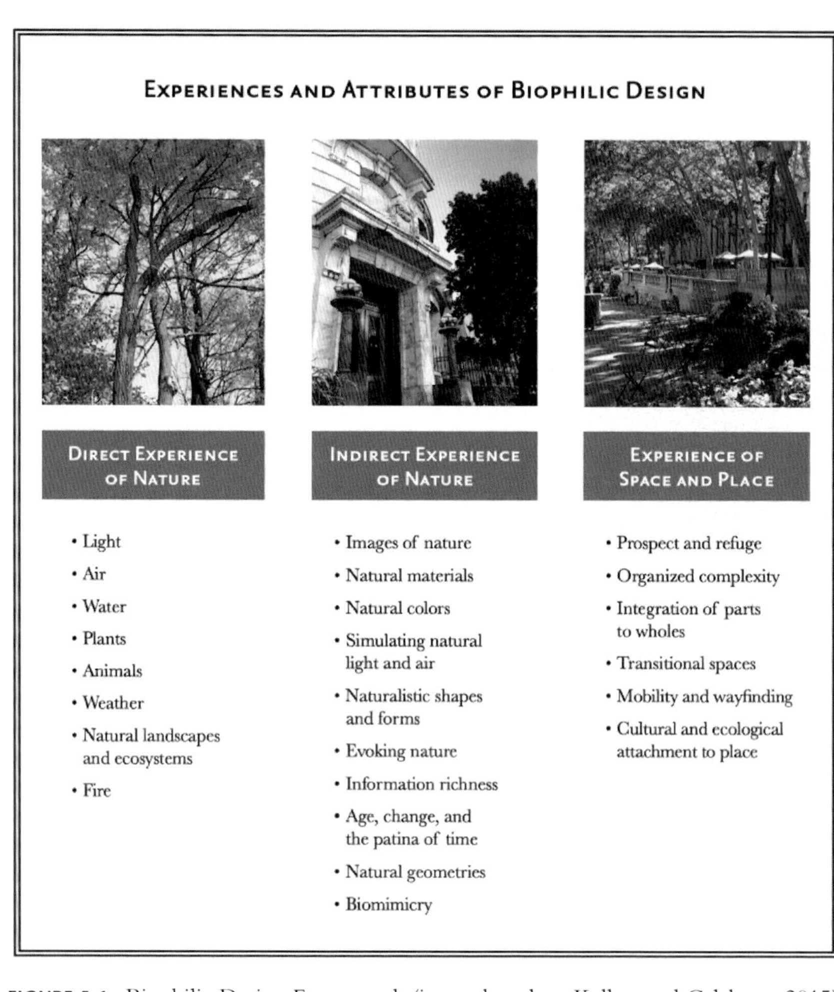

FIGURE 5.6 Biophilic Design Framework (image based on Kellert and Calabrese 2015)

environment and connecting to natural landscapes and the local ecosystem. Buildings and spaces that have abundant natural daylight, fresh air, animal and plant life possess a living and dynamic quality. Urban spaces that include indigenous vegetation and streets and walkways lined with trees and flowers provide habitats for local fauna and can be enjoyed by people directly and from within adjacent interior spaces.

Water is an element that humans seek to be in and near, both for survival and pleasure. There are numerous ways to integrate water in the built environment through fountains, rain gardens, constructed wetlands and views of water that offer a multisensory Experience. The sound of water is soothing, the feel of water on a hot day is cooling and the smell of clean running water is refreshing. Furthermore, property with shoreline frontage or water views is often considered to be more valuable than property without such Attributes (Nichols, 2014).

The San Antonio River Walk features many Attributes of the Direct Experience of Nature and is an excellent example of how blue infrastructure, in this case San Antonio's flood control and storm water system, can be incorporated as an important feature at the heart of San Antonio's downtown. The River Walk is lined

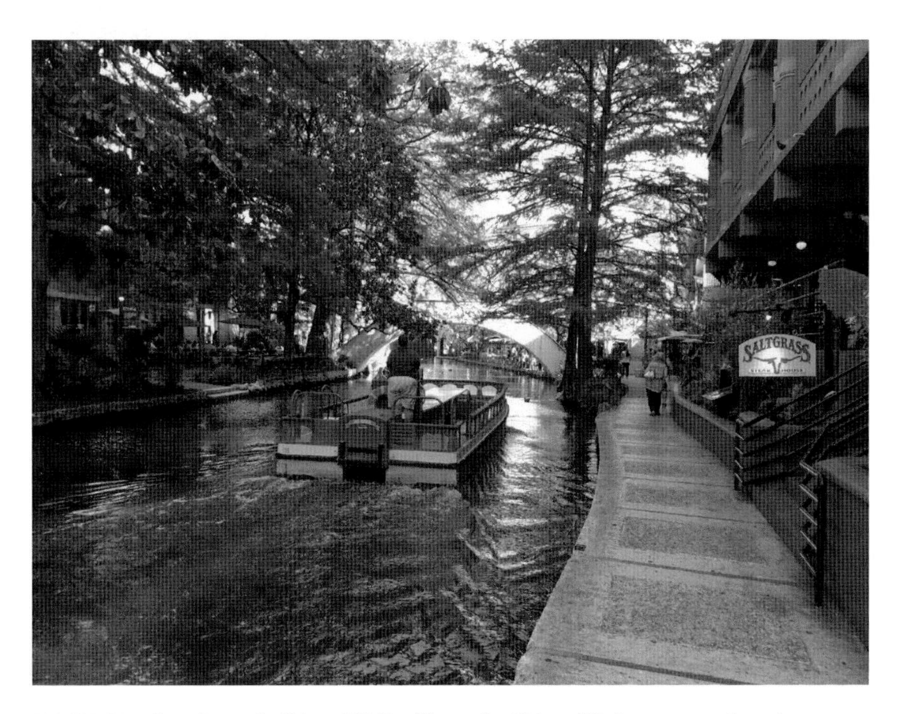

FIGURE 5.7 San Antonio River Walk. Along the River Walk water taxis and tour boats utilise the river for transportation and recreation providing additional biophilic multisensory Experiences (Calabrese)

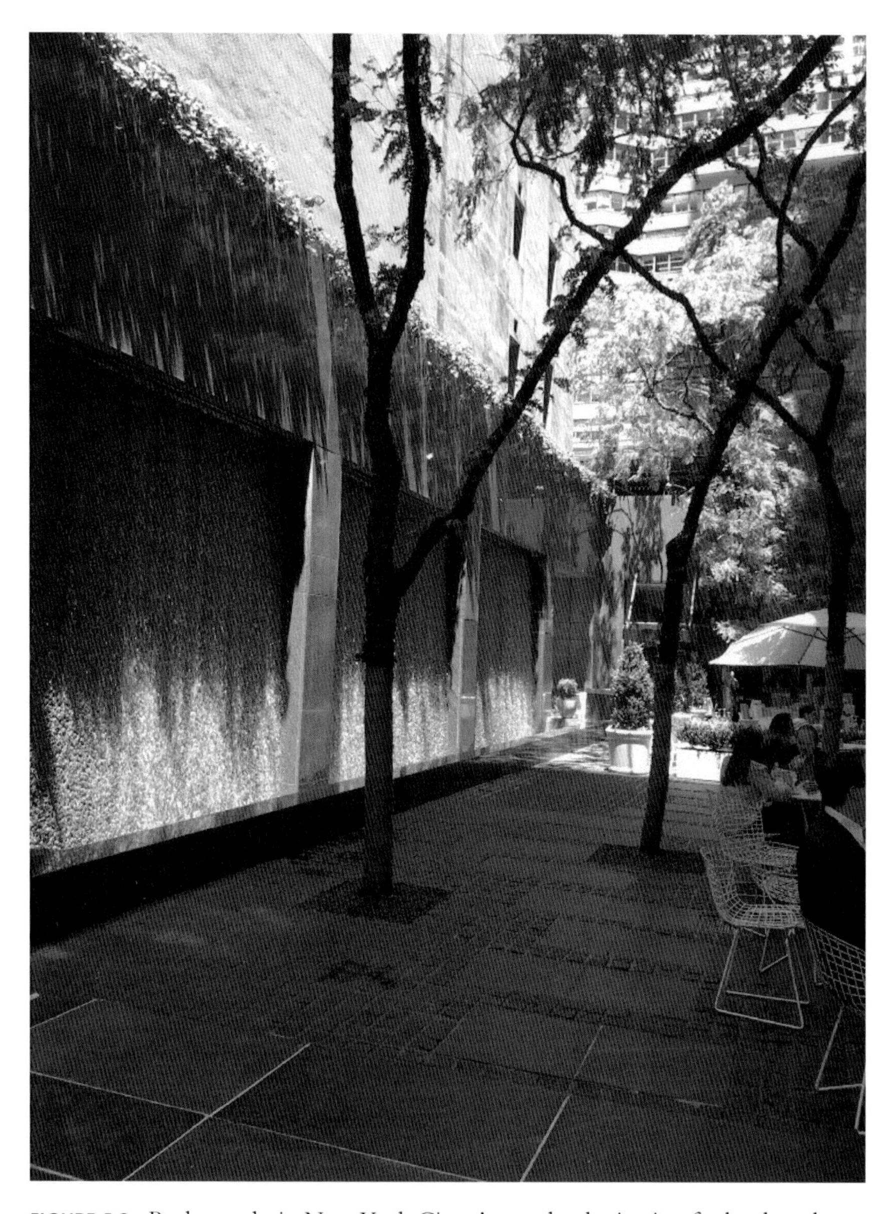

FIGURE 5.8 Pocket parks in New York City. A popular destination for locals and tourists alike. The aerated water and vegetation improve the air quality in the park while the dynamic and filtered daylight streams through the canopy of trees providing much-needed dappled shade on hot summer days (Calabrese)

with cypress trees and other assorted local vegetation, attracting visitors young and old to meander along the shaded river's edge, enjoy the views of water and nature while dining at umbrella-topped tables under vine-covered trellises or pause at the pocket parks.

The abundance of cafes, pathways, benches and nodes support pedestrian mobility and foster a sense of community. Pocket parks with natural landscapes along the River Walk provide rich habitats for animals including squirrels and a large variety of birds, insects, butterflies and bees; ducks and waterfowl dive after schools of fish swimming about. The presence of animals is indicative of a healthy environment and creating spaces that allow wildlife to thrive as part of a balanced urban ecosystem is beneficial for both people and the local ecology (Beatley, 2011, 2016).

Plants have been critical for human survival – for nutrients, medicines, building materials and protection from the elements and predators. In addition, the presence of greenspace and natural landscapes is linked to positive social behaviours. Studies in Baltimore, Portland and Philadelphia, showed that neighbourhoods with more trees and greenspace were associated with lower crime rates (Troy et al., 2012). Forest bathing originated in Japan during the 1980s as the practice of spending time under the canopy of a living forest and has become a cornerstone of preventive health care and healing with health benefits including lower blood pressure, reduced stress and elevated moods (Chun et al., 2016; Han et al., 2016).

Exposure to natural daylight is another Direct Experience of Nature and is fundamental to human health and well-being. The colour spectrum, intensity, angles and timing of sunlight change throughout the day depending on the weather and seasons. Dynamic sunlight is especially engaging, such as filtered light dancing below a tree canopy, streams of light and shadows moving throughout the day, and the ever-changing colours of light varying from sunrise to sunset. These changes help orient us in time and place and dictate our circadian rhythms which influence our sleep patterns and our moods (Howarth, 1984). Natural daylight is also required for our bodies to naturally make vitamin D and regulate hormones (Cama, 2009).

Before modern meteorological forecasting, humans relied on their innate intuition and observation of the weather, seasons and behaviour patterns of plants and animals in order to predict and prepare for inclement weather. Although our survival no longer relies on such keen observations, many people continue to celebrate the changing of the seasons, hunt for familiar shapes in cloud formations or pause to watch a dramatic sunrise or sunset. It is during these times that we feel connected to something greater than ourselves and to each other (McHarg, 1995).

Many buildings open to the natural environment through doors, windows, skylights and light wells. The low E coatings often used on window glazing for energy efficiency can change the colour spectrum of daylight; therefore, both the quality and quantity of natural daylight should be considered in the design process. In addition, many structures built over the past several decades with modern air handling systems have increasingly eliminated operable windows preventing occupants from having control over the regulation of the temperature, natural air flow and daylight. While these strategies may have been initiated for energy efficiency, adapted solutions can be created to meet human needs and energy concerns (Browning et al., 2012; ILFI, 2018; IWBS, 2018).

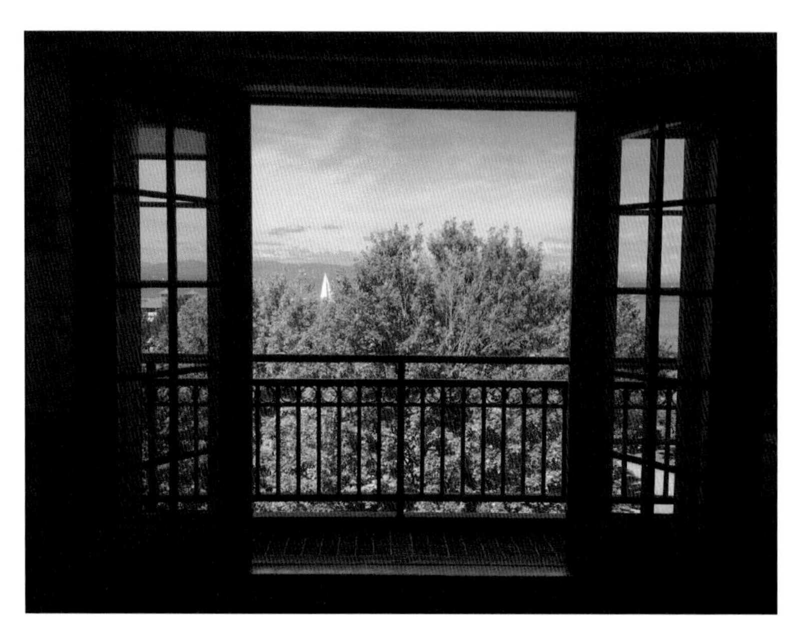

FIGURE 5.9 This conference room offers direct access and views of plants, animals and birds, water, weather, sunlight and air. We are empowered by the ability to regulate the amount of daylight and flow of natural air around us (Calabrese)

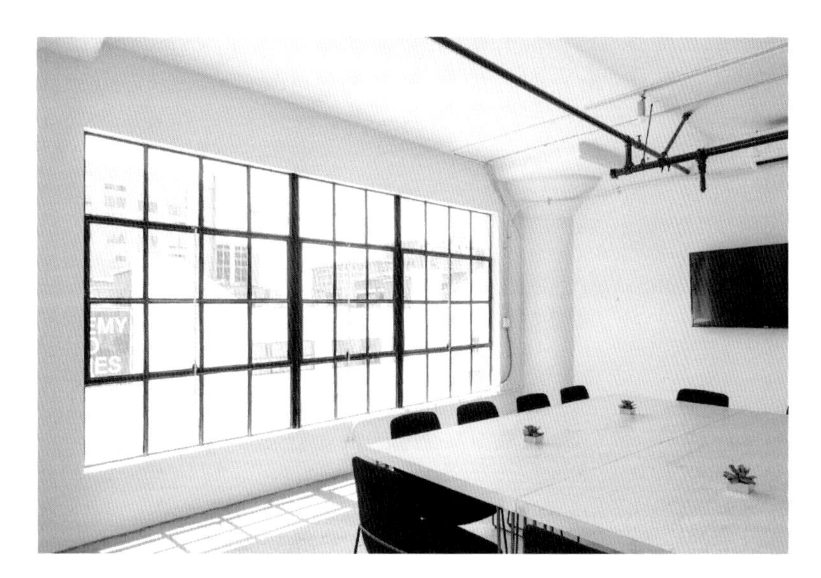

FIGURE 5.10 Employees are happier and healthier when they have access to high quality natural daylight, minimal glare and the ability to control the temperature and airflow of their workspace (Browning et al., 2012; ILBC, 2018; IWBS, 2018) (via UNSPLASH)

Fire is another important biophilic Attribute of the Direct Experience of Nature and has long been associated with rituals, folklore, gathering, nourishment, wayfinding and protection at night (Harari, 2015). We have warmed ourselves physically and emotionally by a fire and hearth. Studies show sitting by a fire induces evolutionary responses of safety and community causing our blood pressure to drop and leaves us feeling more at ease and social (Dana Lynn, 2014).

The element of fire was added to the Providence, Rhode Island waterfront in 1994 with an installation of bonfires, by artist Barnaby Evans, to the riverfront in what continues today as WaterFire Providence. There are now almost one hundred sparkling bonfires along the path of Waterplace Park engaging the senses and emotions of over 10 million visitors – the scent of wood smoke, the flickering firelight on the arched bridges and the torch-lit vessels on the water. This festival has revitalised the urban experience, fostered community engagement and has become the crown jewel of the downtown Providence renaissance.

Our relationship with nature is complex and – like fire – can be comforting or devastating depending on the intensity and circumstance. The spirit of Biophilic Design is intended to embrace the positive aspects of the Direct Experience of Nature while respecting our aversions to what may frighten or hurts us with the hope that in reconnecting us to nature, we may fear it less and love it more.

The Indirect Experience of Nature

The Indirect Experience of Nature celebrates nature through images, natural materials, colours, shapes, forms and geometries that represent nature and natural systems and processes. Grand Central Terminal, a much-beloved structure in New York City, is a classic example of the effective incorporation of an Indirect Experience Of Nature (Figure 5.12). The main concourse responds like a clearing in a forest of trees opening up to the sky above with a cerulean blue 125-foot high barrel vault ceiling. It is adorned with an expansive zodiac mural painted in gold leaf punctuated by LED lighting that mimics the intensity of the corresponding stars. Information-richness is achieved with these Attributes in addition to the use of stone and ironwork in naturalistic shapes and forms.

Images of nature and their representation were evident in the oldest known cave paintings. Over millennia, paintings and sculptures of nature have been discovered in ancient temples, chapels and burial chambers. Greek and Roman column capitals were carved with shell and plant motifs. Textiles over the ages have been adorned with natural patterns and colours. Images of nature are emotionally and intellectually satisfying and continue to be represented further in photographs, murals and video as design elements in the modern built environment (Figure 5.13)

Historically buildings were made from local natural materials. Organic matter like wood, stone, iron, clay, rammed earth, lime, animal hides, plant matter, grasses, wool, silk, cotton, hemp and melted sand all became the materials of the built environment in adaptive response to the stresses and challenges of human

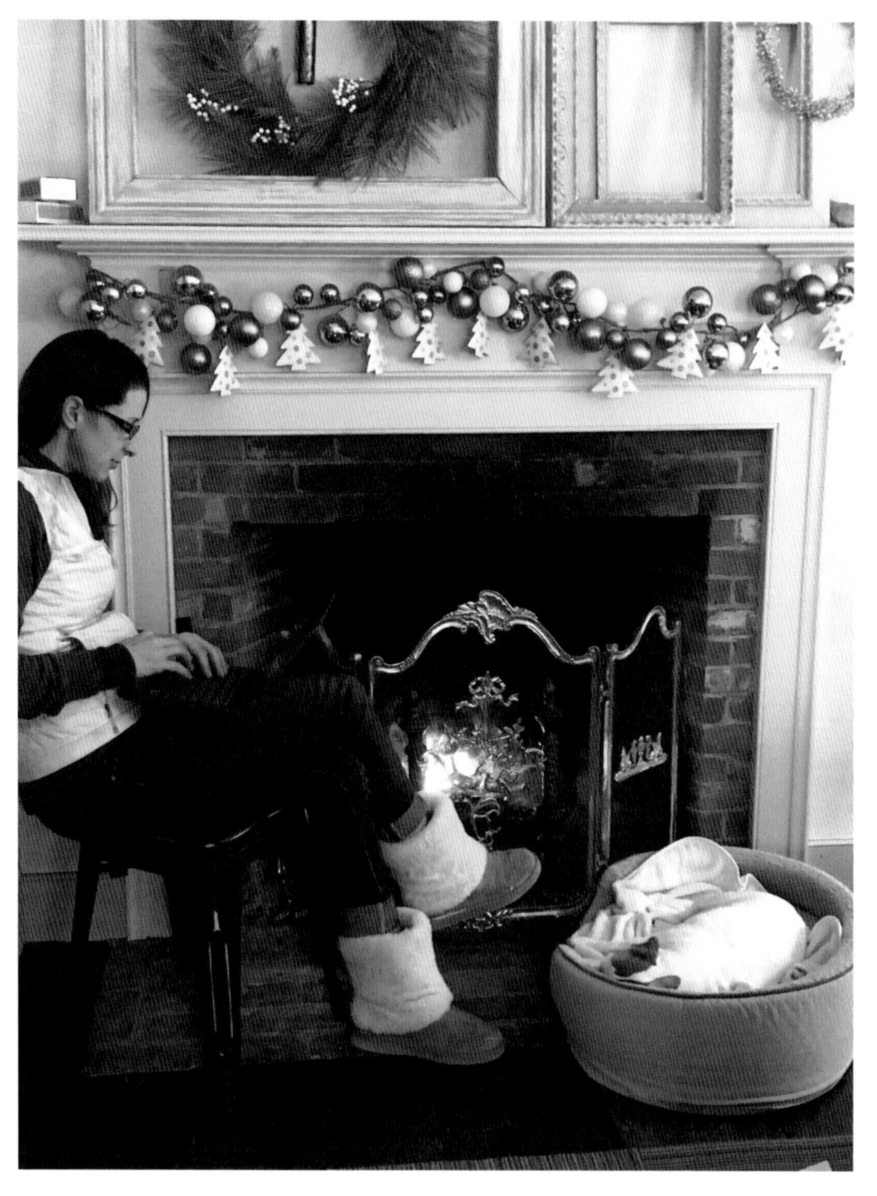

FIGURE 5.11 Fireplaces, wood stoves, campfires, kitchens and hearths are often special gathering spots and we associate a warm glowing light bulb with firelight, warmth and a sense of welcome (courtesy Lisa Rourke)

survival over time. These natural materials both are pleasing to the eye and to the touch in a way that artificial materials lack.

Our preference for natural materials has continued to evolve with high-end homes, resorts and buildings including wood trim and cabinetry, heavy wood

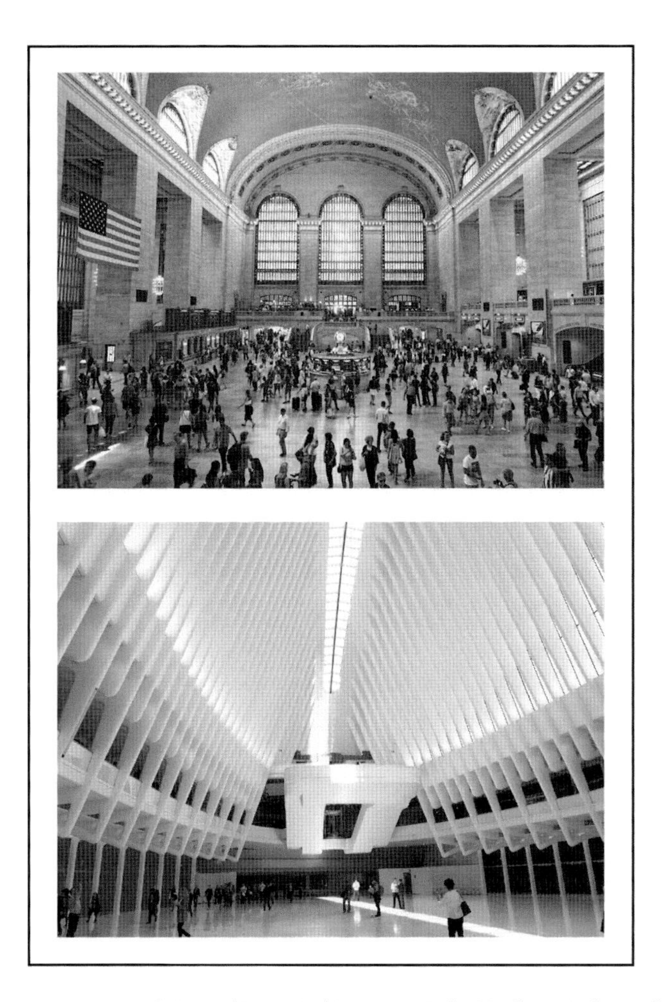

FIGURE 5.12 Top – Grand Central Terminal in New York City botanical motifs are carved into the natural stone cornices and archways that reach like branches and foliage beyond the massive trunk-like pillars. Natural daylight filters in through the high arched windows further supporting an implied tree canopy (Rob Bye via UNSPLASH). Bottom – Santiago Calatrava's Transit Hub in New York City is quite sculptural and organic in form, yet contrasts with the shear "aliveness" Grand Central Terminal embodies. Sculptural and organic designs do not necessarily follow Biophilic Principles (Calabrese)

timbers, fine metals, smooth and textured plaster, natural textiles and fabrics, and stone floors, terraces and countertops.

Throughout our evolution as hunter-gatherers, natural colour has played a vital role providing information that aided our survival as a species (Humphrey, 1976). Using colour we were able to locate ripe and safe fruit, berries and nuts, and interpret the impending weather based on the colour of the sky, water and landscape.

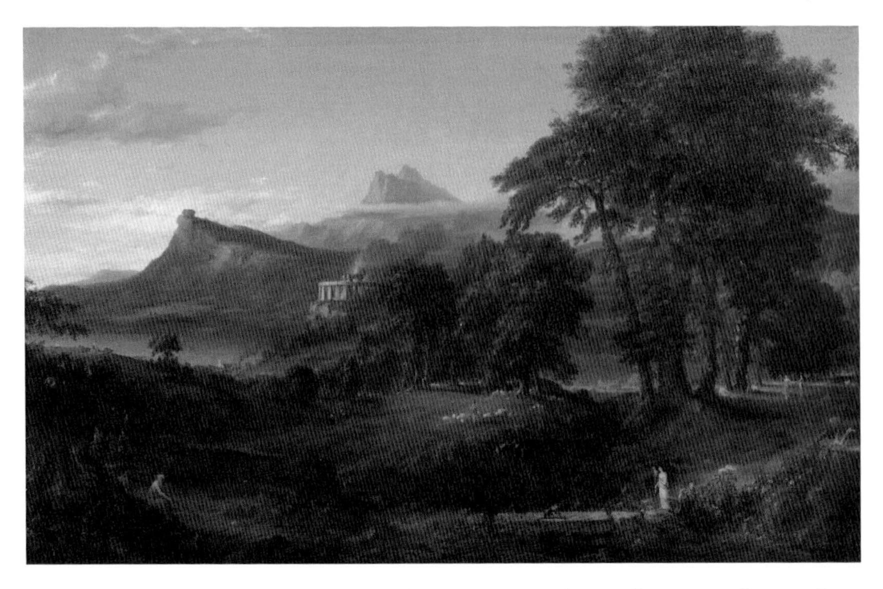

FIGURE 5.13 Many of our most revered paintings are of natural scenes and research shows that we have a universal affinity for landscape scenes that have rolling green fields, trees with a canopy, low arched branching patterns, water in the distance and a path. Such images are believed to intuitively connect us to the African savannah, our original home as a species (Balling & Falk, 1982) (Public domain)

Research shows our colour preferences have to do with an effective response to environmental objects and situations associated with each colour. Natural colours like blue, become associated with a clear sky and clean water and elicit positive reactions (Palmer & Schloss, 2010).

Simulated natural light and air are necessary within modern buildings. This advancement in technology and construction has helped achieve higher levels of energy efficiency. However, these advancements have also fostered some environments with extreme static conditions that can be physically and psychologically detrimental to occupants. The quality and quantities of simulated light and air are crucial to how we feel in a space (IWBI, 2015).

The colour spectrum of artificial light can range from cool to warm light, mimicking sunlight from various times of the day and firelight. Warm coloured light is associated with the evening sun or firelight and is often used in bedrooms, living rooms, studies, cafes and more formal restaurants. Cool coloured light is bluer on the spectrum, associated with rigorous activities, and is often used in kitchens, bathrooms, workshops, gymnasiums, hospitals and fast food restaurants. LED lights allow for many colour variations and can mimic a more natural circadian lighting. Hospital patients and staff, including premature infants in neonatal units, are benefiting from the introduction of circadian lighting, as are passengers travelling on airplanes traversing multiple time zones (Küller & Lindsten, 1992).

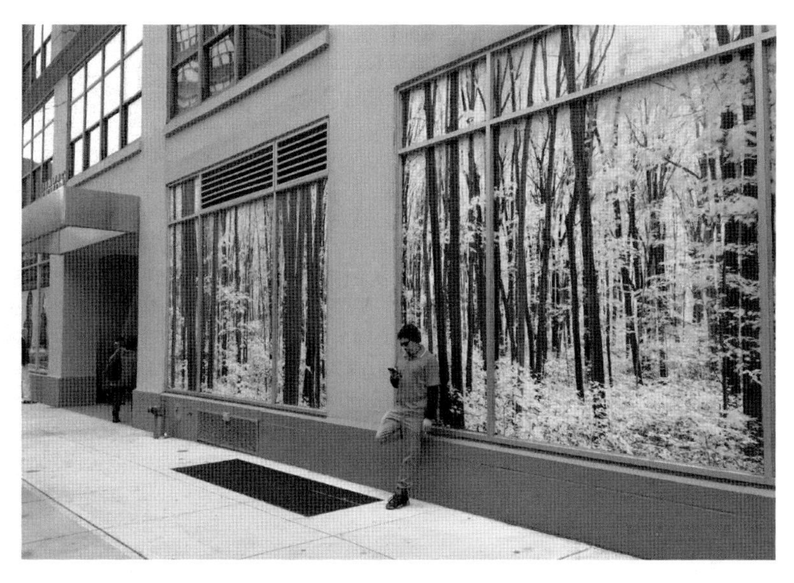

FIGURE 5.14 Images of nature can be brought into unlikely environments such as this urban setting. Subterranean and windowless spaces can also benefit from natural images (Calabrese)

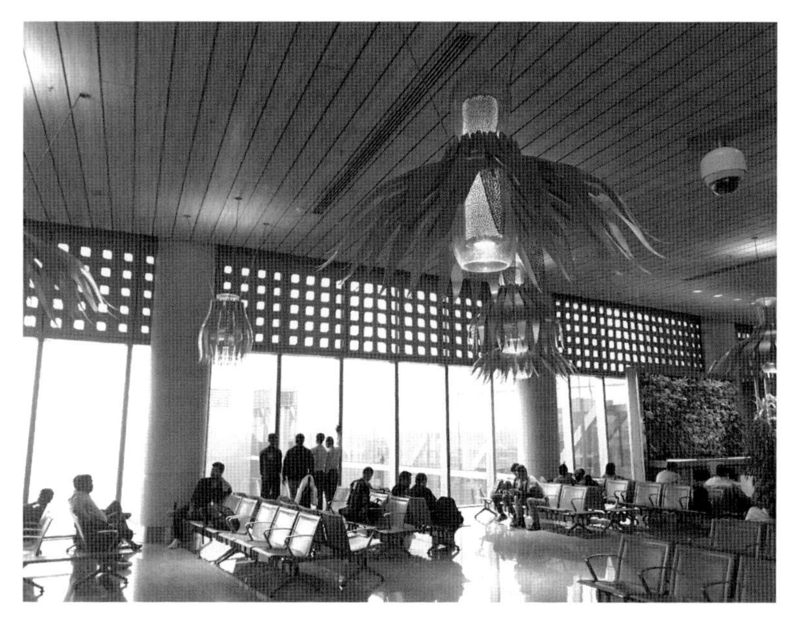

FIGURE 5.15 The ambiance of the Mumbai Airport is culturally rich and connected to place. The ceilings are a warm coloured wood, patterns of light and shadows filter through leaf shaped openings above the glazing, and light fixtures offer a golden glow with the suggestion of blossoming flowers (Calabrese)

Many ancient and historic structures possess natural shapes and forms that respond to or were influenced by the natural processes we can easily detect such as erosion and growth—the sinuous meandering curves created by rivers and land formations and the organic and biological shapes of plants and animals. Evoking nature, another indirect experience is an imaginative and fantastical expression inspired by nature and is evident in art, sculpture and many beloved buildings. The Sydney Opera House in Australia, a designated World Heritage site, is one of the twentieth century's most distinctive structures with stacked opera shells resembling sails. Not only does this masterful structure evoke nature, it integrates natural systems and processes holistically by utilising a seawater cooling system, LED lights that maintain a warm glow, and comprehensive waste and water efficiency programs.

The natural world, with its diversity and variety, has been described as the most information-rich environment people will ever encounter. While it is complex, it

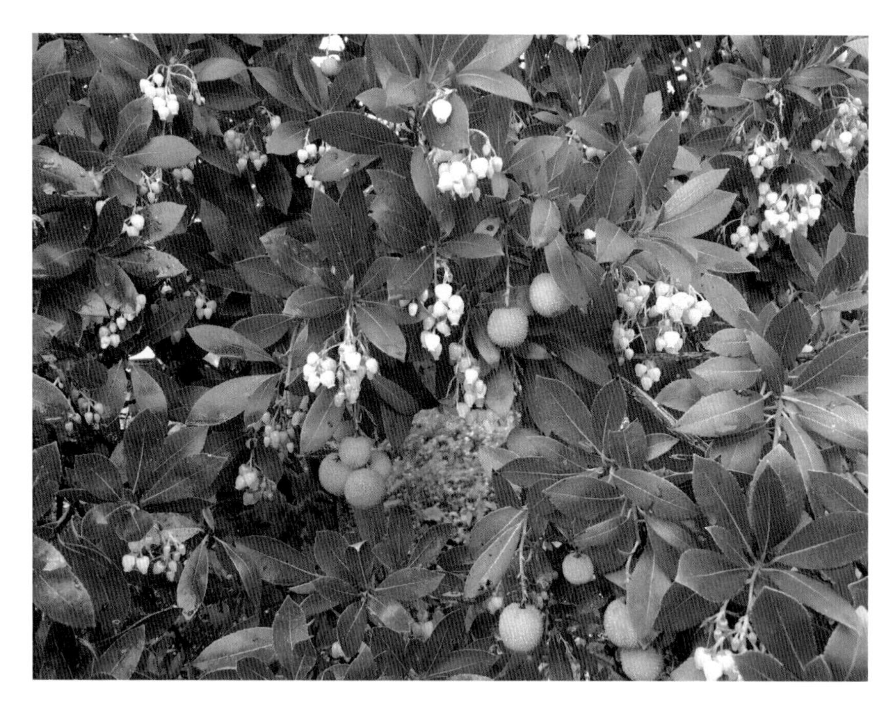

FIGURE 5.16 We are swayed by an evolutionary bias as well as a situational response to colour, in the absence of colour this feedback regarding the appeal of the brightly coloured fruits is absent. Colours of ripe fruit make it easier to locate from a distance and inform of its ripeness. Research has shown that women prefer redder colours while men prefer blue-green colours which supports an evolutionary/behaviourally adaptive hypothesis based on our hunting and gathering past (Hurlbert & Ling, 2007) (Calabrese)

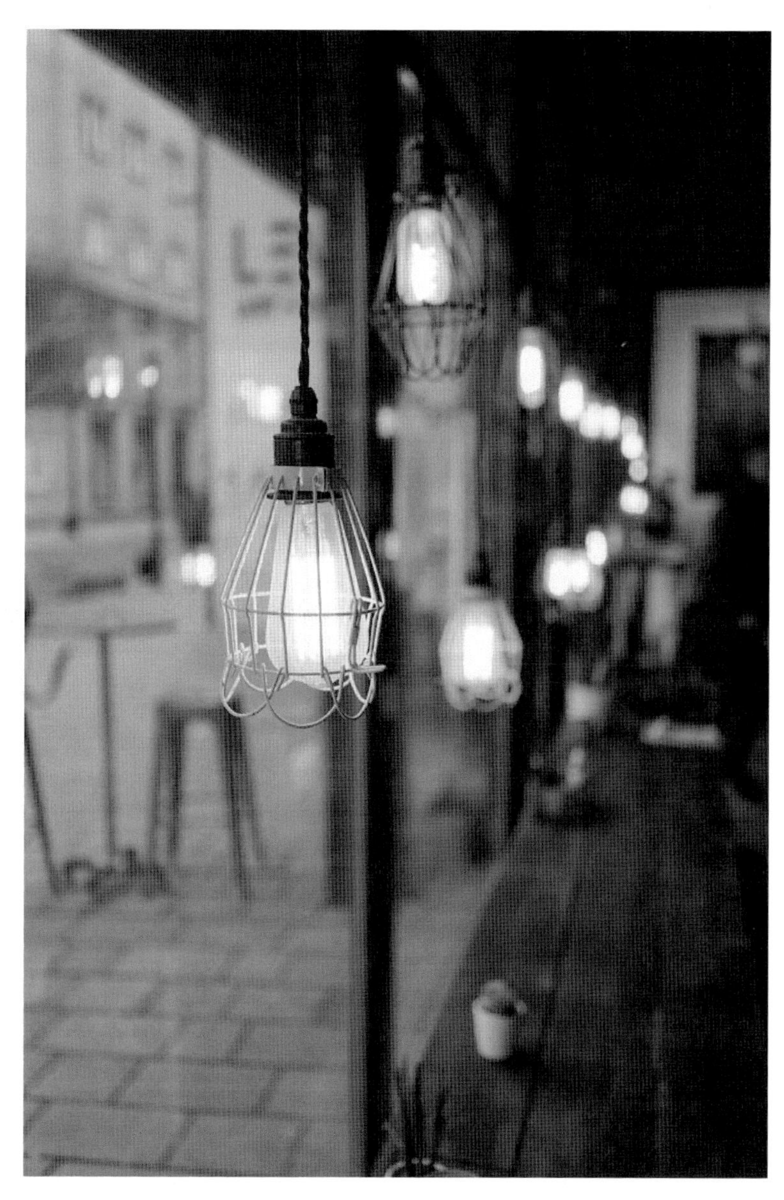

FIGURE 5.17 Lighting in a space should consider how the fixtures may or may not work in combination with some natural daylight. In a restaurant, the lighting may be used at one level during the day and a different quantity and setting for the evenings. The colour rendition of the bulbs is important and can have a positive or negative impact on the resulting ambiance (Tomas Jasovsky via UNSPLASH)

also functions as a brilliant and meticulous working system, with each piece a synergistic part of the working whole. Natural geometries, like fractals, are mathematical repetitions that repeat with an ordered variety. The Golden Ratio and Fibonacci Sequence are other systems based on natural geometries. Humans respond positively to information-richness in the built environment that is created in a coherent way of natural geometries. It engages the innate skills that were used by early humans to survive and represents a wealth of options and opportunities

Buildings and materials, like humans, change over time. Nature is in constant flux – some elements in growth and expansion while others fade. The age, change and the patina of time Attribute encourages the use of natural materials that endure gracefully over time and exude a sense of "aliveness". We tend to gravitate to the older places that embrace the elegance of bygone time – like Stonehenge, the Greek ruins and Roman aqueducts, and meandering cobblestoned streets in medieval cities. Time is also reflected in the darkening of wood and cut stone, the green patina of copper spires and lustre of bronze statues, and moss growing on stone walls, facades and roofs.

The last Indirect Experience of Nature, biomimicry, occurs when nature is used to inspire, inform and solve contemporary problems (Benyus, 1997). Velcro,

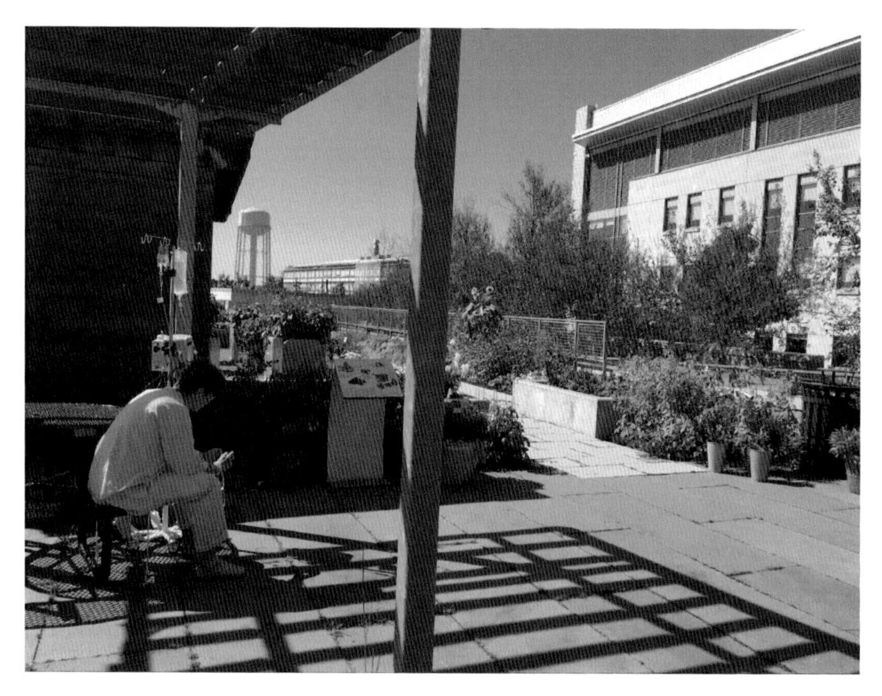

FIGURE 5.18 Hospital rooftop gardens are part of a greater human constructed ecomimetic system with multiple benefits that include providing outdoor park-like space for patients and staff, fostering biodiversity of plant and animal life while reducing the heat island effect associated with traditional impervious roofs (Dommert)

invented in 1941, is an example of biomimicry. George De Mestral, a Swiss Electrical Engineer, observed Burdock seed clinging to his coat and his dog after a walk in the woods and then engineered the Velcro system from his observations. Lofted winter coats and dual pane glazing are other examples of biomimicry since both rely on the insulating qualities of air-space achieved in down feathers and animal fur. Eco-mimicry is biomimicry at a larger ecosystem scale, where each component supports the others in a holistic, synergistic and symbiotic way. A closed loop rainwater catchment system on a roof structure is an eco-mimetic system solution. Water is captured on a green roof, used to hydrate wildflowers and other plants that attract birds and insects while increasing the roof's insulation value and reducing the heat island effect created by an otherwise bare black membrane roof.

Experience of Space and Place

Experience of Space and Place addresses the quality, proportions and order of both natural and built environments. Historically, the ecology, climate, geology and geography of a specific area has had a significant impact on the culture of a region and its unique sense of place. Most human constructs were made of local materials by local craftspeople. These connections provided a strong authenticity of place and promoted a sense of belonging to a greater whole.

Over the years due to the globalization of goods, services, building materials, architectural styles and mass media, our cultural and ecological attachment to place has diminished. However, many of the most celebrated cities, towns and buildings have attempted to retain a strong sense of place. The historic French Quarter in New Orleans is a good example of a rich Experience of Space and Place. The vernacular architecture has a patina of time and responds well to the climate, ecology and culture of New Orleans, attracting tourists from all over the world.

Many of the building facades in the French Quarter are constructed of terracotta coloured brickwork with decorative nature-inspired wrought ironwork supporting wraparound balconies. Prospect and refuge spaces offer a sense of protection while allowing for a vantage point overlooking a view or activity (Hildebrand, 1991; Appleton, 1996). Transitional spaces such as balconies, porches, colonnades, terraces and roof gardens feel safe and relaxing because they often provide prospect and refuge while connecting the indoors to the outdoors, and bridge one level of social interaction to another. Other examples of transitional space are cafes, pubs and restaurants with walls that can open to the exterior and patrons can enjoy both the protection being inside while also being connected to the streetscape and outdoors.

Humans enjoy visual patterns and textures, pleasant sounds and smell when they are part of a dynamic and complex system. Nature can seem chaotic on the surface, yet the universal laws of nature provide order as demonstrated in the many examples of organised complexity that nature provides (Alexander et al., 1977;

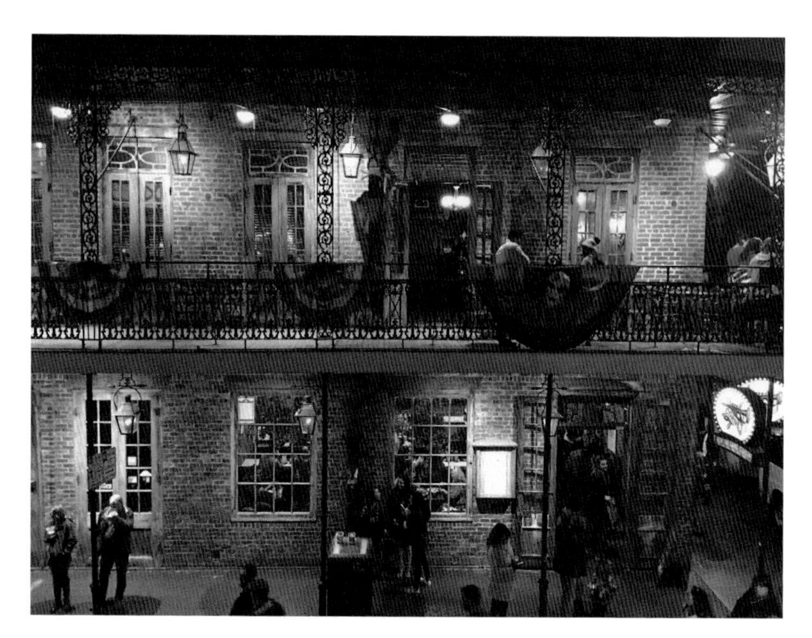

FIGURE 5.19 Balconies offer prospect and refuge and a connection to the weather and community. The brick facade, cypress doors and windows are of a human scale and the copper roof sheds the rain and provides much-needed shade. The lights have a warm flickering glow, while native ferns hang in baskets (Calabrese)

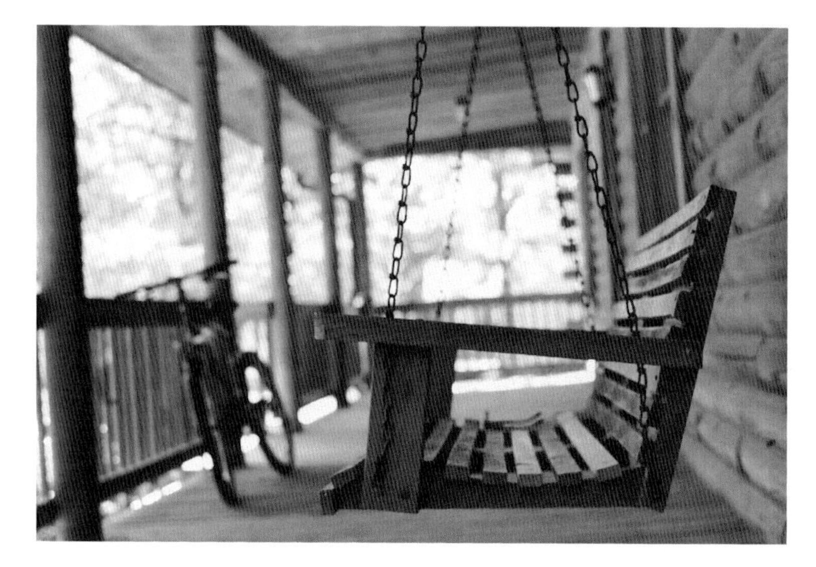

FIGURE 5.20 This porch is an example of a prospect and refuge located in a transition space as it offers visual and social connectivity beyond the more private spaces of the house. Porches have historically been a place to socialise (James Garcia via UNSPLASH)

Browning et al., 2014; Salingaros, 2015). Pebbles washing up onto a beach can appear to be random, though they are in part a result of the mass of the pebble and the velocity of the wave. The same may be said for Manarola (Figure 5.21), a seaside town of stacked vibrant coloured structures along the cliffs of northern Italy. Dating back to 1338, the town has grown somewhat organically over hundreds of years responding to its geography, ecology, local resources, sea and climate. Manarola displays the essence of organised complexity and embodies the balance and harmony achieved between random chaos and static mechanical order.

We have innate needs for privacy and solitude and the need to feel safe and secure with others in small groups and as we gather as part of a larger community. Integration of parts to whole addresses the spatial connectivity and boundaries we crave as biological and social creatures. Offices are an example of a changing trend. In the past, the model was for executives' offices to be located on the perimeter of the building, enjoying the abundant natural light and views, while administrative and support staff worked at cubicles in the centre of the

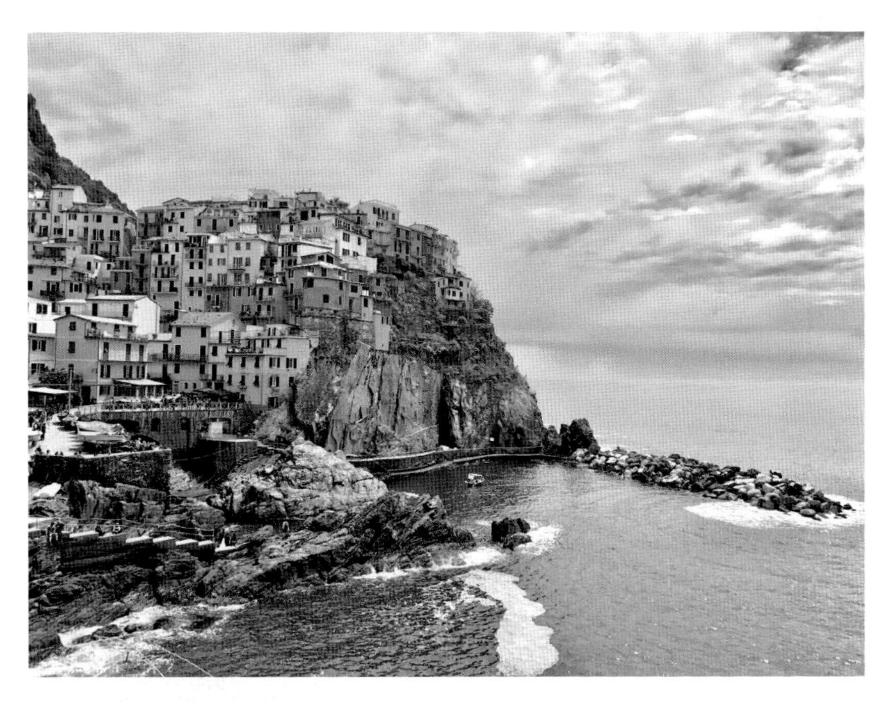

FIGURE 5.21 The seaside town of Manarola in northern Italy dates back to 1338 and is a favourite among tourists. At first glance the town may seem chaotic, however, there is an overarching order in which the buildings interact and respond to the geography, ecology, local resources, sea and climate. Such places resonate with us as pleasing and familiar – steeped in the organised complexity of natural systems and processes (Carlos Santiago via UNSPLASH)

building. More recently office spaces have adopted open floor plans that allow natural light to penetrate to the core of the office. Finding a balance of the integration of parts to the whole, such as private territory and common space, is an important aspect of designing environments that support individuals and the entire community alike.

As hunter-gatherers, one of the most fundamental survival skills was the ability to travel and navigate – mobility and wayfinding. Without the navigation tools of today, humans had to use all of their senses to be keenly attuned to their surroundings by mentally mapping the landscape features or tracking the direction of the sun and stars. Over time and with advances in technology-based navigation tools, humans have become less connected with nature and our sensory attunement has atrophied. Our sense of orientation, grounding and connection to place has suffered and is reflected in the increase of stress due to the sense of feeling lost, disconnected and disoriented.

Within the natural environment, mountains and other geological features provide reference points that offer a sense of physical and emotional orientation. Church steeples or a central town plaza are examples of focal points for social orientation within a community. In hospitals where visitors and patients may already

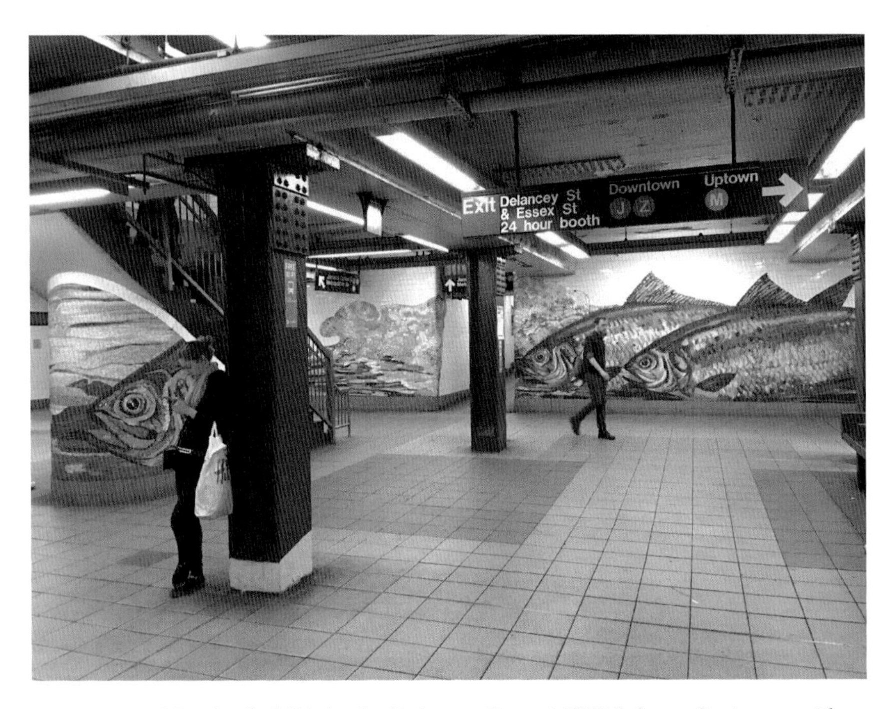

FIGURE 5.22 Mosaic tiled fish in the Delancey Street NYC Subway Station provide effective and playful wayfinding. The images of nature and use of vibrant natural colours create a strong sense of place. Many locals are enthusiastic about "their" subway stop. Mosaic and tile artwork is proliferating throughout the NYC subway system (Calabrese)

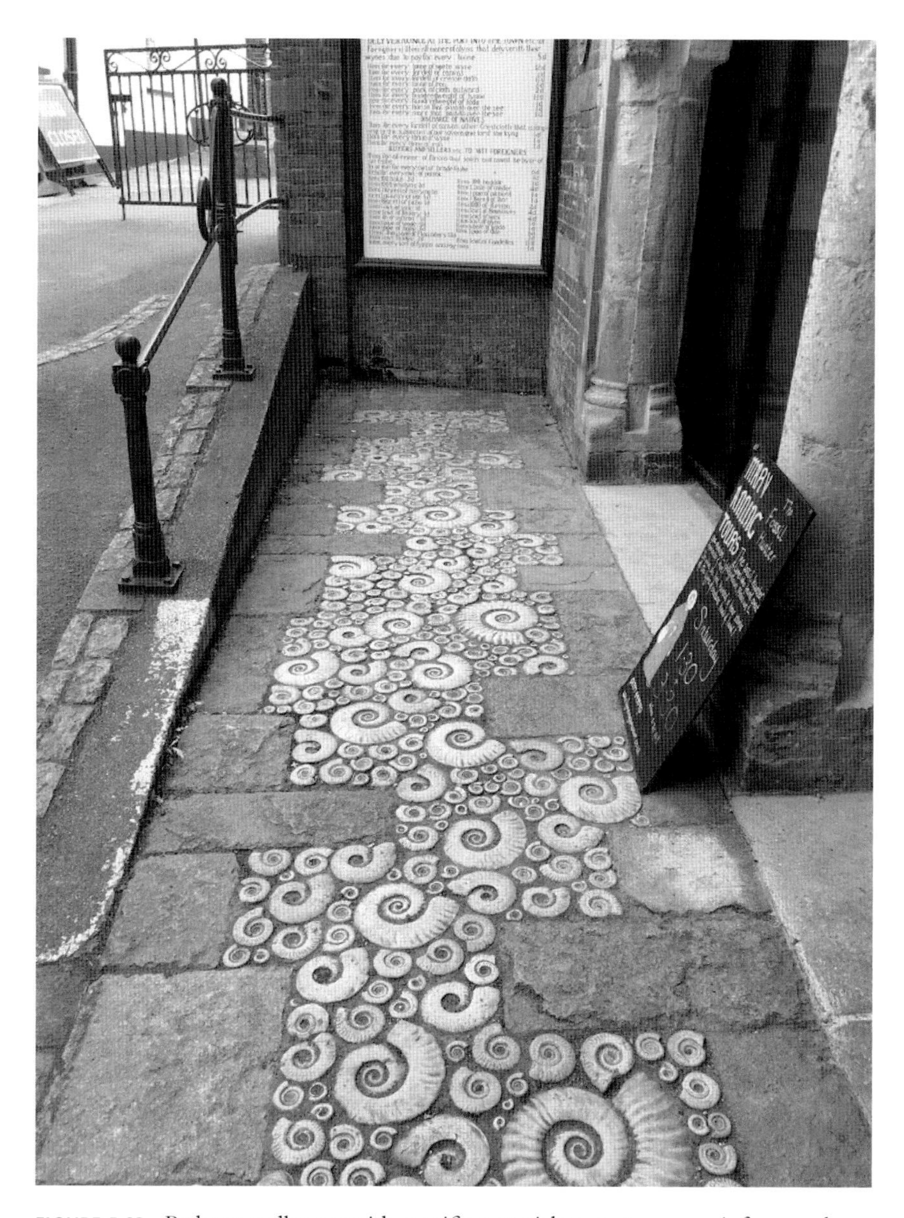

FIGURE 5.23 Paths or walkways with specific materials or patterns can inform and help provide wayfinding like this entryway where people meet for fossil walks outside of the Lyme Regis Museum, UK. The images of nature, natural materials and textures provide information-richness and cultural and ecological connection to place (Calabrese)

be overwhelmed, different wings or floors can be themed to help provide orientation and an ease of wayfinding. Themes can include natural colours, images and textures that incorporate the soothing and comforting Direct and Indirect Experiences of Nature.

Towards a Biophilic Design ecology

Our biocentric evolution has influenced how we perceive and respond to the places and spaces around us, both natural and built environments whether they are relaxing or stressful, lush or sparse. Although each individual responds differently to situations based on their experiences, preferences and culture, underlying evolutionary bonds to nature remain. Upon seeing the world through a biophilic lens, the complexity and interconnectedness of our health and well-being with our physical environment become more obvious. We have unintentionally designed stress, obesity, aggression, hostility, disease, fear and environmental degradation into our lives. Quoting the late Dr Stephen Kellert, "We designed ourselves into this predicament and we can design ourselves out of it with the help of biophilic design" (Kellert & Finnegan, 2011).

Biophilic Design can have a positive impact on urban planning, new construction and the renovation of existing buildings. The Biophilic Principles, Experiences and Attributes offer a Framework for designers to employ their own

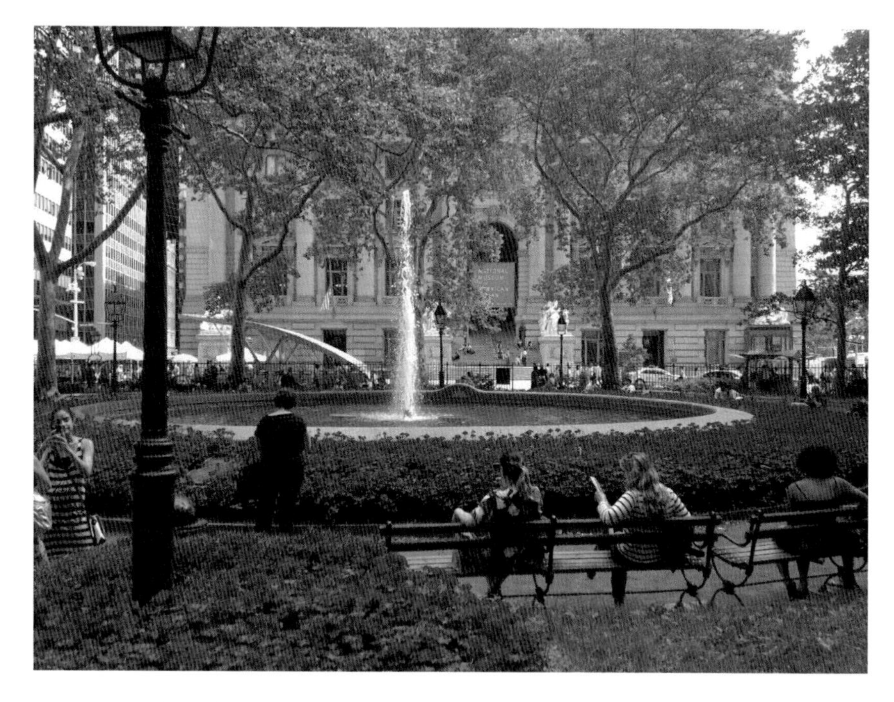

FIGURE 5.24 Bowling Green Park in New York City brings together all three Biophilic Design Experiences and Attributes, a Direct Experience of Nature as people relax among the water, trees, flowers and sunshine and Indirect Experience of Nature with the curved benches, circular fountain and the natural stone and detailing of the facade across the park. When used holistically, the Experiences and Attributes create a powerful Experience of Space and Place (Calabrese)

innate wisdom and expertise to create unique design solutions that can range from simple to complex. When nature and natural systems and processes are consciously integrated into the design process there is the potential for profound impacts – a built environment where we feel connected and safe, healthy and whole.

References

Alexander, C. (1979) *The Timeless Way of Building*, New York: Oxford University Press.

Alexander, C., Ishikawa, S., Silverstein, M., Jacobson, M., Fiksdahl-King, I. & Angel, S. (1977) *A Pattern Language*, New York: Oxford University Press.

Annerstedt, M. & Währborg, P. (2011) Nature-assisted therapy: systematic review of controlled and observational studies, *Scandinavian Journal of Public Health* 39 (4): 371–388.

Appleton, J. (1996) *The Experience of Landscape*, Chichester: Wiley.

Balling, J. D. & Falk, J. H. (1982) Development of visual preference for natural environments, *Environment and Behavior* 14: 5–28.

Beatley, T. (2011) *Biophilic Cities*, Washington, DC: Island Press.

Beatley, T. (2016) *Handbook of Biophilic City Planning and Design*, Washington, DC: Island Press.

Benyus, J. (2002) *Biomimicry*, New York: Perennial.

Bowler, D. E., Buyung-Ali, L. M., Knight, T. M. & Pulin, A. S. (2010) A systematic review of evidence for the added benefits to health of exposures to natural environments, *BMC Public Health* 10: 456.

Browning, W. D., Ryan, C. & Clancy, J. (2014) *Patterns of Biophilic Design, Improving Health & Well-Being in the Built Environment*, New York: Terrapin Bright Green.

Browning, W. D., Ryan, C., Kallianpurkar, N., Laburto, L., Watson, S. & Knop, T. (2012) *The Economics of Biophilia, Why Designing with Nature in Mind Makes Financial Sense*, New York: Terrapin Bright Green.

Cama, R. (2009) *Evidence-Based Healthcare Design*, Hoboken, NJ: John Wiley.

Chun, M., Chang, M. & Lee, S. (2016) The effects of forest therapy on depression and anxiety in patients with chronic stroke, *International Journal of Neuroscience* 127 (3): 199–203.

Dana Lynn, C. (2014) Hearth and campfire influences on arterial blood pressure: defraying the costs of the social brain through fireside relaxation, *Evolutionary Psychology* 12 (5): 983–1003.

Dubos, R. (1980) *The Wooing of Earth*, New York: Charles Scribner's Sons.

Fitwel.org (2018) https://fitwel.org/, last accessed 17 February 2018.

Frumkin, H. (2001) Beyond toxicity: human health and the natural environment, *American Journal of Preventive Medicine* 20 (3): 234–240.

Frumkin, H. (2008) Nature contact and human health: building the evidence base, in S. R. Kellert, J. Heerwagen, & M. Mador (eds.), *Biophilic Design: The Theory, Science, and Practice of Bringing Buildings to Life*, Hoboken, NJ: John Wiley.

Frumkin, H., Bratman, G. N., Breslow, S. J., Cochran, B., Kahn, P. H., Lawler, J. J., Levin, P. S., Tandon, P. S., Varanasi, U. & Wolf, K. L. (2017) Nature contact and human health: a research agenda, *Environ Health Perspect.* 125 (7). Available at doi: 10.1289/EHP1663.

Han, J., Choi, H., Jeon, Y., Yoon, C., Woo, J. & Kim, W. (2016) The effects of forest therapy on coping with chronic widespread pain: physiological and psychological differences between participants in a forest therapy program and a control group, *International Journal of Environmental Research and Public Health* 13 (12): 255.

Harari, Y. N. (2015) *Sapiens: A Brief History of Humankind*, New York: HarperCollins.

Heerwagen, J. H. & Orians, G. H. (1986) Adaptations to windowlessness, *Environment and Behavior* 18 (5): 623–639.

Heerwagen, J. H. & Orians, G. H. (1993) Human's, habitats and aesthetics, in S. R. Kellert & E. O. Wilson (eds.), *The Biophilia Hypothesis*, Washington, DC: Island Press, Shearwater Books.

HermanMiller.com (2018) Nature-based design. Available at www.hermanmiller.com/research/categories/white-papers/nature-based-design-the-new-green/, last accessed 17 February 2018.

Hildebrand, G. (1991) *The Wright Space*, Seattle: University of Washington Press.

Howarth, E. & Hoffman, M. (1984) A multidimensional approach to the relationship between mood and weather, *British Journal of Psychology* 75 (1): 15–23.

Human Spaces (2018) The global impact of Biophilic Design in the workplace. Available at http://humanspaces.com/global-report/the-global-impact-of-biophilic-design-in-the-workplace/, last accessed 17 February 2018.

Humphrey, N. (1976) The colour currency of nature, in T. Porter & B. Mikellides (eds.), *Colour for Architecture*, London: Studio-Vista, pp.95–98.

Hurlbert, A. & Ling, Y. (2007) Biological components of sex differences in color preference, *Current Biology* 17 (16): R623–R625.

International Living Future Institute (2018) https://living-future.org/lbc/, last accessed 17 February 2018.

International WELL Building Institute (2018) www.wellcertified.com/, last accessed 17 February 2018.

Kaplan, S. & Kaplan, R. (1983) *Cognition and Environment: Functioning in an Uncertain World*, Ann Arbor, MI: Ulrich's Books.

Kellert, S. (1997) *Kinship to Mastery: Biophilia in Human Evolution and Development*, Washington, DC: Island Press.

Kellert, S. (2005) *Building for Life: Understanding and Designing the Human-Nature Connection*, Washington, DC: Island Press.

Kellert, S. (2012) *Birthright: People and Nature in the Modern World*, New Haven, CT: Yale University Press.

Kellert, S. & Wilson, E. O. (1993) (eds.) *The Biophilia Hypothesis*, Washington, DC: Island Press.

Kellert, S. & Heerwagen, J. (2007) Nature and healing: the science, theory, and promise of biophilic design, in R. Guenther & G. Vittori (eds.), *Sustainable Healthcare Architecture*, Hoboken, NJ: John Wiley.

Kellert, S. & Calabrese, E. (2015) The practice of biophilic design. Available at www.biophilic-design.com.

Kellert, S. & Finnegan, B. (2011) *Biophilic Design: The Architecture of Life* (a 60 minute video). Available at www.bullfrogfilms.com.

Kellert, S., Heerwagen, J. & Mador, M. (2008) (eds.) *Biophilic Design: The Theory, Science, and Practice of Bringing Buildings to Life*, Hoboken, NJ: John Wiley.

Küller, R. & Lindsten, C. (1992) Health and behavior of children in classrooms with and without windows, *Journal of Environmental Psychology* 12 (4): 305–317.

Kuo, F. (2010) *Parks and Other Green Environments: Essential Components of a Health Human Habitat*, Washington, DC: National Recreation and Parks Association.

Louv, R. (2005) *Last Child in the Woods*, Chapel Hill, NC: Algonquin Books of Chapel Hill.

Louv, R. (2012) *The Nature Principle: Reconnecting with Life in a Virtual Age*, Chapel Hill, NC: Algonquin Press.

Marcus, C. M. & Sachs, N. A. (2014) *Therapeutic Landscapes: An Evidence-based Approach to Designing Healing Gardens and Restorative Outdoor Spaces*, Hoboken, NJ: John Wiley.

McHarg, I. (1995) *Design with Nature*, New York: John Wiley.

Nichols, W. (2015) *Blue Mind*, New York: Back Bay Books, Little Brown.

Öhman, A. (1986), Face the beast and fear the face: animal and social fears as prototypes for evolutionary analyses of emotion, *Psychophysiology* 23 (2): 123–145.

Palmer, S. & Schloss, K. (2010) An ecological valence theory of human color preference, *Proceedings of the National Academy of Sciences* 107 (19): 8877–8882.

Salingaros, N. A. (2015) *Biophilia and Healing Environments: Healthy Principles for Designing the Built World*, New York: Terrapin Bright Green, LLC.

Shepley, M. M. & Pasha, S. (2017) *Design for Mental and Behavioral Health*, New York: Routledge.

Taylor, A., Kuo, F. & Sullivan, W. (2001) Coping with ADD, *Environment and Behavior* 33 (1): 54–77.

Todd, N. J. & Todd, J. (1993) *From Eco-Cities to Living Machines: Principles of Ecological Design*, Berkeley, CA: North Atlantic Books.

Townsend M. & Weerasuriya R. (2010) *Beyond Blue to Green: The Benefits of Contact with Nature for Mental Health and Well-Being*, Melbourne: Beyond Blue Limited. Available at www.Beyondblue.org.au.

Troy, A., Morgan Grove, J. & O'Neil-Dunne, J. (2012) The relationship between tree canopy and crime rates across an urban – rural gradient in the greater Baltimore region, *Landscape and Urban Planning* 106 (3): 262–270.

Ulrich, R. (1984) View through a window may influence recovery from surgery, *Science* 224 (4647): 420–421. PubMed PMID: 6143402.

Ulrich, R. (1993) Biophilia, biophobia, and natural landscapes, in Kellert, S. R. & Wilson, E. O. (eds), *The Biophilia Hypothesis*, Washington, DC: Island Press, Shearwater Books.

Ulrich, R. (2008) Biophilic theory and research for healthcare design, in S. R. Kellert J. Heerwagen & M. Mador (eds.), *Biophilic Design: The Theory, Science, and Practice of Bringing Buildings to Life*, Hoboken, NJ: John Wiley.

Wells, N. & Rollings, K. (2012) The natural environment: influences on human health and function, in Clayton, S. (ed.), *The Oxford Handbook of Environmental and Conservation Psychology*, London: Oxford University Press.

Wilson, E. O. (1984) *Biophilia: The Human Bond with Other Species*, Cambridge, MA: Harvard University Press.

6

"ON EMPATHY" AND WELL-BEING IN DESIGN EDUCATION

Amrit Phull

Introduction

An awakening global effort towards more conscious and ethical human behaviour has encouraged a change in the realm of design. Practices of engaging publics in their built environment are increasing in number, innovation, and inclusivity, from grassroots urbanist leagues to artistic public interventions, from YIMBY boards to Little Free Libraries. Citizens are looking carefully at their surroundings in the interest of collective betterment, an indication that publics truly see and believe in their ability to intervene in the established processes and bureaucratic structures that shape our cities. This presents challenges of incorporating ethics and accountability, alongside other professional remits in addressing the education of professionals involved in the design of built environments. Fostering educational experiences within positive collective spaces for learning will facilitate conversations surrounding both the impact and wider context of professional action. These are processes with which the architect can find space for reflection in her or his internal worlds.

Accordingly, this chapter explores the idea of movement towards an "Empathic Design response", which has a natural synergy with well-being. The ideas considered advance an alternative framework for learning within architectural education. Discussion concerns "On Empathy", a student-driven initiative at the University of Waterloo, School of Architecture, Canada. This chapter focuses on the collaborative structure of On Empathy and lessons gleaned from its inclusive, informal blend of discussions and workshops which were initiated following changes in the academic curriculum and the resulting disparate opinions and practices within the school environment. Outcomes are discussed in relation to the sensitive reflection of architectural work sustained by the initiative and the resulting relationships fostered between the University, its local community, and between peers within the programme.

Re-centring of architectural education

On Empathy is a student-led ethics initiative at the University of Waterloo which specifically responds to the wider debate regarding professional responsibilities and is set within a consciousness regarding the re-centring of architectural education through initiatives that engender an empathic response and lead to a heightened awareness. As a demonstration project, this initiative has sought to continually carve out space within the finely-tuned, rigorous, academic structure of the school for reflective conversation on the educational climate of architecture and the impacts of experiences gleaned within it (Phull 2014a).

Historically, architects were commissioned by the privileged few who could afford to build. While access to an education and profession in architecture is still greatly impaired by gender, racial, and economic biases, the sense today is that architects are as much designers of as participants in the built environment. In his brief for the 2016 Venice Biennale of Architecture, "Reporting from the front", Architect, Festival Director and Pritzker Prize Laureate, Alejandro Aravena asked participating designers to carefully reflect on the impacts of their ideas and curate thoughtful spatial responses for the public festival. The design brief used words like "need, awareness, opportunity", and "choice" to describe the act of creating architecture (Biennale Architettura, 2016). Aravena sought to challenge the privileged voices that shape our shared environments, instead giving space to social issues and topics less represented in the field. Forming the entrance to the Biennale was his personal response: a series of installations incorporating waste material from the 2014 Festival. In a literal sense, this design framed the event with the less visible impacts of architectural work in order to bring ideas of accountability, sustainability, and consequence to the immediate foreground.

Today, architects confront spatialized problems beyond the building envelope, tackling issues of ecologies, social conditions and scales. With the arrival of the Anthropocene has come a global shift of attention towards environmentally conscientious, human-centred design choices in response to the failed practices of utopian modernism (Steffen et al., 2011). There is increasing motivation in the contemporary practice of design to ensure that spaces are sensitive and adaptable, ones in which those who are oppressed due to issues of gender, sexuality, ethnicity, culture, religion and so forth, can occupy without fear. In short, contemporary crises are fuelling a broad investigation of inherited practices in architecture and urban design.

In an open, collaborative, student-led lab at the University of Waterloo School of Architecture, students from diverse backgrounds and outlooks come together to explore the matters that incite their spirits, where, at their best, schools like this can encourage students to approach design in an open-hearted way, because fear and deep learning rarely, if ever, coexist.

On Empathy

On Empathy is an ongoing, participatory series of discussions and presentations founded in the midst of a transitioning architectural curriculum in 2013 at the

University of Waterloo School of Architecture. With a change in faculty, structure, and class content, the school found itself representing a disparate array of philosophies and approaches to architecture segregated by course code. In response to the lack of collective discussion between the range of academic methodologies operating within the school, the group aimed to facilitate a more sensitive understanding and encourage a more open flow of ideas. The group took particular inspiration from the writings of Richard Shaull and Paulo Freire, who argued for a freedom of programming within education:

> There is no such thing as a neutral education process. Education either functions as an instrument which is used to facilitate the integration of generations into the logic of the present system and bring about conformity to it, or it becomes the "practice of freedom", the means by which men and women deal critically with reality and discover how to participate in the transformation of their world.
>
> *(Shaull, 1970, p.34)*

Supporting one another through their graduate thesis work, Fernie Lai, Currim Suteria, Connor O'Grady and Amrit Phull sought to create a "practice of freedom" accessible to all participants in the school and its immediate community. In their respective research practices, which collectively represented the diversity of design approaches and aesthetics at play within the school, they noticed a common thread of empathy and a shared interest in place-making and place-makers. At the foundation of their work, beyond representational aesthetics and mapping methods, was the simple intention to learn how people carried out their lives.

Within the collaborative event series, students, faculty, local community members and invited guests share and discuss personal viewpoints on ethics and accountability within the practice of architecture. On Empathy acts as a non-physical agora within the school where the diversity of perspectives can be safely expressed and explored within a respectful and open-hearted community. In line with Shaull and Freire's call for criticality and freedom, the act of sharing experiences beyond the confines of fear and apprehension fosters creative freedom and innovation: two principles that are often at the core of all educational institutions.

The question posed to the University of Waterloo School of Architecture community was unadorned: How does an architect do good work? Beyond beautiful, but good? In the intensity of studio courses and deadlines that typify the experience of architectural education, students are often exploring an impressive range of design approaches and methodologies. However, this seemingly obvious question about how to negotiate between these approaches, especially how they perform in the practice of architecture versus the education of architecture, is rarely given space for collective discussion within schools. The success of On Empathy is simply rooted in giving time and space to this simple reflection.

Orientations and Conversations

On Empathy sessions take two forms: *Orientations* and *Conversations*. An *Orientation* is a presentation facilitated by one or a few participants, often of works-in-progress rather than completed products (be they buildings, designs, or theories), and are distinct from typical lectures. Janna Levitt of LGA Architectural Partners in Toronto departed from the usual presentation of her firm's work in the interest of sharing a personal account of her home environment and its evolution over time. Architect Lola Sheppard described what she would do differently, given the opportunity to revisit the work of her acclaimed practice Lateral Office. Joanne Yau, a fourth year student at Waterloo, spent the winter season working with architect Uno Tomaki and presented stories on morning conversations with her mentor, photographs of details and construction sites, and insights into working with a craftsman (Figure 6.1). By virtue of its grounding in the fundamental question of ethics, On Empathy is a safe, supportive and enlightening space in the school – not without criticality. However, it naturally fosters a tone distinct from the traditional critique, PechaKucha or academic presentation and encourages participants to learn about each other as humans, first and foremost.

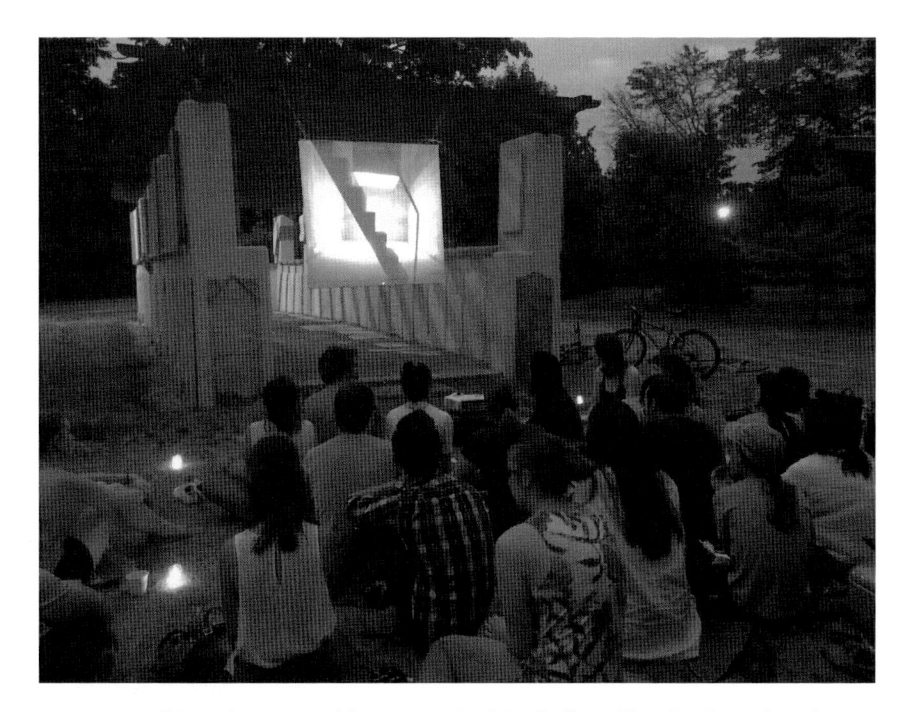

FIGURE 6.1 Discussions on architecture and ethics facilitated by On Empathy take place in key public spaces within the community. Fourth year students give a talk about craftsmanship

Where *Orientations* are intended as opportunities to listen, *Conversations* are opportunities to reflect. They are intended to be a site for co-mentorship, foundational learning and the collective mining of ethical and social issues. From these sessions, students at the University established a series of guidelines to inform the growth of the architect.

Why empathy

On Empathy was established in order to promote a more accessible forum within the school for the learning, teaching and execution of design. The intention is to let this forum be guided by the experiences unique to each participant, experiences that often take place beyond the walls of the school. In his book, *The Empathic Civilization*, Jeremy Rifkin explains, "When we empathize with another being, there is an unconscious understanding that their very existence, like our own, is a fragile affair, which is made possible by the continuous flow of energy through their being." In this vein, On Empathy creates opportunities for human connection that may not occur otherwise.

Rifkin describes empathy as "the mental process by which one person enters into another's being and comes to know how they feel and think" (Rifkin, 2009, p.39). He writes that "[u]nlike sympathy, which is more passive, empathy conjures up active engagement" (Rifkin, 2009, p.12).

The On Empathy sessions are a proven safe space, where students that otherwise might not share their personal outlooks and experiences have found a place to openly develop their spirit in conjunction with their peers and access this innate place of that Rifkin considers common to all (Figure 6.2).

At a fundamental level, architects form the places where people carry out their lives. In this sense, it is an incredibly intimate art. The connections between people and their fellow humans, as well as their environments, are sacred. Describing this bond, in *The Phenomenom of Man*, Pierre Teilhard de Chardin writes, "Man is unable to see himself entirely unrelated to mankind, neither is he able to see mankind unrelated to life, nor life untreated to the universe" (Teilhard, 1959, p.34).

With global connectivity reaching a new historic peak each passing day, human interaction is no longer limited by geographical location or blood ties. As more individuals identify with other "strangers", linked together by common desires, collective awareness grows. By offering a common space, On Empathy builds relationships between participants founded upon the desire to share and express personal values. In the words of cognitive science and philosophy Professor Evan Thompson: "The individual human subject is the encultured bodily subject. In this way the knowing and feeling subject is not the brain in the head . . . but the socially and culturally situated person, the encultured human being" (Thompson, 2007, p.411).

The social bonds fortified by an open forum for discussion within the school community not only helps to unite the student body but also encourages participants to recognise the larger, collective pursuit of which they are a part.

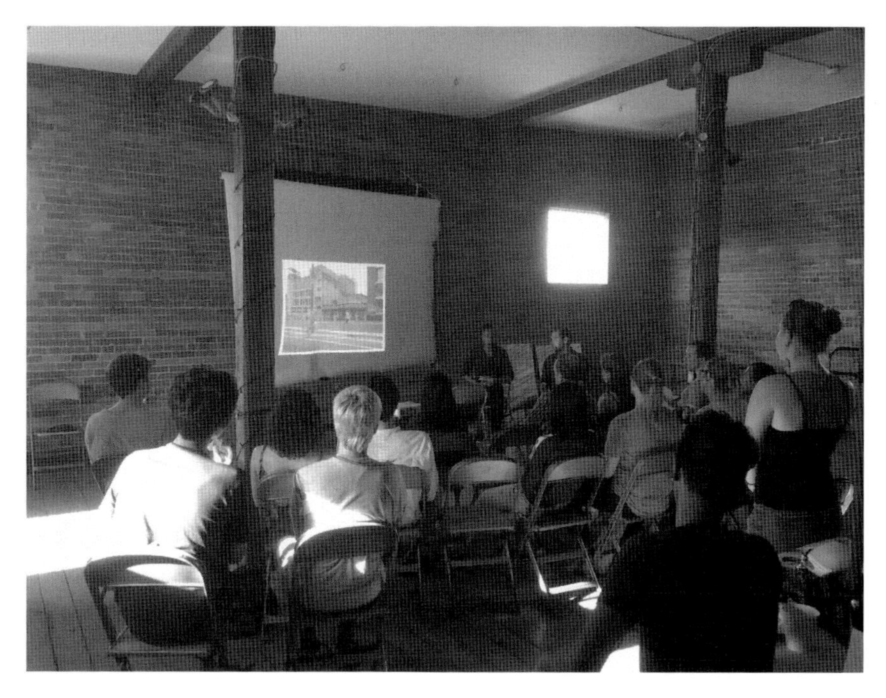

FIGURE 6.2 At the centre of all On Empathy events are shared conversations in which students collectively mine issues that inspire diverse opinions

Guiding principles

Participants of On Empathy have developed a core structure of beliefs that frame all of the organisation's events. What follows is an in-progress synopsis of these tenets, as well as examples of events that demonstrate them in action:

1. Architecture is not just for architects

The community of On Empathy extends beyond the walls of the School of Architecture, the social and academic climate of which has been historically insulated. On Empathy supports voices from outside the field, with topics of broad and inclusive concern. As a result, it performs as a conduit between the school community and the greater culture it is sited within. In 2014, Canadian writer Laura Legge encouraged participants to contemplate the design of a space of connection and amnesty in her talk "Call and response" on the Canadian criminal justice system and the role of the architect in facilitating restorative justice practices. Community members not enrolled in the school have shared their every passion, from photography to letter writing to home renovations. A designer may not always consider additional opinions or impacts beyond the research they conduct within a studio environment. However, On Empathy seeks to challenge and to complement this practice by offering an experiential transaction between the designer and those they are hypothetically designing for.

In addition to promoting connections between people, the initiative seeks to promote empathy for one's self. Continually emerging studies on the mental health of students within architecture reveal bleak statistics: "1 in 4 architecture students are suffering from mental health issues, with a further 26% stating that they would likely seek treatment and professional help in the future." The School of Architecture's resident counsellor has held several On Empathy workshops on resiliency, stress hardiness and self-care-topics that are rarely openly addressed in architecture schools. Similarly, architecture Professor Andrew Levitt, has led guided meditations on creativity without fear and group discussions on dealing with stress. Certainly, forms of support already existed at the school prior to On Empathy. However, the stigma around accessing such services inhibits students from giving proper value and attention to their well-being. On Empathy creates gentle opportunities for students to learn about issues of mental health particular to their school while reducing the stigma and conveying that well-being can and should be an open conversation.

2. Craft and care give dignity to a space and its participants

On Empathy sessions offer a space of decompression, often outside the school building, where collective reflection on work and ideas stimulated by experiences from education can safely take place. Emphasis is placed on the close relationships between design, labour and craft. Lessons on observation and local craft are mined from the philosophies of Peter Zumthor, Bijoy Jain, MASS design group and similar architects. In one such discussion, Glen Murcutt's studio course was raised as an example of learned observation within education:

> I'm teaching students how to observe. For example . . . when we were on Lightning Ridge, there were about three trees. Everybody went to the trees, to the biggest one in the area of shade . . . I asked the students, 'Why are we all standing under this tree?' What else can you observe? Nobody could say a thing. I said, "We're at the lowest point of the site. Look at it!" . . . "What about water collection? What about the water table? Why is this tree this big? . . . They realized they were learning to see!"
>
> *(Godsell, 2012, p.17)*

In this vein, On Empathy supports a mindfulness approach to design, whereby the act of gathering and meditating on a simple lesson can both nourish and activate the human imagination. Students apply these lessons to their own school experiences and once they recognise their desire to further explore alternative modes of learning, they initiate supplementary group initiatives and projects (Figure 6.3). An additional student-led initiative, "Treat lands, global stories", precipitated from On Empathy activities in the interest of creating workshops and discussions challenging the Western framework of the school, addressing the curriculum's failure to represent the diverse cultures that make up the student body, and acknowledging Canada's Indigenous heritage (Phull 2014b). One particular workshop looked closely at syllabi as a crowd-sourced, activist-generated framework rather than a standard document. Together, students looked at how dominant modes of thought and cannons of education could be unpacked, challenged, and re-designed.

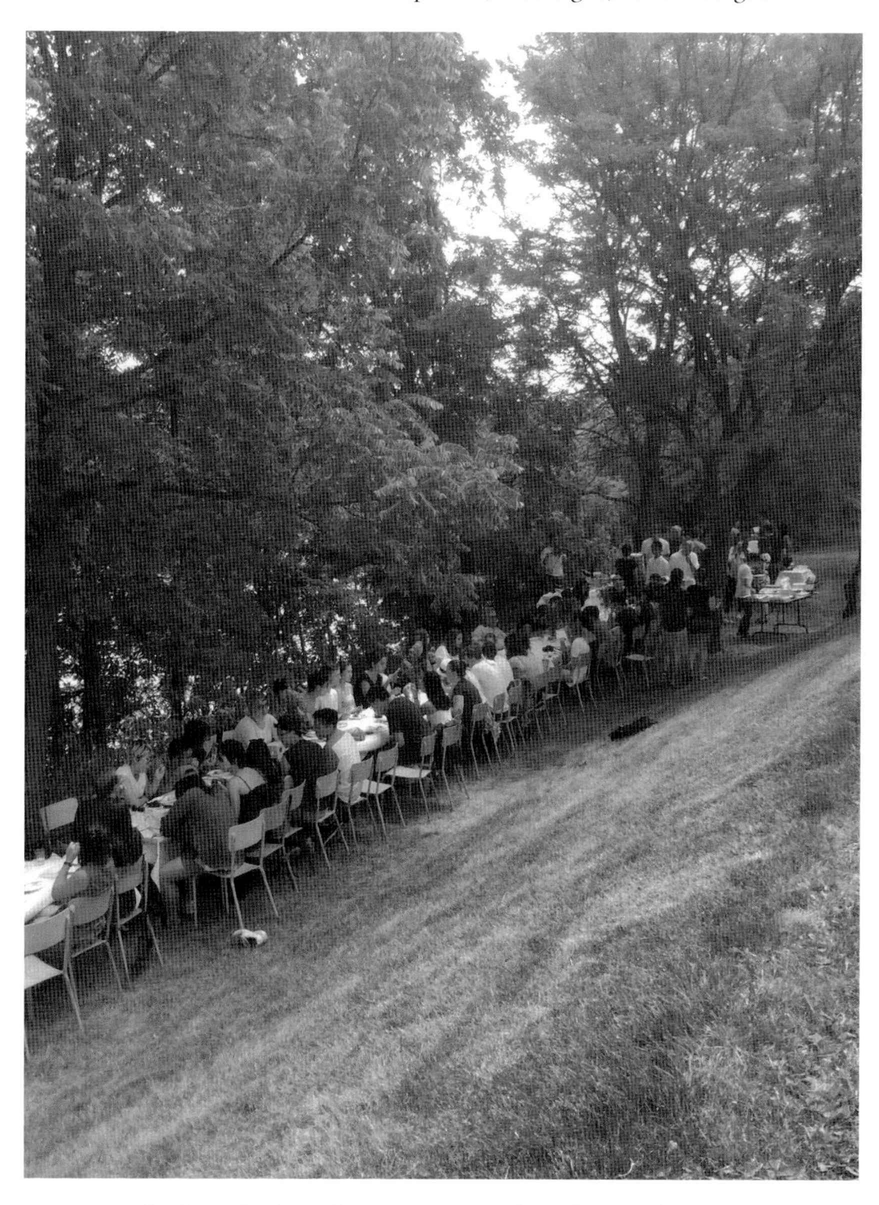

FIGURE 6.3 Students, faculty and community members dine together as part of Twelve Pavilions, a 2B student project

3. The architect is a community member

In the same way that On Empathy intends to openly include the local community within the school, members of the school community are also encouraged to mine their identity as community members. Events are sited in favourite parks and coffee shops around Cambridge, Ontario, such that the activities of the group are publicly advertised and anyone can join, regardless of their condition or creed. The School of Architecture has several additional student-run initiatives that are focused on creating public events, be they art installations, competitions, exhibitions or markets. In these forums, academic and community-oriented work coalesce (Figure 6.4).

4. Self-reflection is an essential practice

On Empathy sustains an ongoing and school-wide discussion on the ethical role of the architect where students can learn to express how they position their values within the profession and can observe their peers doing the same, events are sometimes organised after a guest lecture or symposium as a debriefing session for students to collectively reflect on the material being disseminated within the school.

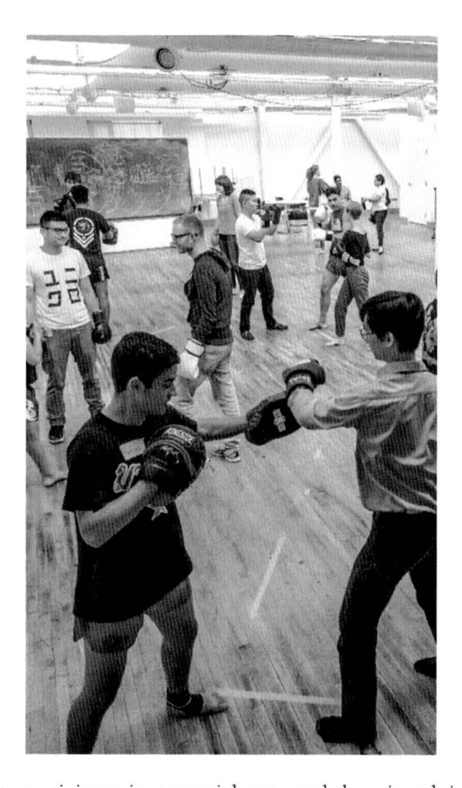

FIGURE 6.4 Students participate in a martial arts workshop involving wider "community-oriented" experience

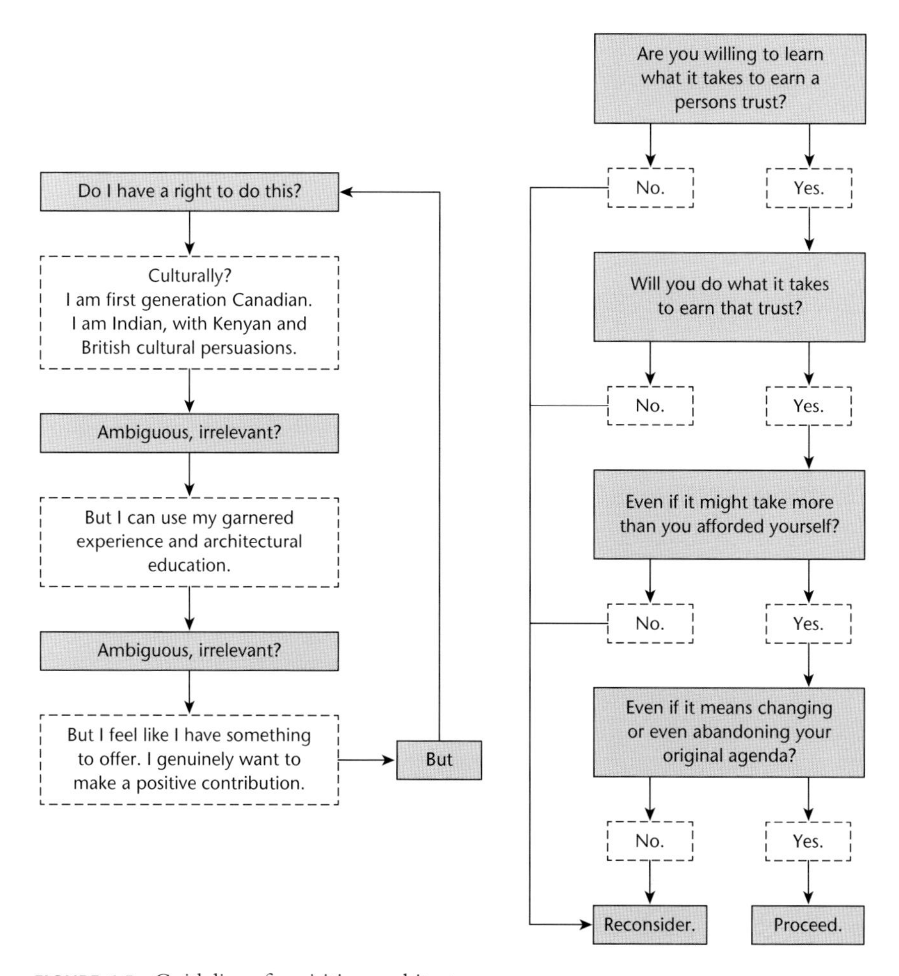

FIGURE 6.5 Guidelines for visiting architects

Lola Sheppard's discussion raised a specific conversation about the experiences gained from working in First Nations communities, particularly with Inuit groups in Northern Canada. The succeeding event involved a debate on the risks involved in assuming the role of visiting architect. Similarly, a discussion session was organised following a guest lecture by Danish firm Henning Lassen, where students queried the social, economic and environmental issues at play when building in remote places. The implications of internationally manufactured products, foreign architects and an ailing Icelandic economy were discussed in a way that a typical lecture may not facilitate. Students contemplated how an architectural project might, in its construction, stimulate local economies and empower local identities. On Empathy conversations often return to this fundamental matter of the architect's role. Events like these resulted in a proposal of guidelines for visiting architects operating within unfamiliar geographies, economies and cultures (Figure 6.5).

Conclusion

As the initiative continues at the University of Waterloo, the community mindfully stitches together a fabric of ideas and principles inspired by diverse theorists, architects, films and lived experiences. The aim continues to be to explore, with honesty and sensitivity, the question: How does an architect do good work? Although On Empathy began within a specific geography, school environment and academic, the method and approach is valuable for anyone looking to move further on their empathic journey. On Empathy is concerned with individual well-being and with the well-being of others; we honour both by reflecting on our work and actions, ultimately contributing positively to an empathic community.

The guiding principles that emerge in an alternate profession or context may differ greatly, but the approach can still enrich the well-being of those participating and facilitate development of an inclusive, empathic group. Through this "educational" method, everyone has an opportunity to lead and share, to participate and listen – it dismantles, even if only for a short while, the common "apprenticeship" model typical of North American universities.

Although, empirical results can often be difficult to place, certain gauges allow us to see beneficial outcomes from the work carried out so far. Over 75 sessions have occurred over the span of 4 years, and facilitation of the collective has passed through several students' hands. Through On Empathy, the school as a whole has strengthened its ties to the surrounding community, while empowered students reflect sensitively on their own work and on the balance they are or are not receiving in their architectural education. These actions reduce topic generalisations, break down stereotypes and allow participants to expand their comfort zones.

The simple design of the group has allowed for an open discussion of well-being at the university, and for each individual to feel as if they can have agency within creating it. These future designers of buildings, cities and landscapes will benefit from the establishment of this continual, evaluative "practice of freedom" (Shaull, 1970) which announces one important fact in the craft of place-making. We are responsible for the spaces and environments in which people carry out their lives.

Acknowledgements

Connor O'Grady, Currim Suteria, Fernie Lai, Bradley Paddock, Jaliya Fonseka, Kunaal Mohan, Kemal Alladin, Peter Bohdal, Samuel Ganton, Joanne Yau, Daniel Abad, and Jonas Chin.

References

Biennale Architettura (2016) Architecture Biennale 2016. Available at www.labiennale.org/en/architecture/exhibition/15/, last accessed 13 July 2016.

Godsell, S. (2012) A conversation with Glenn Murcutt, *El Croquis*, 163/164: 17.

Phull, A. (2014a) On Empathy – recap & coming events. Bridge Waterloo Architecture. Available at http://waterlooarchitecture.com/bridge/blog/2014/10/23/empathy-recap-upcoming-events/, last accessed 14 July 2016.

Phull, A. (2014b) Hunting for ourselves: lessons on architecture in Cree Territory, MArch thesis, University of Waterloo.

Rifkin, J. (2009) *The Empathic Civilization: The Race to Global Consciousness in a World in Crisis*, New York: J. P. Tarcher/Penguin (2009 print).

Shaull, R. (1970) Foreword, in Paulo Freire, *Pedagogy of the Oppressed*, New York: The Continuum International Publishing Group Inc., pp.29–34.

Steffen, W., Persson, Å., Deutsch, L., Zalasiewicz, J., Williams, M., Richardson, K., Crumley, C., Crutzen, P., Folke, C., Gordon, L. & Molina, M. (2011) The Anthropocene: from global change to planetary stewardship, *Ambio* 40 (7): 739–761.

Teilhard de Chardin, P. & Huxley, J. (1959) Foreword: Seeing, *The Phenomenon of Man*, New York: Harper.

Thompson, E. (2007) Empathy and enculturation, *Mind in Life: Biology, Phenomenology, and the Sciences of Mind*, Cambridge, MA/London: Belknap Press of Harvard University Press, p.411.

7

EMOTIONAL TRANSITION AND THE INTERNET WORLD

Implications for well-being

John Sparrow

Our understanding of the need for, and mechanisms of, designing our physical world in order to enhance well-being has grown considerably in recent years. This chapter aims to add to our understanding of how the non-physical, virtual or internet world can be designed to enhance well-being. Specifically, it explores the role of emotions in well-being, and how they can be influenced by our online activities.

The role of emotion in cognition and action

Much of the early research on emotion focused upon associated negative impact upon the thinking process. Emotion was seen as impeding rational thought, and hence effective decision-making. More recently, emotion has been seen to be inherent in thinking processes, and its contribution more fully considered. It has been argued that decision-making with implicit emotions is assuming greater import in a modern world with increased uncertainty. Emotion in social interaction has also been found to play a central role (Chervonsky & Hunt, 2017).

Increasingly, research is examining the impact of explicit attempts to incorporate distinct emotions in decisions and action. Sparrow (2008) demonstrated how strategic decision-making could be enhanced through engaging in different emotions in the course of strategic visioning. Sparrow (2009) demonstrated that personal reflection upon one's efforts in the course of reflective practice, could benefit from explicitly seeking information of an alternative emotional tone.

Engagement in the non-physical "internet world" also has emotion implications. The following sections will consider these implications in three regards: how emotion can be engendered through generic and extensive internet activity; how material on the internet can have a distinct emotional tone; and, how social media engagement relates to emotion. In all three areas, evidence concerning movement, change or transition in emotion can occur.

Emotion engendered through intensive internet activity

Sanders et al. (2000) identified a correlation between depression and level of internet usage. They argued that the relative social isolation of time spent online as opposed to in company may be associated with depression. There may be an addictive element in internet usage. Stavropoulos et al. (2016), for example, identified relationships between role-playing gaming and internet addiction, although these effects were ameliorated to some extent, where the person's physical social world included other gamers, as opposed to a more solitary and isolated usage context. Van Rooij et al. (2017) highlight that different forms of internet usage (browsing, gaming, social media etc.) are associated with different processes and outcomes. It may be useful therefore, to distinguish between the cognitive and social-cognitive processes involved in engaging with the internet world.

Emotional correlates of social media usage

Pantic et al. (2012) identified a correlation between time spent in online social networks and depression. Are the emotional correlates of social media engagement the same for all individuals? Feinstein et al. (2012, p.372), in a longitudinal study of social media usage concluded, "people who report greater depressive symptoms are not using social network mediums more. Rather, they are engaging in more problematic social networking interactions and they are experiencing more negative affect following those interactions". Huang (2017) in a meta-analysis of the overall published studies of generic usage, concluded that the overall effect sizes were quite small.

There are however, different forms of social media usage and there is evidence that they differ with regard to associated emotions. Rosen et al. (2013) identified different effects for different forms of Facebook usage. Those engaged more in impression management (frequency of checking in, updating their profile, with more friends that they haven't met) had higher depression scores than participants making more general use of Facebook (liking, commenting etc.). In reviewing studies, Verduyn et al. (2017) distinguish between active and passive use of social media, and identify different correlates. They argue that active use can enhance one's assessment of personal social capital, feelings of social connectedness and self-esteem, whereas passive use (browsing) may emphasise social comparison and envy and be associated with lower subjective well-being.

It was noted earlier that designed content on the internet can consider emotional tone. Social interaction is inherently dynamic. As a social process there is evidence of emotional contagion in social media engagement. These have been considered in both naturalistic contexts, and as designed or orchestrated endeavours.

Lewis (2014) reports an experiment undertaken by Facebook whereby a proportion of positive emotion news feed items or negative emotion items were removed from the posts users saw in their feeds. They found that people who had positive words removed from their feeds made fewer positive posts. People who had had negative words removed made fewer negative posts. Additionally, people who received overall less emotionally-expressive posts, contributed less emotionally in their own subsequent posts. Sunstein (2001) established that the "argument pool" can be qualitatively different within different communities. If one is "restricted" to, say, negatively-framed discussion, then the pool of arguments is more uniformly negative. It is, as Sunstein (2001) puts it, an "echo chamber" where one hears the same form of information reverberating within a community. The impact of this upon personal opinions is polarisation. Del Vicario et al. (2016) demonstrated however that polarisation in online communities may progressively drift to a more *negative* tone. In addition, the speed with which a participant's own posts manifest a negative tone is related to the volume of posts that he/she makes. One key question therefore is who and what sets the tone? Bessi (2016) found a statistical relationship between the number of posts made by an individual and their personality characteristics. Brady et al. (2017) found that re-tweet rates were greater with tweets with words that had both a higher emotional and moral tone.

Sentiment provocation is also being more explicitly managed. In the marketing context, attention has recently turned towards the impact of explicit attempts to provoke sentiment. Hassan (2014) explored how brand messages on social media may use an "emotions strategy" concentrating on influencing affective beliefs. Abdullah and Zolkepli (2017) in an analysis of Starbucks' use of social media, identified how posts and tweets on Facebook, Instagram and Twitter can provoke predictable emotional reactions among the virtual community. A message such as "Feeling exhausted from a busy week? Let us give you a little boost today!", provokes sharing with accompanying sentiments. Research in artificial intelligence has explored characteristics of visual images that invoke distinct emotions (You et al., 2016).

It is clear that internet engagement can have emotion connotations. There is a need however, for further research upon how well-being can be enhanced through the design of encounters. It is towards our understanding of the mechanisms through which activity in the internet world affects emotion and well-being that this chapter now turns.

Informational and therapeutic design and emotion

Picard (1997, p.3) defined affective computing as "computing that relates to, arises from, or deliberately influences emotions". Klein et al. (1999) reported a study where "supportive" messages were able to mitigate some of the frustration experienced by computer users. Tzeng (2004) found that computer "apologies" using emoticons were more effective than text alone. Sparrow (2006) highlighted the potential for managing emotional tone in online material. He demonstrated that where users were experiencing a specific emotion, that online information that had a complementary tone was felt to be more valuable than information with the same emotional tone. Sparrow (2006) highlighted that encounters with online material could engender emotional transitions towards the tone of the online material. Kim and Doh (2017) demonstrated that commercially successful computer games entail significantly larger emotional transitions than less successful games. It seems clear that there is considerable potential within information design to manage emotional tone adaptively.

Therapeutic support can be provided by computerised counselling (Newman, 2004). Maxwell's (1992) indicators of service quality can be used to summarise overall evidence upon computerised support. The criteria are effectiveness, safety, equity, efficiency, accessibility and acceptability. Meta-analyses of computer-aided psychotherapy have found that it had a small to moderate effect on quality of life (Kaltenthaler et al., 2008). Computerised cognitive behavioural therapy (CBT) support has been found to be an effective alternative overall (Ferriter et al., 2008). With regard to safety, Yeung et al. (2009) report that 85% of clinicians refer clients to self-help sources for support with mild disorders, with no major reported issues. Computerised support addresses many aspects of equity such as geographic inequity (Shapiro et al., 2003). Efficiency has primarily been evaluated through cost-benefit studies. Gerhards et al. (2010) concluded that computerised support constitutes the most efficient treatment strategy. Accessibility in terms of availability is better with computerised support. It is available 24 hours a day. On the other hand, it may be less accessible for people with visual impairment, poor IT skills or a lower educational level (Waller & Gilbody, 2009). Williams and Garland (2002) for example, found that cognitive behaviour therapy typically had a mean reading age of 17 years. In terms of acceptability and satisfaction, Kaltenthaler et al.'s (2008) systematic review of computerised CBT services found overwhelmingly positive expectancies and high levels of client satisfaction. Sentiment provocation has long been recognised as a goal in therapeutic contexts (Greenberg et al., 1993). Computerised CBT has been found to be effective in the treatment of common mental health disorders, (Grist & Cavanagh, 2013), where clients are encouraged to challenge their cognitions around current emotions.

Researching the links between emotion, self-talk, self-efficacy, well-being and e-coaching

A key element in the impact of informational and interpersonal encounters upon well-being is self-talk. Self-talk can be key element in one's narratives of well-being. Furthermore, it is possible to alter self-talk through "design" processes such as coaching. The following section considers these elements and looks at evidence on the use of computer-supported therapeutic interventions.

Self-talk

Hackfort and Schwenkmezger (1993) defined self-talk as "dialogue through which the individual interprets feelings and perceptions, regulates and changes evaluations and convictions, and gives him/herself instructions and reinforcement" (p.355). Hardy (2006) defines self-talk as: "(a) verbalizations or statements addressed to the self; (b) multidimensional in nature; (c) having interpretive elements association with the content of statements employed; (d) is somewhat dynamic; and (e) serving at least two functions; instructional and motivational" (p.84). Neck and Houghton (2006) detail the range of outcomes associated with self-talk as including commitment, independence, creativity/innovation, trust, potency, positive affect, job satisfaction, psychological empowerment and self-efficacy. Rogelberg et al. (2013) demonstrate how constructive self-talk positively related to effective leadership of others and was negatively related to job strain. Dysfunctional self-talk related negatively to creativity/originality. In summary, self-talk can have a dynamic positive or negative effect upon performance.

Narratives of self

Self-talk can include narratives of our lives, in general. Hedonism reflects the view that well-being consists of pleasure or happiness. Eudaimonism considers well-being to consist of more than just happiness. It lies instead in the actualisation of human potentials. Well-being consists of fulfilling or realising one's daimon or true nature (Ryan & Deci, 2001). Bauer et al. (2008) highlight how the narratives of individuals with higher or lower levels of eudaimonic well-being differ. People with high levels of eudaimonic well-being tend to emphasise personal growth in their life stories, and tend to frame difficult life experiences as transformative experiences in line with a culturally-shaped script highlighting pain, upward social mobility, liberation, recovery, atonement and actualisation.

The use of narrative is well-established in therapeutic situations. McLeod (1997, pp.28–53) itemises a number of ways in which narrative knowing and story-telling generally, are helpful in therapeutic situations. Flintham (2011) highlights how McLeod argues that our narratives:

> Give us our own personal myths, helping us to handle the multiplicity of our of selves; they offer ambiguity, allowing space for interpretive and imaginative acts, and as such they are liminal, offering "threshold" experiences which can be personally transformative or cathartic; they have sequentiality and thus impel events into an order, reducing apparent chaos, helping us to solve problems and assimilate the exceptional; and they are shared experiences, opening windows into each other's lives, forging social bonds and implying a moral landscape where they emerge around sites of social conflict.

Writing about stressful or traumatic events has been shown to improve several health-related outcomes. Smyth et al. (1999) for example, found that structured writing about stressful events improved symptomatology in 112 patients with rheumatoid arthritis and asthma relative to patients who did not write. Pennebaker (1990) theorised about a positive effect due to disclosure of trauma-related emotions and memories, and an integration of emotions and thoughts associated with stressful events as reducing harmful ruminations. More recently, it has been suggested that it is the narrative function of meaning-making that is therapeutic (Freda & Martino, 2015).

Self-efficacy

One potential consequence of positive or negative self-talk may be perceptions of self-efficacy. Perceived self-efficacy is concerned with people's beliefs in their capabilities to produce given attainments (Bandura, 1977) and has been reliably assessed and consistently related to causal and consequential factors. There has been considerable research into self-beliefs about capability in numerous specific domains. Bandura (2006) details specific self-efficacy scales concerning regulating exercise, eating habits, driving, problem-solving, pain management and many other areas. Scale development has continued in specific domains, e.g. technology self-efficacy (Huffman et al., 2013); leadership self-efficacy (Ng et al., 2008); yoga self-efficacy (Birdee et al., 2016). The highest proportion of studies however investigate relationships with a general measure of self-efficacy. The most cited scale is the general self-efficacy scale developed by Sherer et al. (1982). Scores on this scale have been related to many variables including emotional leadership (Yoon & Lee, 2015), leadership effectiveness (Mesterova et al., 2015); stress and well-being (Soysa & Wilcomb, 2015); hope and ethical climate (Swanepoel et al., 2015).

The impact of positive or negative self-talk in emotional self-reflection may be moderated by general skills of emotion self-appraisal. Self-emotion appraisal relates to the individual's ability to understand their own emotions and be able to express these emotions naturally (Wong & Law, 2002). For example, individuals who have greater self-emotion appraisal skills may manifest greater impact of emotional self-reflection upon subsequent thinking and action. Self-emotion appraisal is one of four aspects of emotional intelligence identified by Mayer and Salovey (1997).

The Wong and Law Emotional Intelligence Scale (WLEIS; Wong & Law, 2002) is based on Mayer and Salovey's (1997) EI model and measures four dimensions: self emotional appraisal (SEA) measures the individual's ability to understand their emotions, others' emotional appraisal (OEA) is the ability to recognise and understand other people's emotions, use of emotion (UOE) is the tendency to motivate oneself to enhance performance and regulation of emotion (ROE) assesses the ability to regulate emotions (Fukuda et al., 2011).

Well-being as flourishing

Finally, one might hypothesise that positive or negative self-talk might have differential impact upon flourishing. "Flourishing refers to the experience of life going well. It is a combination of feeling good and functioning effectively. Flourishing is synonymous with a high-level of mental wellbeing, and it epitomises mental health" (Huppert & So, 2011, p.838). Accordingly, Huppert and So (2011) identify ten features of flourishing. These features combine feeling and functioning, i.e. hedonic and eudaimonic aspects of well-being: competence, emotional stability, engagement, meaning, optimism, positive emotion, positive relationships, resilience, self-esteem and vitality. The authors use items from the European Social Survey (ESS; Jowell & The Central Co-ordinating Team, 2003) to develop an assessment.

Coaching and e-coaching

So, where does coaching fit in the chain of events from dynamic self-talk, general narratives of self, self-efficacy and well-being? Coaching has been defined as "a customised, collaborative relationship that elicits the client's potential for self-awareness, for understanding the meaning of his or her unique situation, for visualising change, and for making choices and plans to achieve a goal" (Hayes & Kalmakis, 2007, p.556). Coaching is a learning process that is widely used in the contemporary workplace (CIPD, 2013). Although coaching research is still at its infancy, a number of studies have demonstrated its relation to important workplace outcomes, such as employee performance (Agarwal et al., 2009; Liu & Batt, 2010), satisfaction (Kim et al., 2013; Kim, 2014), feedback ratings (Smither, et al., 2003) and entrepreneurial behaviour (Wakkee et al., 2010). A number of studies have attempted to identify and distinguish the various types of workplace coaching in order to offer a more comprehensive understanding of the practice (e.g. D'Abate et al., 2003; Segers et al., 2011). More specifically, Segers, et al. (2011) categorised the numerous types of workplace coaching on a three-dimensional cube based on the agenda of the intervention, the type of the coach and the adopted methodology.

Cognitive behavioural coaching extends CBT to non-clinical populations (Kearns et al., 2007). It focuses upon the cognitions and beliefs that a coachee has and helps the coachee appraise them and where appropriate, re-frame them. Coaching can also place an emphasis upon emotionality. Segers et al. (2011) classified under the "emotionality" label all the coaching approaches that focus on "the importance of phenomenological experiencing and personal feelings" (p.207). Emotional cognitions are a major element in learning and coaching (Dryden, 2011). Coaching can highlight key aspects of emotion in the workplace (Cox & Patrick, 2012). The need for coaches to understand the connection between emotions and change, leadership and motivation has been identified (Cremona, 2010). There is a need for greater understanding of the means through which framing situations (and associated self-talk) engender emotion, and impact upon coaching outcomes. One theory that considers how positive and negative framing affect thinking and learning has been developed by Boyatsis (2006). In conceptualising learning from a complexity perspective, Boyatsis (2006) argues that two attractors, positive emotional and negative emotional attractors, determine whether learning operates as an adaptation to existing conditions or adaptation to new, emergent conditions. Positive emotional attractors (PEA), he argues, "pull the person toward their ideal self . . . focusing the person on future possibilities and filling them with hope" (pp.615–616). In contrast, negative emotional attractors (NEA) "pull a person toward defensive protection" (p.616). Howard (2015) applied these ideas to executive coaching. She structured coaching around these two alternative attractors and identified measurable differences in the expressed emotion of the two groups of coachees in the course of the coaching session. Howard (2015) hypothesised that there may be differential impacts after the coaching sessions upon levels of stress between the two groups, but was unable to identify any significant effect. An alternative potential impact of these different emphases in coaching might however be perceived self-efficacy.

Kamphorst (2017) defines e-coaching systems as "a set of computerized components that . . . engages proactively in an ongoing collaborative conversation with the user in order to aid planning and promote effective goal striving through the use of persuasive techniques" (p.629). Frazee (2008) found that e-coaching (with extensive use of online resources) in the workplace was perceived as particularly valuable for geographically dispersed groups or when scheduling conflicts otherwise presenting logistical challenges. Poepsel (2011) reports positive findings with an online evidence-based coaching system upon goal striving, subjective well-being and level of hope. Sparrow (2013) undertook a review of e-coaching in life coaching and identified clear potential for enhancing well-being. Automated coaching software has been developed to assist coachees in life coaching decisions and actions (Sparrow, 2014).

Objectives of the current study

Research is needed to understand the impact of framing e-coaching questions upon subsequent self-talk, self-esteem and assessments of well-being. An empirical study of these relationships is reported here. The study hypothesises that an e-coaching process invoking different emotional self-talk will impact differentially upon perceived self-efficacy, which will, in turn, impact upon well-being (flourishing). The study also sought to establish that any observed differences in self-talk, self-efficacy and self-assessments of well-being were not attributable to general differences in ability to self-appraise, but rather were associated with the emotional framing of coaching questions.

Methodology

Assessments

E-coaching and self-reflection accounts

Standardisation of coaching through automated e-coaching is increasing. The use of computerised alternatively emotionally-charged scenarios in reflecting upon past experiences was used by Sparrow (2009). Sparrow analysed the emotional tone of personal reflections with the Dictionary of Affect in Language (DAL) developed by Whissell (1989).

Mylifecoachapp and *messagemycoachfriend* (www.visualsolve.com) are self-help coaching applications that draw upon self-assessments of personality, strengths, ways of coping, age, gender and current emotions to focus computer-generated coaching questions upon parallel issues (using clean language and metaphor therapy) in order to help users address current issues. The rationale for the applications is outlined by Sparrow (2014). The "strengths assessment" questions prompt users to consider valuable strengths and the positive role they play. Six items were used in the current study. These were:

> Please think about one of your longstanding attributes that you value that has served you well in your life. Please write down an example instance where you used this attribute to good effect.
>
> Please think about one of your more recently acquired attributes that you value that has served you well in the last six months. Please write down an example instance where you used this attribute to good effect.
>
> What would you consider to be the attribute you have, that you value that has the broadest positive effect? Please indicate the attribute and why you consider it to have a broad positive effect.
>
> What would you consider to be the attribute you have that you value, that while quite specific, has positive effect? Please indicate the specific attribute and give an example of where you used it to good effect.
>
> Of all your attributes, which one do you consider to be the most valuable, and why?
>
> Of all your attributes, which one do you think is most appreciated by others, and why?

Six contrasting items were developed for the current study utilising a more negative framing. These items are not used in *mylifecoachapp* or *messagemycoachfriend* but serve to examine the differential impact of positive and negative framing. The six parallel negatively-framed items were:

> Please think about one of your longstanding attributes that you feel has impeded you in your life. Please write down an example instance where this attribute has had a negative effect.
>
> Please think about one of your more recently acquired attributes that you feel has impeded you in the last six months. Please write down an example instance where you this attribute has had a negative effect.
>
> What would you consider to be the attribute you have that you dislike, that has the broadest negative effect? Please indicate the attribute and why you consider it to have a broad negative effect.
>
> What would you consider to be the attribute you have that you dislike, that while quite specific, has negative effect? Please indicate the specific attribute and give an example of where it has had a negative effect.

Of all your attributes, which one do you consider to be the one you like the least, and why?

Of all your attributes, which one do you think is most disliked by others, and why?

1. Self-emotion appraisal

   The four items from the self-emotion appraisal subscale of the Wong and Law Emotional Intelligences Scale (2002) were administered.
2. General self-efficacy

   The 17 items from the general self-efficacy subscale developed by Sherer et al. (1982) were administered.
3. Flourishing

   The ten items from the European Social Survey and the Huppert and So (2011) scale were administered.

Participants

The study worked with 2 independent groups of 11 part-time postgraduate students on professional human resource management programmes. The first group received the automated standardised positively-framed strengths exploration questions followed by the assessment items. The second group received the automated standardised negatively-framed strengths exploration questions followed by the assessment items.

Analyses and findings

Self-emotion appraisal scores

Scores on the self-emotion appraisal subscale were contrasted to see if the impacts of self-reflection upon assessments of self-efficacy and flourishing were moderated by different levels of competence in self-emotion appraisal. The scores upon the four items assessing self-emotion appraisal for the two groups were compared using one-tailed independent groups t-tests with equal variances not assumed. Table 7.1 details the results. There were no statistically significant differences between the two groups. The results concerning self-talk, self-efficacy and well-being are not due to any difference in the two groups of participants concerning a general ability to appraise their own emotions.

Emotional tone of self-reflections

The responses to the automated standardised positively and negatively-framed strengths exploration questions were analysed to determine if they had successfully invoked 'self-talk' with statistically significantly different emotional tones.

TABLE 7.1 Differences between the two experimental groups in general self-emotion appraisal

	Mean for positively-framed question group	*Mean for negatively-framed question group*	*t*	*df*	*Sig*
Self-emotion appraisal "good sense of why I have certain feelings"	6.18	6.00	0.339	17.350	0.369
Self-emotion appraisal "good understanding of my own emotions"	6.18	6.00	0.282	19.974	0.391
Self-emotion appraisal "really understand what I feel"	5.91	5.64	0.343	18.520	0.368
Self-emotion appraisal "always know whether or not I am happy"	6.00	6.09	– 0.129	19.830	0.449

A number of analytical tools can be used to analyse text to yield an emotional profile (see Pennebaker, Mehl & Niederhoffer, 2003 for a review). The written responses of the coachees were analysed using the DAL (to identify relative emphases upon positive and negative valence). The DAL developed by Whissell (1989) has 8,742 emotion-related words within a computer program that can be used to assess the proportion of words in a text that have positive/negative valence and high/low levels of activation. The DAL has been used in many studies of emotion in textual analysis (e.g. Mossholder et al., 1995; Whissell, 2006).

The responses from the eleven participants receiving positively-framed first question were combined for the first question and contrasted with the combined responses to the first question from the eleven participants receiving the negatively-framed question. A similar procedure was used for the other five questions.

The six pairs of pleasantness scores calculated by the DAL software were analysed using a paired t-test. The results are presented in Table 7.2.

Table 7.2 shows that there was a significant difference in the pleasantness scores ($t=10.356$, df (5), $p<0.001$). The question framings had successfully prompted significantly different emotional tones in the self-reflections of the two groups of participants.

The strength of feeling invoked by the negatively-expressed questions was notable. Some examples of negative self-talk included:

> "I doubt myself and my ability to do things especially at work."
> "[I suffer from] a lack of organisation and ability to plan."

TABLE 7.2 Significant difference in Mean DAL pleasantness scores in narrative responses for the groups with positively vs negatively worded strengths questions

Positive frame mean	*Negative frame mean*	*t*	*df*	*Sig*
2.033	1.844	10.356	5	$p<0.001$

"People now don't consider me to be open or welcoming anymore."
"My inability to focus has a negative effect."
"[I am] shy and reserved and I am not able to articulate who I actually am and what I am like."
"[I have an] indecisive nature."

If one imagines the above statements for a moment as chants, and repeated each of them to oneself, one has a clear sense of their potential negative impact upon self-efficacy and well-being.

The statements above can be contrasted with those invoked by the positively-oriented questions. Some examples of the concomitant positive self-talk included:

"I always pride myself on my ability to be compassionate to others and their needs."
"I have improved my influencing skills – explaining to people the benefits of why they should complete tasks."
"When others feel they have nobody to talk or lean on. I have been told I am an approachable person and often find others seeking counsel."
"[I have] resilience as if things go wrong I don't allow it to affect other aspects of my life negatively and I learn from these experiences."
"[I have] positivity and always smiling helps me in all situations as people comment on my upbeat approach to situations."
"[I am] trustworthy. People are able to confide in me."

Again, if one imagines the above positive statements as chants, and repeated each of them to oneself, one has a clear sense of their potential positive impact upon self-efficacy and well-being.

General self-efficacy scores

The scores upon the 17 items of the general self-efficacy scale for the two groups were compared using one-tailed independent groups t-tests with equal variances not assumed. Table 7.3 details the results.

Table 7.3 shows that statistically significantly differences were identified in terms of tending to avoid difficulties ($t=1.722$, df(17.444, $p<0.05$) and self-reliance ($t=1.754$, df(14.858), $p<0.05$).

TABLE 7.3 Significant differences in the mean general self-efficacy scores for the groups with positively vs negatively worded strengths questions

	Mean for positively-framed question group	*Mean for negatively-framed question group*	*t*	*df*	*Sig*
Self-efficacy Tend to avoid difficulties	5.73	8.27	−1.722	17.444	p<0.05
Self-efficacy Self-reliance	12.50	10.27	1.754	14.858	p<0.05

Well-being (flourishing) scores

The scores upon the ten items assessing flourishing for the two groups were compared using one-tailed independent groups t-tests with equal variances not assumed. Table 7.4 details the results. A statistically significantly difference was identified in terms of vitality ($t=2.252$, df(18.792), $p<0.05$).

Discussion and conclusions

The study presented in this chapter sought to explore relationships between e-coaching processes invoking positive or negative self-reflection (self-talk) and subsequent perceived self-efficacy and well-being.

The analyses indicate that e-coaching software such as *mylifecoachapp* or *message-mycoachfriend* can prompt self-talk with statistically significantly different emotional valence. The potential power of such self-talk was evident from some of the examples detailed in the results. Self-talk with different emotional valences impacts upon general self-efficacy both in beliefs about tending to avoid difficulties and one's overall self-reliance. Self-talk can impact upon one's self-assessments of vitality. This is an important aspect of flourishing and well-being.

Self-talk can be linked to the increasingly popular concept of self-compassion. According to Neff (2003), self-compassion is comprised of three interconnected aspects exhibited at times of failure and pain: (a) self-kindness (i.e. being understanding and kind towards Self rather than being self-critical); (b) common humanity (i.e. seeing one's shortcomings as part of the broader human condition

TABLE 7.4 Significant difference in flourishing score for the groups with positively vs negatively worded strengths questions

	Mean for positively-framed question group	*Mean for negatively-framed question group*	*t*	*df*	*Sig*
Flourishing Vitality	3.82	2.73	2.606	17.104	p<0.05

rather than unique to self and isolating); and (c) mindfulness (i.e. holding one's distress in mindful awareness rather than over-identifying with or avoiding it). Self-compassion has been found to promote well-being and protect against psychological distress (Sutherland et al., 2014). A key role for coaching therefore, is to help coachees appreciate where they are being perhaps excessively self-critical, and to consider the impact of associated negative self-talk.

Clearly, the study has only been conducted with a small sample of professionals. There would be clear value in increasing the sample size to consider the robustness of the findings and increase statistical power. Nevertheless, the potential of e-coaching software to prompt reflection and facilitate positive self-talk and associated beliefs about self-efficacy and well-being is an important finding.

More broadly, this chapter has illustrated how internet content carries an emotional tone. Encountering and reflecting upon internet material invokes self-talk. This may involve social comparison as noted in research upon social media contexts as described, or, as reported here, it may stem from invoking memories with distinct emotional tones. Self-talk, in itself, has an emotional valence (positive vs negative). The dynamic impact of self-talk upon self-belief and self-efficacy has been established. These effects extend to self-appraisals of well-being. One might hypothesise that these effects could affect current assessments of well-being, and potentially future assessments. Interestingly, the current study has shown that retrospective assessments are affected. This may be a small element in explaining the deeper mental health effects reported in other research, as a negative (and potentially depressive) negative interpretation of both the present and the past, can be invoked.

It is clear that the online world needs to be designed with well-being in mind. The research reported in this chapter has highlighted how content can be designed to promote positive self-talk, self-efficacy and well-being. Other research summarised in the chapter indicates that emotional transitions can be supported. It may be possible to dynamically alter the emotional tone of online material to complement a user's current emotion and support them in a transition towards a desired emotion.

References

Abdullah, N. S. D. & Zolkepli, I. A. (2017) Sentiment analysis of online crowd input towards brand provocation in Facebook, Twitter, and Instagram. Available at www.researchgate.net/profile/Izzal_Zolkepli/publication/319207393_Sentiment_Analysis_of_Online_Crowd_Input_towards_Brand_Provocation_in_Facebook_Twitter_and_Instagram/links/599bc03345851574f4ac7836/Sentiment-Analysis-of-Online-Crowd-Input-towards-Brand-Provocation-in-Facebook-Twitter-and-Instagram.pdf, last accessed 20 July 2017.

Agarwal, R., Angst, C. M. & Magni, M. (2009) The performance effects of coaching: a multilevel analysis using hierarchical linear modelling, *The International Journal of Human Resource Management* 20 (10): 2110–2134.

Bandura, A. (1977) Self-efficacy: toward a unifying theory of behavioural change, *Psychological Review* 84 (2): 191.

Bandura, A. (2006) Guide for constructing self-efficacy scales, *Self-Efficacy Beliefs of Adolescents* 5: 307–337.

Bauer, J. J., MacAdams D. P. & Pals J. L. (2008) Narrative identity and eudaimonic well-being, *Journal of Happiness Studies* 9: 81–104.

Bessi, A. (2016) Personality traits and echo chambers on Facebook, *Computers in Human Behavior* 65: 319–324.

Birdee, G. S., Sohl, S. J. & Wallston, K. (2016) Development and psychometric properties of the yoga self-efficacy scale (YSES), *BMC Complementary and Alternative Medicine* 16 (1): 1.

Boyatzis, R. E. (2006) An overview of intentional change from a complexity perspective, *Journal of Management Development* 25: 607–623.

Brady, W. J., Wills, J. A., Jost, J. T., Tucker, J. A. & Van Bavel, J. J. (2017) Emotion shapes the diffusion of moralized content in social networks, *Proceedings of the National Academy of Sciences* 114 (28): 7313–7318.

Chervonsky, E. & Hunt, C. (2017) Suppression and expression of emotion in social and interpersonal outcomes: a meta-analysis, *Emotion* 17 (4): 669–683.

CIPD (2013) *Learning & Talent Development 2013*, London: CIPD. Available at Available at www.cipd.co.uk/hr-resources/survey-reports/learning-talent-development-2013.aspx, last accessed 17 May 2013.

Cox, E. & Patrick, C. (2012) Managing emotions at work: How coaching affects retail support workers' performance and motivation, *International Journal of Evidence Based Coaching & Mentoring* 10 (2): 34–51.

Cremona, K. (2010) Coaching and emotions: an exploration of how coaches engage and think about emotion, *Coaching: An International Journal of Theory, Research and Practice* 3 (1): 46–59.

D'Abate, C. P., Eddy, E. R. & Tannenbaum, S. I. (2003) What's in a name? A literature-based approach to understanding mentoring, coaching, and other constructs that describe developmental interactions, *Human Resource Development Review* 2 (4): 360–384.

Del Vicario, M., Vivaldo, G., Bessi, A., Zollo, F., Scala, A., Caldarelli, G. & Quattrociocchi, W. (2016) Echo chambers: emotional contagion and group polarization on Facebook, *Scientific Reports* 6.

Dryden, W. (2011) *Dealing with Clients' Emotional Problems in Life Coaching: A Rational-Emotive and Cognitive Behaviour Therapy (RECBT) Approach*, London: Routledge.

Feinstein, B. A., Bhatia, V., Hershenberg, R. & Davila, J. (2012) Another venue for problematic interpersonal behavior: the effects of depressive and anxious symptoms on social networking experiences, *Journal of Social and Clinical Psychology* 31 (4): 356–382.

Ferriter, M., Kaltenthaler, E., Parry, G. & Beverley, C. (2008) Computerised CBT: a review, *Mental Health Today* October: 30–31.

Flintham, J. (2011) Narrative approaches to wellbeing, *Paper presented at WELL-BEING 2011: The First International Conference Exploring the Multi-dimensions of Well-being*, Birmingham City University, 18–19 July 2011.

Freda, M. F. & Martino, M. L. (2015) Health and writing: meaning-making processes in the narratives of parents of children with leukemia, *Qualitative Health Research* 25 (3): 348–359.

Gerhards, S. A., de Graff, L. E., Jacobs, L. E., Severens, J. L., Huibers, M. J., Arntz, A., Riper, H., Widdershoven, G., Metsemakers, J. F. & Evers, S. M. (2010) Economic evaluation of online computerized cognitive-behavioural therapy without support for depression in primary care: randomized trial, *British Journal of Psychiatry* 196 (4): 310–318.

Greenberg, L. S., Rice, L. N. & Elliot, R. (1993) *Facilitating Emotional Change: The Moment by Moment Process*, New York: Guildford Press.

Grist, R. & Cavanagh, K. (2013) Computerised cognitive behavioural therapy for common mental health disorders, what works, for whom under what circumstances? A systematic review and meta-analysis, *Journal of Contemporary Psychotherapy*, 43 (4): 243–251.

Hackfort, D. & Schwenkmezger, P. (1993) Anxiety, in R. N. Singer, M. Murphy & L. K. Tennant (eds.), *Handbook of Research on Sport Psychology*, New York: Scientific Research Publishing, pp.328–364.

Hardy, J. (2006) Speaking clearly: a critical review of the self-talk literature, *Psychology of Sport and Exercise* 7 (1): 81–97.

Hassan, A. (2014) Do brands targeting women use instamarketing differently: a content analysis, *Marketing Management Association Spring 2014 Proceedings*, pp.62–65.

Hayes, E. & Kalmakis, K. A. (2007) From the sidelines: coaching as a nurse practitioner strategy for improving health outcomes, *Journal of the American Association of Nurse Practitioners* 19 (11): 555–562.

Howard, A. R. (2015) Coaching to vision versus coaching to improvement needs: a preliminary investigation on the differential impacts of fostering positive and negative emotion during real time executive coaching sessions, *Frontiers in Psychology* 6: 1–15.

Huang, C. (2017) Time spent on social network sites and psychological well-being: a meta-analysis, *Cyberpsychology, Behavior, and Social Networking* 20 (6): 346–354.

Huffman, A. H., Whetten, J. & Huffman, W. H. (2013) Using technology in higher education: the influence of gender roles on technology self-efficacy, *Computers in Human Behavior 29* (4): 1779–1786.

Huppert, F. A. & So, T. C. (2013) Flourishing across Europe: application of a new conceptual framework for defining well-being, *Social Indicators Research* 110 (3): 837–861. Available at http://dx.doi.org/10.1007/s11205-011-9966-7.

Jowell, R. & The Central Co-ordinating Team (2003) *European Social Survey 2002/2003: Technical Report.* London: Centre for Comparative Social Surveys, City University.

Kaltenthaler, E., Parry, G., Beveley, C. & Ferriter, M. (2008) Computerised cognitive-behavioural therapy for depression: systematic review, *The British Journal of Psychiatry* 193 (3): 181–184.

Kamphorst, B. A. (2017) E-coaching systems: what are they, and what are they not? *Personal and Ubiquitous Computing* 21 (4): 625–632.

Kearns, H., Forbes, A. & Gardiner, M. (2007) A cognitive behavioural coaching intervention for the treatment of perfectionism and self-handicapping in a non-clinical population, *Behaviour Change* 24 (3): 157–172.

Kim, M. & Doh, Y. Y. (2017) Computational Modeling of players' emotional response patterns to the story events of video games, *IEEE Transactions on Affective Computing* 8 (2): 216–227.

Kim, S. (2014) Assessing the influence of managerial coaching on employee outcomes, *Human Resource Development Quarterly* 25 (1): 59–85.

Kim, S., Egan, T. M., Kim, W. & Kim, J. (2013) The impact of managerial coaching behavior on employee work-related reactions, *Journal of Business and Psychology* 28 (3): 315–330.

Klein, J., Moon, Y. & Picard, R. W. (1999) This computer responds to user frustration, in *CHI '99 Extended Abstracts on Human Factors in Computing Systems*, New York: ACM, pp.242–243.

Lewis, T. (2014) Emotions can be contagious on online social networks, *Scientific American*, 1 July 2014. Available at www.scientificamerican.com/article/facebook-emotions-are-contagious/.

Liu, X. & Batt, R. (2010) How supervisors influence performance: a multilevel study of coaching and group management in technology-mediated services, *Personnel Psychology* 63 (2): 265–298.

Maxwell, R. J. (1992) Dimensions of quality revisited: from thought to action, *Quality in Health Care* 1: 171–177.

Mayer, J. D. & Salovey, P. (1997) What is emotional intelligence? In P. Salovey & D. Sluyter (eds.), *Emotional development And Emotional Intelligence: Educational Implications*, New York: Basic Books, pp.3–34.

McLeod, J. (1997) *Narrative and Psychotherapy*, London: Sage.

Mesterova, J., Prochazka, J., Vaculik, M. & Smutny, P. (2015) Relationship between self-efficacy, transformational leadership and leader effectiveness, *Journal of Advanced Management Science* 3 (2): 109–122.

Mossholder, K. W., Settoon, R. P., Harris, S. G. & Armenakis, A. A. (1995) Measuring emotion in open-ended survey responses: An application of textual data analysis, *Journal of Management* 21 (2): 335–355.

Neck, C. P. & Houghton, J. D. (2006) Two decades of self-leadership theory and research: Past developments, present trends, and future possibilities, *Journal of Managerial Psychology* 21 (4): 270–295.

Neff, K. (2003) Self-Compassion: an alternative conceptualization of a healthy attitude towards oneself, *Self and Identity* 2 (2): 85–101.

Newman M. (2014) What's the good of counselling and psychotherapy? The benefits explained, *Child and Adolescent Mental Health* 9 (2): 92–93.

Ng, K. Y., Ang, S. & Chan, K. Y. (2008) Personality and leader effectiveness: A moderated mediation model of leadership self-efficacy, job demands, and job autonomy, *Journal of Applied Psychology* 93 (4): 733.

Pantic, I., Damjanovic, A., Todorovic, J., Topalovic, D., Bojovic-Jovic, D., Ristic, S. & Pantic, S. (2012) Association between online social networking and depression in high school students: Behavioral physiology viewpoint, *Psychiatria Danubina* 24 (1): 90–93.

Pennebaker, J. W. (1990) *Opening Up: The Healing Power of Expressing Emotion*, New York: Guilford Press.

Pennebaker, J. W., Segers, J., Vloeberghs, D., Henderickx, E. & Inceoglu, I. (2011) Structuring and understanding the coaching industry: the coaching cube, *Academy of Management Learning & Education* 10 (2): 204–221.

Picard, R. W. (1997) *Affective Computing*, Cambridge, MA: MIT Press.

Poepsel, M. A. (2011) The impact of an online evidence-based coaching program on goal striving, subjective well-being, and level of hope, Dissertation, Capella University. Available at https://pqdtopen.proquest.com.

Rogelberg, S. G., Justice, L., Braddy, P. W., Paustian-Underdahl, S. C., Heggestad, E., Shanock, L., Baran, B. E., Beck, T., Long, S., Andrew, A. & Altman, D. G. (2013) The executive mind: leader self-talk, effectiveness and strain, *Journal of Managerial Psychology* 28 (2): 183–201.

Rosen, L. D., Whaling, K., Rab, S., Carrier, L. M. & Cheever, N. A. (2013) Is Facebook creating "iDisorders"? The link between clinical symptoms of psychiatric disorders and technology use, attitudes and anxiety, *Computers in Human Behavior* 29 (3): 1243–1254.

Ryan, R. M. & Deci, E. L. (2001) On happiness and human potentials: review of research on hedonic and eudaimonic well-being, *Annual Review of Psychology* 52: 141–166.

Sanders, C. E., Field, T. M., Miguel, D. & Kaplan, M. (2000) The relationship of internet use to depression and social isolation among adolescents, *Adolescence* 35 (138): 237.

Segers, J., Vloeberghs, D., Henderickx, E. & Inceoglu, I. (2011) Structuring and understanding the coaching industry: the coaching cube, *Academy of Management Learning & Education* 10 (2): 204–221.

Shapiro, D. A., Cavanagh, K. & Lomas, H. (2003) Geographic inequity in the availability of cognitive behavioural therapy in England and Wales, *Behavioural and Cognitive Psychotherapy* 31 (2): 185–192.

Sherer, M., Maddux, J. E., Mercandante, B., Prentice-Dunn, S., Jacobs, B. & Rogers, R. W. (1982) The self-efficacy scale: construction and validation, *Psychological Reports* (2): 663–671.

Smither, J. W., London, M., Flautt, R., Vargas, Y. & Kucine, I. (2003) Can working with an executive coach improve multisource feedback ratings over time? A quasi-experimental field study, *Personnel Psychology* 56 (1): 23–44.

Smyth, J. M., Stone, A. A., Hurewitz, A. & Kaeli A. (1999) Effects of writing about stressful experiences on symptom reduction in patients with asthma or rheumatoid arthritis, *The Journal of the American Medical Association* 281 (14): 1304–1309.

Soysa, C. K. & Wilcomb, C. J. (2015) Mindfulness, self-compassion, self-efficacy, and gender as predictors of depression, anxiety, stress, and well-being, *Mindfulness* 6 (2): 217–226.

Sparrow, J. (2006) Addressing emotional tone in retrieval and browsing applications, Paper presented at the 3rd Operational Research Society Conference on Knowledge Management, Aston University, 17–18 July 2006.

Sparrow, J. (2008) Enhancing emotional range in strategic visioning, *International Journal of Business Innovation and Research* 2 (4): 437–448.

Sparrow, J. (2009) Impact of emotions associated with reflecting upon the past, *Reflective Practice* 10 (50): 567–576.

Sparrow, J. (2013) Enhancing wellbeing with an e-coach, *Proceedings of the 2nd International Wellbeing Conference 2013*, Birmingham City University, 24–25 July 2013.

Sparrow, J. (2014) Computerised life coaching, *Paper presented to the Euro Coach List Conference*, Eastwood Park, Gloucestershire, 8–9 November 2014.

Speier, C. & Frese, M. (1997) Generalized self-efficacy as a mediator and moderator between control and complexity at work and personal initiative: a longitudinal field study in East Germany, *Human Performance* 10 (2): 171–192.

Stavropoulos, V., Gentile, D. & Motti-Stefanidi, F. (2016) A multilevel longitudinal study of adolescent internet addiction: the role of obsessive – compulsive symptoms and classroom openness to experience, *European Journal of Developmental Psychology* 13 (1): 99–114.

Sunstein, C. R. (2001) *Echo Chambers: Bush v. Gore, Impeachment, And Beyond*, Princeton, NJ: Princeton University Press.

Sutherland, O., Peräkylä, A. & Elliott, R. (2014) Conversation analysis of the two-chair self-soothing task in emotion focused therapy, *Psychotherapy Research* 24 (6): 738–751.

Swanepoel, S., Botha, P. & Rose-Innes, R. (2015) Organizational behaviour: exploring the relationship between ethical climate, self-efficacy and hope, *Journal of Applied Business Research* 31 (4): 1419.

Tzeng, J. I. (2004) Toward a more civilized design: studying the effects of computers that apologize, *International Journal of Human–Computer Studies* 61 (3): 319–345.

Van Rooij, A. J., Ferguson, C. J., Van de Mheen, D. & Schoenmakers, T. M. (2017) Time to abandon internet addiction? Predicting problematic internet, game, and social media use from psychosocial well-being and application use, *Clinical Neuropsychiatry* 14 (1): 113–121.

Verduyn, P., Ybarra, O., Résibois, M., Jonides, J. & Kross, E. (2017) Do social network sites enhance or undermine subjective well-being? A critical review, *Social Issues and Policy Review* 11 (1): 274–302.

Wakkee, I., Elfring, T. & Monoghan, S. (2010) Creating entrepreneurial employees in traditional service sectors: the role of coaching and self-efficacy. *International Entrepreneurship and Management Journal* 6 (1): 1–21.

Waller, R. & Gilbody, S. (2009) Barriers to the uptake of computerized cognitive behavioural therapy: a systematic review of the quantitative and qualitative evidence, *Psychological Medicine* 39 (5): 705–712.

Whissell, C. M. (1989) The dictionary of affect in language, in R. Plutchik & H. Kellerman (eds.), *Emotion: Theory, Research and Experience, Vol. 4, The Measurement of Emotions*, San Diego, CA: Academic Press, pp.113–131.

Williams, C. & Garland, A. (2002) A cognitive-behavioural therapy assessment model for use in everyday clinical practice, *Advances in Psychiatric Treatment* 8 (3).

Wong, C. S. & Law, K. S. (2002) The effects of leader and follower emotional intelligence on performance and attitude: an exploratory study, *Leadership Quarterly* 13: 243–274.

Yeung, A., Feldman, G. & Fava, M. (2009) *Self-Management of Depression: A Manual for Mental Health and Primary Care Professionals*, Cambridge: Cambridge University Press.

Yoon, M. H. & Lee, C. S. (2015) Impacts of emotional leadership, self-efficacy and self-image of employees on organizational effectiveness, *Indian Journal of Science and Technology* 8 (S7): 512–519.

You, Q., Luo, J., Jin, H. & Yang, J. (2016) Building a large scale dataset for image emotion recognition: the fine print and the benchmark, in *Proceedings of the Thirtieth AAAI Conference on Artificial Intelligence (AAAI-16)*, pp.308–314.

8

THE LEGAL PROTECTION OF THE WELL-BEING OF FUTURE GENERATIONS

Haydn Davies

Introduction

Recently the Welsh Government passed into law the *Well-Being of Future Generations Act 2015* which enshrines in law a duty on public bodies to safeguard the interests of future generations in Wales. The well-being duty in the *Act* is a proxy for sustainable development and this is the first such legislative initiative in the world. It requires public bodies to take account of sustainable development (in terms of environmental, social, economic and cultural well-being) in all its strategic decision-making in order to maximise the public bodies' contributions to the achievement of the well-being goals set out by the Welsh Ministers. As such it raises fundamental questions about the precise legal nature of the duty and whether it amounts to a right enforceable on behalf of those who do not yet exist – which would be a considerable departure from classic rights theory. This chapter will explore the philosophical and legal issues that surround the creating of rights and obligations in respect of future generations and the extent to which the *Act* has overcome these issues and creates a plausible and extendable model for safeguarding the well-being of future generations more generally.

The legal protection of the interests of future generations

Since the creation of the Universal Declaration on Human Rights 1948 (UDHR) there has been an increasing reliance on the use of rights to protect the fundamental interests of individuals or classes of individuals. The use of fundamental rights as a means of protecting fundamental human interests, such as the right to life, rights to own property, freedom of speech and association and so on, reflects the natural law origins of the UDHR and is an expression of the sanctity of human autonomy and the idea, promulgated most famously by Immanuel Kant, that every human individual is an end in themselves (Kant, 1785, 1788). These ideas were subsequently developed by a great many philosophers and jurists and underpin the modern legal mechanisms by which Kant's Categorical Imperative is realised, at least in respect of certain fundamental rights.

However, in classical rights theory the creation of a legally enforceable right from a moral imperative requires that there should exist a relationship of reciprocity between the right-holder and those charged with the duty to the right-holder to uphold that right (or not to interfere with its exercise). This is the modern manifestation of the "golden rule" of classical philosophy, which also forms one of the main tenets of most of the major world religions, namely that you should do unto others as you would have them do unto you. In order for this relationship to subsist, both parties to the right must be extant. Classical theory holds that "a right cannot exist without a right-holder". This requirement is thought to underpin one of the principal theories for the existence of rights, the "status" theory. Wenar (2015), quoting Quinn (1993), states that "morality recognizes [a person's] existence as an individual with ends of his own—an independent *being* [emphasis in original]. Since that is what he is, he deserves this recognition." Here the terms "being" and "what he is" both presume existence as a *sine qua non* for the holding of rights. This is not the same as stating that a right-holder need be capable of asserting their legal rights; the law makes provision for enforcing rights "by proxy" for those who exist but are unable, either through immaturity or incapacity to enforce their rights for themselves. Hence the creation of the Court of Protection, which oversees the rights, especially property rights, of those who have lost the capacity to do for themselves, and the statutory creation of various Commissioners, such as for the elderly and children whose role it is to protect the rights and interests of those groups in society.

However, the limitations of the classical reciprocal model for rights have been demonstrated by the rise of the concept of sustainable development. Commonly attributed to the *Report of the World Commission on Environment and Development* (UN, 1987, known as the *Brundtland Report*), sustainable development is the idea that "Humanity has the ability to make development sustainable to ensure that it meets the needs of the present without compromising the ability of future generations to meet their own needs" (ibid., para 27). This idea has been incorporated into a very large number of policy documents by many of the world's governments but until recently it has not formed the basis of a directly enforcement legal obligation towards future generations. This legislative lassitude is partly attributable to a lack of political will (the need for which was explicitly recognised in the *Brundtland Report*, see ibid., para 30) and partly because of disagreements as to where the emphasis should be placed – sustainability or development (which is usually interpreted as economic development) – a debate which has divided developing and developed countries for 30 years. However, it also owes something to the legal difficulties of formulating a right to sustainable development in favour of future generations, precisely because they do not exist and cannot therefore engage in reciprocity in respect of their rights. There is also the inherent, and very significant, difficulty of balancing the needs of current generations (who have the advantage of being tangible and quantifiable) against those of future generations (who do not). The principal, and most influential theory of justice in the twentieth century, the "justice as fairness" theory of John Rawls (1971), paid extensive attention to the plight of the disadvantaged in society, and did attempt to assess intergenerational justice as part of this analysis. Rawls' "just savings" principle suggested that current generations have a relationship of indirect reciprocity with future generations, though he conceded that this was at best a "virtual" relationship (see Lawrence, 2014, pp.51–52) and to that extent was a somewhat theoretical relationship and one that has been subject to considerable criticism in terms of its potential to be realised.

In the vanguard of attempts to correct the defects of Rawls' conception and to create a sound ethical and legal basis for the protection of the interests of future generations, have been the communitarian ethicists (readers are referred to the excellent introduction by Selznick, 1987). A number of fairly recent texts have attempted to harness this philosophy, particularly the capacity-based theories of Amarta Sen (2009) and Martha Nussbaum (2006), in the service of future generations (see in particular Hiskes, 2009; Lawrence, 2014). Communitarianism emphasises responsibility towards community as a counterbalance to what is seen as the over-emphasis on the individual – as opposed to the "person" – that characterises liberalism, even "welfare liberalism" (Selznick, 1987, pp.447–448; Glendon, 1991). At the heart of communitarianism in this context are the concepts of duty and responsibility, not only to our fellow citizens who comprise current generations, but also to those yet to come. Thus, those who espouse communitarianism as an ethical basis for the protection of future generations, including Hiskes and Lawrence – both of whom are particularly concerned with the effects of climate change on future generations – use the language of obligation, rather than that of rights *per se*, to press their argument. Moreover, they stress the collective nature of this obligation, since climate change is ultimately caused by collective behaviour. This emphasis on duty enables communitarianism to avoid, or refute most of the traditional rights-based objections to consideration of future generations, albeit on the basis of the moral rights to be protected, rather than legal ones.

However, the emphasis on the obligations of current generations to those yet unborn also permits a consideration of legal obligations – but based on duties rather than rights. This is significant because the predominant model for the creation of legal rights, developed by Wesley Hohfeld (1913, 1917) insists that a right cannot exist without a corresponding duty – the so-called "correlative pairs" model (see also Campbell & Thomas, 2001). This is problematic in that the right must come first, and, as we have seen, meaningful legal rights are very difficult to create for non-existent entities since they cannot enforce them. However, there is nothing in Hohfeld's model that prevents the creation of a duty without a corresponding right. Obviously, to be meaningful the duty must be enforced by someone, but there is no necessity for that enforcement to be undertaken by the beneficiary of the duty. It is precisely this emphasis on duty that characterises the world's first attempt to make the well-being of future generations legally enforceable.

The remainder of this chapter discusses this initiative and the extent to which it might achieve its aspirations.

The Well-Being of Future Generations (Wales) Act 2015

The Well-Being of Future Generations (Wales) Act 2015 (WFGA) became law in Wales on 29 April 2015, and most of its provisions entered into force on 1 April 2016. The *Act* is one of the first of its kind anywhere in the world and, for the first time, creates a legal duty on public bodies in Wales to take account of the needs of future generations in every aspect of their decision-making. In effect this is a duty to implement sustainable development.

What follows will trace the origins and policy background to the *Act* before examining in more detail the exact nature of the duty which has been created and the extent to which it can truly be described as a legally enforceable duty (as opposed to a political duty) together with the possible implications of the duty – whatever its nature – for public governance in Wales. This in turn leads to some conclusions about the extent to which it is possible to create legally enforceable duties for future generations and the extent to which the Welsh initiative realises this possibility.

Origins and background in policy

Wales received a measure of devolved power as a result of the manifesto promises of Tony Blair's Labour government implemented in the *Government of Wales Act 1998*. However, it was s.79 of the subsequent *Government of Wales Act 2006* which was to lead to the creation of the WFGA. Section 79(1) stated that: "The Welsh Ministers must make a scheme ('the sustainable development scheme') setting out how they propose, in the exercise of their functions, to promote sustainable development."

This requirement led to a series of consultation documents between 2009 and 2012 (see Davies 2016, p.47) culminating in a green paper, *Proposals for a Sustainable Development Bill* (Welsh Government, 2012a) and, later in the same year, a white paper, *A Sustainable Wales: Better Choices for a Better Future* (Welsh Government, 2012b). *The Sustainable Development Bill* was introduced to the Welsh Assembly on 7 July 2014. Following several ministerial reshuffles and changes in the names of Welsh Government departments, the bill was renamed the *Well-Being of Future Generations (Wales) Act 2015* and was piloted through the Assembly by the late Carl Sargeant AM, Minister for Natural Resources (see Davies, 2016, p.48).

The progression of this policy development and the consultation process that accompanied it have been discussed elsewhere (Davies, 2013) but the thrust of the initiative was to make sustainable development the "central organising principle" of governance in Wales (Welsh Government, 2009, p.9). However, the Welsh Government chose to use "well-being" – specifically the setting of national well-being goals and local well-being objectives – as the vehicles by which to implement sustainable development. This was undoubtedly partly influenced by the *Fitoussi Report* (Stiglitz et al., 2009) which had worldwide effects in placing well-being at the heart of international and domestic policy as an alternative to the reliance on GDP as the sole measure of the "happiness" of a nation – happiness not necessarily being predicated on wealth. The ongoing, and extensive, well-being initiative of the UK Office of National Statistics was another result of this influence (Office of National Statistics, UK, n.d.).

Of course, the classic Brundtland Commission's definition of sustainable development (United Nations, 1987, para 27) makes perfectly clear that its purpose is to protect the interests of future generations while satisfying the needs of our own generation and hence the WFGA is premised on the notion of a well-being duty which considers long-term effects as well as those in the short-term.

The nature and scope of the well-being duty in the WFGA

The well-being duty is relatively straightforward in concept but legally quite complex. Section 3 of WFGA states that:

(1) Each public body must carry out sustainable development.
(2) The action a public body takes in carrying out sustainable development must include:

   (a) Setting and publishing objectives ("well-being objectives") that are designed to maximise its contribution to achieving each of the well-being goals, and
   (b) Taking all reasonable steps (in exercising its functions) to meet those objectives.

Thus, to understand the precise nature of the duty requires the answers to several further questions, the first of these being: what is a public body? These are listed by s.6 of WFGA as:

(a) the Welsh Ministers;
(b) a local authority;
(c) a Local Health Board;
(d) the following NHS Trusts –

   (i) Public Health Wales;
   (ii) Velindre;

(e) a National Park authority for a National Park in Wales;
(f) a Welsh fire and rescue authority;
(g) the Natural Resources Body for Wales;
(h) the Higher Education Funding Council for Wales;
(i) the Arts Council of Wales;
(j) the Sports Council for Wales;
(k) the National Library of Wales; and
(l) the National Museum of Wales.

The statutory guidance issued to guide stakeholders in interpreting the new *Act* (Welsh Government, 2016a, 2016b, 2016c, 2016d) estimates that this list will initially capture 43 public bodies in Wales, though the Welsh Ministers have the power to extend or amend the list at any time by virtue of s.52 WFGA. The list clearly includes all local authorities in Wales and thus affects all elements of public governance at the local level. The list also includes several bodies with national (Welsh) functions and thus also encompasses national governance.

Secondly: what is meant by "carry[ing] out sustainable development"? To answer this one must turn to s.2 WFGA which defines sustainable development as a process of "improving the economic, social, environmental and cultural well-being of Wales by taking action, in accordance with the sustainable development principle (see section 5), aimed at achieving the well-being goals (see section 4)". Unfortunately, this makes reference to two further definitions, which in turn leads to two further questions: what is acting "in accordance with the sustainable development principle" and, what are the well-being goals? It is easiest to deal with these in reverse order.

The well-being goals may be summarised as: a prosperous Wales; a resilient Wales; a healthier Wales; a more equal Wales; a Wales of cohesive communities; a Wales of vibrant culture and thriving Welsh language; a globally responsible Wales (see WFGA, section 4, Table 1 for the full definitions of the goals).

The definition of acting "in accordance with the sustainable development principle", appears in s.5 WFGA, and means that "the [public] body must act in a manner which seeks to ensure that the needs of the present are met without compromising the ability of future generations to meet their own needs". In doing so a public body must take account of:

(a) the importance of balancing short-term needs with the need to safeguard the ability to meet long-term needs, especially where things done to meet short-term needs may have detrimental long-term effect;
(b) the need to take an integrated approach, by considering how–

    (i) the body's well-being objectives may impact upon each of the well-being goals;
    (ii) the body's well-being objectives impact upon each other or upon other public bodies' objectives, in particular where steps taken by the body may contribute to meeting one objective but may be detrimental to meeting another;

(c) the importance of involving other persons with an interest in achieving the well-being goals and of ensuring those persons reflect the diversity of the population of–

    (i) Wales (where the body exercises functions in relation to the whole of Wales), or
    (ii) the part of Wales in relation to which the body exercises functions;

(d) how acting in collaboration with any other person (or how different parts of the body acting together) could assist the body to meet its well-being objectives, or assist another body to meet its objectives; and
(e) how deploying resources to prevent problems occurring or getting worse may contribute to meeting the body's well-being objectives, or another body's objectives.

(WFGA, s.5(2))

However, all the analysis so far derives from section 6, subsection 1. Subsection 2 goes on to indicate how the process of carrying out sustainable development is to be undertaken and it is here that the specific requirements with respect to well-being arise. The requirement is that the relevant public bodies draw up a set of well-being objectives "designed to maximise [the public body's] contribution to achieving each of the well-being goals" and to take "all reasonable steps" to meet those objectives.

Moreover, the duty is exercised at three levels in order to attempt to ensure the integration of efforts across Wales. This has been described extensively elsewhere (Davies, 2016, pp.51–52). As stated each public body has a duty to set well-being objectives and take all reasonable steps to achieve them, but each public body is also a member of a Public Services Board (PSB; see WFGA, ss.29–45; Welsh Government, 2016c) which is formulated locally and made up of a number of public bodies which are also subject to the duty. Each PSB is subject to the well-being duty in its own right (WFGA, s.36). Also, in certain areas local community councils are under a duty to contribute to the PSB's achievement of its duties (WFGA, s.40; Welsh Government, 2016d). Thus, there is a requirement for all public bodies to cooperate with one another in setting objectives and taking steps to achieve them.

Is the well-being duty a legal duty?

The classic view is that a duty enshrined in legislation is always a legal duty precisely because it is enshrined in law and can, in principle, be enforced. This is in contrast to a moral duty, which may be widely observed (or ignored) but does not have the imprimatur of the legislative process and hence cannot be enforced by the courts. Of course, like most classic views this is idealistic and in practice the situation is a good deal more complicated. A duty can be enshrined in law but whether in practice it amounts to a legal duty depends entirely on the mechanisms for enforcement which accompany the measure and the nature of the penalties for non-compliance. There are many duties imposed upon public bodies by legislation but not all of them give rise to corresponding rights for individuals in society, or even classes of individuals, which they can rely on directly and in person, before a court. In many cases the duty is a duty to "try" or "aspire" or "seek to achieve" etc. and does not give rise to an individual right. Often there will be a supervisory body which assesses the extent to which such a duty has been discharged and it will sometimes have regulatory powers which it can exercise to encourage, or even force compliance. However, such a mechanism will seldom result in litigation. Such duties have been described as "political duties" (Wade & Forsyth, 2009, p.499; Reid, 2012, p.754) and are characterised by enforcement by internal political mechanisms rather than by recourse to litigation in the courts or tribunals. Such duties tend have a collective character rather than an individual one (by contrast, for example, with the duty to prevent torture).

Enforcement of the well-being duty in the WFGA, falls to a number of individuals and institutions. The Auditor General for Wales (AGW) is empowered and required (WFGA, s.12) to carry out examinations of public bodies in Wales in respect of their discharge of the well-being duty. However, the AGW's powers of enforcement are limited to laying a report before the Welsh Ministers (Davies, 2016, p.53) and the *Act* and the statutory guidance is silent on what penalties might apply in the event of non-compliance. The *Act* also created the position of the Future Generations Commissioner (FGC) and Sophie Howe was appointed as the first FGC on 3 November 2015. Her role is to act as the "guardian" of the interests of future generations (WFGA, s.18) and to that end the *Act* confers powers to make recommendations to public bodies on the objectives they have set and the steps taken to meet them. However, a public body is not necessarily bound by those recommendations and may depart from them provided that reasons are given. Finally, the performance of PSBs in the discharge of their duty is overseen by local scrutiny committees who may also make recommendations to the PSB. As with the AGW's powers the *Act* is silent on the matter of sanctions which might follow a failure to abide by recommendations given by the FGC or a local scrutiny committee.

Hence the well-being duty is much closer to a "political duty" than a legal one. Nothing in the *Act* itself creates anything even approaching a right for an aggrieved citizen of Wales to take court action to force a failing public body to discharge its duty properly. Such a citizen would of course have recourse to judicial review under the normal principles of public law, since all public bodies charged with the duty are emanations of the state. However, judicial review (JR) is well beyond the means of all but the wealthiest and most determined of citizens. Of course, there is a possibility that the well-being duty could, in certain circumstances, be considered an "environmental matter" and hence may come within the remit of the Aarhus Convention, and thus be amenable to a Protective Costs Order (PCO, see R on the Application of Edwards v The Environment Agency and Others (No. 2) 2013 UKSC 78). This may make JR a more attractive option for individuals and NGOs. However, even this mechanism (where it is in fact considered applicable) would only cover costs at first instance under the Civil Procedure Rules.

On the other hand, political duties such as this are not without effect and most such duties in other areas of the law (such as welfare law) are, in general, diligently observed by the bodies subject to them and the mechanisms of accountability within local and national government can be highly effective in ensuring that public duties are discharged (the public sector equality duty is a good example, albeit one that does have a more robust system of penalties for failure, see ss.1 and ss.149 of the *Equality Act 2010*). Internal scrutiny bodies and the Public Services Ombudsman for Wales (PSOW) have an overarching remit and may contribute to the enforcement of this duty beyond the explicit mechanism built into the WFGA itself (though even the PSOW's recommendations do not *have* to be followed). However, these institutions have a vast additional remit and it is open to question whether they have the capacity to make a significant contribution to this new duty. Having said that, the recommendations of Commissioners and Ombudsmen in the UK are usually followed by the public bodies to whom they are addressed, though ultimately the decision-makers discretion receives considerable deference by the courts (see Davies, 2017).

However, it is clear that the enforcement mechanisms accompanying this important and ground-breaking duty are not as transparent and as public-facing as they might have been and the rigorous enforcement of the duty will be dependent on political will to an extent which is larger than for other important public sector duties such as those related to discrimination.

Conclusion

It is early days for the WFGA and it remains to be seen whether the efforts of the public bodies in Wales do indeed result in more robust protection for the well-being of future generations (see City and County of Swansea, 2015). The FGC has already demonstrated her willingness to take on vested interests in Wales and to publicise what she considers their lack of consideration for the interests of future generations in the context of the controversial proposed M4 relief bypass which is due to pass to the south of Newport in South Wales; a scheme that is likely to compromise considerably the wetland habitat in that part of the Gwent levels (see Davies, 2017). Whatever the long-term success of this legislation we should not under-estimate the achievement of the Welsh Government in promulgating legislation which attempts to protect the well-being of those generations as yet unborn. As discussed earlier, the question of creating rights and associated duties for non-legal and non-existent entities has been the source of intense academic debate for many years (Brown-Weiss, 1992; Westra, 2008; Hiskes, 2009; Lawrence, 2014) and the Welsh Government is one of very few that has been able to turn academic theorising into reality in recognising that a duty can indeed be created without a right provided that individuals and institutions are created to ensure that the duty is discharged on behalf of those who cannot speak for themselves. It is true that this measure does not create any individual rights for anyone (not even existing citizens) over and above those already available in administrative and public law, but nevertheless public bodies are now constrained to take a much longer view of public governance than was the case previously. The Welsh

Government is also to be commended for basing this legislation on the concept of measurable well-being objectives as a proxy for sustainable development. The legislation is drafted such that the setting of objectives is perforce part of a nation-wide initiative to achieve national well-being goals and the use of Public Service Boards should ensure that authorities do not undermine one another's efforts in setting their goals and taking all reasonable steps to meeting them. This is a fine example of how to coordinate local action with national target setting. Some misgivings have been expressed about the resources that the Welsh Government have been able to devote to this initiative and in particular the budget of the FGC (see Davies, 2017). We can only hope that that this is the first of many such initiatives aimed at improving the well-being both of ourselves and our descendants and that the expressed hope of Nihkil Seth (Director of the Division for Sustainable Development, Department of Economic and Social Affairs at the United Nations), that "What Wales is doing today the world will do tomorrow", is realised (Future Generation Commissioner, 2016).

References

Brown-Weiss, E. (1992) In fairness to future generations and sustainable development, *American University International Law Review* 8 (1): 19–26.

Campbell, D. & Thomas P. (2001) (eds.) *Fundamental Legal Conceptions as Applied in Judicial Reasoning by Wesley Newcomb Hohfeld*, Classical Jurisprudence Series, London: Dartmouth Publishing Company.

City and County of Swansea (2015) The one Swansea plan place, people, challenges and change, Swansea local service board 2015 update. Available at file:///C:/Users/id009833/Downloads/The_One_Swansea_Plan_2015_final_version_august.pdf, last accessed 23 June 2016.

Davies, H. (2013) The Wales Sustainable Development Bill, *Environmental Law and Management* 25: 99–105.

Davies, H. (2016) The Well-being of Future Generations (Wales) Act 2015: Duties or aspirations? *Environmental Law Review* 18: 41–56.

Davies, H. (2017) The Well-being of Future Generations (Wales) Act 2015 – a step change in the legal protection of the interests of future generations? *Journal of Environmental Law* 29 (1): 165–175.

Future Generation Commissioner (2015) The Wales we want. Available at www.thewaleswewant.co.uk/blog/wales-we-want/%E2%80%9Cwhat-wales-doing-today-world-will-do-tomorrow%E2%80%9D-%E2%80%93-united-nations>, last accessed 23 November 2016.

Glendon, M. (1991) *Rights Talk: The Impoverishment of Political Discourse*, New York: Free Press.

Hiskes, R. (2009) *The Human Right to a Green Future*, Cambridge: Cambridge University Press.

Hohfeld W. N. (1913) Some fundamental legal conceptions as applied in legal reasoning, *23 Yale Law Journal* 16.

Hohfeld W. N. (1917) Fundamental Legal Conceptions as Applied to Judicial Reasoning, *26 Yale Law Journal* 710.

Kant, I. (1785) *Groundwork of the Metaphysics of Morals*, H. J. Paton (trans.), New York: Harper & Row, 1964.

Kant I. (1788) *Critique of Practical Reason*, L. White Beck (trans.), Indianapolis: Bobbs-Merrill Co., 1956.

Lawrence, P. (2014) *Justice for Future Generations, Climate Change and International Law*, Cheltenham: Edward Elgar.

Nussbaum, M. C. (2006) *Frontiers of Justice: Disability, Nationality, Species Membership*, Harvard: Harvard University Press.

Office of National Statistics, UK (n.d.) Well-being metrics web pages. Available at www.ons.gov.uk/peoplepopulationandcommunity/wellbeing.

Quinn, W. (1993) *Morality and Action*, Cambridge: Cambridge University Press.

Rawls, J. (1971) *A Theory of Justice*, Harvard: Harvard University Press (revised edition, 1999).

Reid, C. (2012) A new sort of duty? The significance of "outcome" duties in the climate change and child poverty Acts, *Public Law* October 2012: 749–767.

Selznick, P. (1987) The idea of a communitarian morality, *California Law Review* 75 (1): 445–463. Available at http://scholarship.law.berkley.edu/californialawreview/vol75/iss1/19.

Sen, A. (2009) *The Idea of Justice*, Cambridge, MA: Belnap Press of Harvard University Press.

Stiglitz, J. E., Sen, A. & Fitoussi, J. P. (2009) *Report by the Commission on the Measurement of Economic Performance and Social Progress. Technical Report September 2009.* Available at www.stiglitz-sen-fitoussi.fr (original in French), last accessed 23 June 2016.

Wade, H. W. R. & Forsyth, C. F. (2014) *Administrative Law*, 11th edition, Oxford: Oxford University Press.

Welsh Government (2009) *One Wales, One Planet.* Available at http://gov.wales/docs/desh/publications/090521susdev1wales1planeten.pdf, last accessed 23 June 2016.

Welsh Government (2012a) *Welsh Government 15440, Proposals for a Sustainable Development Bill.* Available at http://wales.gov.uk/docs/desh/consultation/120508susdevbillconsulten.pdf, last accessed 23 June 2016.

Welsh Government (2012b) *WG17030 A Sustainable Wales Better Choices for a Better Future.* Available at http://gov.wales/docs/desh/consultation/121203asusdevwhitepaperen.pdf, last accessed 23 June 2016.

Welsh Government (2016a) *WG27394, Shared Purpose, Shared Future. Statutory Guidance on the Well-being of Future generations (Wales) Act 2015. SPF1: Core Guidance.*

Welsh Government (2016b) *WG27394, Shared Purpose, Shared Future. Statutory Guidance on the Well-being of Future generations (Wales) Act 2015. SPF2: Individual Role (Public Bodies).*

Welsh Government (2016c) *WG27394, Shared Purpose, Shared Future. Statutory Guidance on the Well-being of Future generations (Wales) Act 2015. SPF3: Collective Role (Public Service Boards).*

Welsh Government (2016d) *WG27394, Shared Purpose, Shared Future. Statutory Guidance on the Well-being of Future generations (Wales) Act 2015. SPF4: Collective Role (Community Councils).*

Wenar, L. (2015) Rights, in *Stanford Encyclopedia of Philosophy*. Available at https://plato.stanford.edu/entries/rights/.

Westra, L. (2008) *Environmental Justice and the Rights of Unborn and Future Generations: Law, Environmental Harm and the Right to Health*, London: Routledge.

United Nations (1987) *Report of the World Commission on Environment and Development, Our Common Future. A/42/427 (The Brundtland Report).* Available at www.un-documents.net/our-common-future.pdf.

Table of statutes

Government of Wales Act 1998, ch.38.
Government of Wales Act 2006, ch. 32.
Well-Being of Future Generations (Wales) Act 2015 anaw 2.

Table of statutory instruments

Well-Being of Future Generation (Wales) Act (Commencement No. 2) Order, 2016 No. 86 (W. 40) (C. 8).

9

WELL-BEING RESTORATION IN THE WORKSPACE

Sukanlaya Sawang and Mirko Guaralda

Introduction

Modern workplaces often have an open-plan office design, clear glass offices or even "superdesks" – one huge, continuous single desk for all staff – designed in order to stimulate communication and ideas among employees. While the benefits of an open-plan workspace are present, individuals no longer have a private space to take their timeout. This chapter examines the positive and negative impacts of open-plan office on employees and explores a proof of concept design remedy for well-being restoration in the workspace.

Perceptions of an open-plan workspace

There has been wide and thorough study of the benefits, and pitfalls of open-plan offices. When first developed, the American open-plan represented a radical reimagining of office space (Kaufmann-Buhler, 2016). Architects and designers of the late 1960s promoted the open-plan office as a spatial solution to the problems of contemporary organisations; in particular, it marked the rejection of bureaucratic and hierarchical conventional post-war corporations. These were abandoned in favour of a more "organic" organisational culture that reduced the conventional symbols of status and hierarchy and fostered communication, collaboration and worker autonomy. These sentiments are echoed by employers of today, as the office design is seen to dismantle barriers between management and staff by doing away with individual offices (Waber, Magnolfi & Lindsay, 2014). Open-plan office layout is commonly assumed to facilitate communication and interaction between co-workers, promoting workplace satisfaction and team-work effectiveness (Kim & de Dear, 2013). Open-plan offices can vary in size from small open-plan offices, for two or three employees, to large spaces where over a hundred persons work (Bergström, Miller & Horneij, 2015).

Although open-plan offices intend to facilitate positive work habits and culture, many scholars find that the negative effects of these office designs outweigh the positive. For example, Begström et al.'s (2015) study of employees shifting from individual offices to working in open-plan offices showed that perceived health, work environment and self-estimated productivity decreased during the 12-month period after relocation. Hedge's (1982) study found that loss of privacy and increased disturbances were consistently the source of negative reactions to open-plan offices. Hedge found that although the office did create a favourable social climate, this did not offset employees' negative reactions to work conditions but rather appeared to exacerbate the problems. Kim and de Dear's (2013) study echoes the notion that the positive effects do not offset the negative. They found that enclosed private offices clearly outperformed open-plan layouts in most aspects of indoor environmental quality, particularly in acoustics, privacy and the proxemics issues. The benefits of enhanced "ease of interaction" were found to be smaller than the penalties of increased noise level and decreased privacy resulting from open-plan office configuration. Another study of the opportunities and challenges of the modern workplace found that the ability to focus without interruption is a top priority for employees when it comes to office design (Oxford Economics, 2016). This study found that nearly two-thirds of executives say employees are equipped with the tools they need to deal with distractions at work, and less than half of employees agree.

Rasila and Rothe's (2012) paper provides a different insight. Their findings suggest that "generation Y" employees in fact liked their open-plan office. They acknowledged most of the issues or problems that past literature suggests, but they did not necessarily see these purely in a negative way. Instead, they often perceived these issues as fair trade-offs for some greater good. This suggests that a change in office design may not increase the net benefits enjoyed by employees, and perhaps an investigation into new ways to mitigate the negative effects of open-plan offices is needed.

Factors influencing mental well-being in an open-plan workspace

The increasingly recurrent open-plan design of modern workplaces leads to a lack of privacy and provides limited opportunities for individuals to find spaces for refocusing. Open-plan offices can thus impact one's performance due to long-term exposure to external noises, aggressive conversation or frequent interruption by others. The purpose of this section is to explore well-being in the context of open-plan workplaces from an environmental interaction point of view through a trans-disciplinary approach.

Sense of being away

Exposure to natural environments and settings proves to successfully mitigate mental fatigue and promote restoration (Jahncke et al., 2011). Natural environments are rich in the characteristics necessary for restorative experiences. One characteristic that is of particular importance is "being away". Natural settings are often the preferred destinations for extended restorative opportunities. The seaside, the mountains, lakes, streams, forests and meadows are all idyllic places for "getting away" (Kaplan, 2001). Attentional fatigue increases preference for the natural over the urban environment (Staats & Hartig, 2004). It is therefore not surprising that stress recovery is faster and more complete when people are exposed to natural rather than urban environments (Ulrich et al., 1991). Berto's (2005) study found that only participants exposed to restorative environments – as opposed to non-restorative environments or geometrical patterns – improved their performance on a final attention test.

The sense of being away does not require that the setting be distant (Kaplan, 1995), additionally, regular access to restorative environments can interrupt processes that negatively affect health and well-being in the short and long-term (Hartig et al., 2003). Jahncke et al. (2011) aimed to mitigate the negative effects of open-plan offices by studying the effects of short restoration periods in open-plan offices. Four treatments were run during the restoration periods: the participants were exposed to a river movie with sound, only river sound, silence and office noise. The participants who saw a movie of a flowing river with corresponding sound reported having more energy compared to the participants who just listened to river sounds, or those who continued to listen to office noise. The participants who listened to office noise during the restoration phase also experienced themselves to be less motivated after this period, compared to the participants who listened to river sounds, and those who saw the nature movie with river sounds. This suggests that restoration periods guided by natural stimuli may be able to mitigate some of the negative effects of open-plan offices. A similar approach was conducted in Sitzer's (2013) study, where clinical staff were exposed to a "rejuvenation room" for 10-minute periods in an attempt to reduce work stress. It was found that sitting for 10 minutes in a simple room with a nature scene, sounds of nature, subdued lighting and a comfortable setting can be effective in reducing subjective work stress in clinical staff. Sitzer suggests that this low cost, high impact room is a strategy employers should consider implementing to rejuvenate their staff.

Colour and light

Colour and light are also significant variables in the promotion of mental restoration. The sense of being away is strongly related to the perceived colour quality of light. Being away is also related to the perceived pleasantness and safety of the lighting environment (Nikunen et al., 2014). In the case of hospital workers, staff require privacy and security in their rest areas even for only a few minutes. A room which is visually different in the colour and lighting levels from their workstations can be most reviving (Dalke et al., 2006). Several scholars agree that exposure to blue or green lighting is most effective in regard to promoting relaxation (Rodrigues & Deuskar, 2016). There are also strong arguments for colours such as white and yellow as effective promoters of relaxation and mental restoration (Klotsche, 1993). Some sources agree that violet and purple also promote well-being (Sembian & Aathi, 2015). However, a study by Rodrigues and Deuskar (2016) shows that violet did not increase relaxation significantly when being used in a meditation environment. Additionally, Nourse and Welch's (1971) study found that galvanic skin response (GSR) was greater to violet than to green – meaning violet proved to be more arousing than green.

Sound

Music, in conjunction with imagery, has proven successful in mitigating work-related stress (Beck, Hansen & Gold, 2015). Listening to music has the ability to promote relaxation and relieve stress and anxiety (Jiang, Rickson & Jiang, 2016) and can be considered a means of stress reduction in daily life (Linnemann et al., 2015). Smith (2008) encourages the use of music relaxation to decrease anxiety levels in occupational environments.

Music's power in everyday use contributes to a heightened and renewed form of agency, which is achieved through the connections that music and musicking (Small, 1999) may afford, and as means of enhancing health and well-being such as: feelings of self-recovery, self-confidence, ice breaking, bridge building, self-efficacy, self-change, pleasure, connection to others; effects of calming, inspiring, motivating, comforting, relaxing, "moving" pain and suffering, triggering memory; provision of vitality, happiness, joy, emotional outlet, energy, relief, strength, wholeness in body/mind, self-stability, coping mechanism, sense of being alive and hope (Batt-Rawden, 2010). Krout (2007) explains the importance of self-selected music for relaxation purposes. The most important factor in reducing stress was the degree of liking for the music, but not the degree of familiarity with the music (Jiang et al., 2016).

Krout (2007) stipulates a time frame of 20–30 minutes of exposure to music as a good time length for a relaxation experience. Krout also notes key musical elements that promote relaxation, such as slow and stable tempo (pace or speed), low volume level and soft dynamics, consistent texture (combination of sounds and instruments), absence of percussive and accented rhythms, gentle timbre (sound or tone colour), legato (connected) melodies, and simple harmonic or chord progressions. Ten minutes of music listening can positively affect the mood of workers (Lesiuk et al., 2012), but does not significantly increase work performance.

Technology

The use of technology to promote well-being and relaxation has been successful in a number of cases (e.g. Stetz et al., 2011; Millegan et al., 2015). Stetz et al.'s (2011) study showed that short amounts of exposure time to virtual reality (VR) relaxation stimuli (three seven-minute-long videos) contributed to lower levels of anxiety. Relaxation training using a combination of VR and MP3 players was effective in improving perceived self-efficacy in eating control, as well as in decreasing depressive symptoms, anxiety and physiological arousal (Manzoni et al., 2008). While Manzoni et al. (2008) found the combination of media to be effective, Villani et al. (2007) found that VR stimulus was more supportive as a relaxation tool compared to DVDs and audio tapes, and highlighted the importance of the "sense of presence" in relaxation stimuli.

Promoting relaxation through touch has been recently been explored (Millegan et al., 2015; Yu et al., 2015). The use of iPads and touch tablets have been found to be an effective mediation tool (Millegan et al., 2015). Yu et al.'s (2015) study explored a tactile interface of a breathing assistance system by using a shape-changing airbag. The results showed that for most participants, the overall heart rate variability (HRV) was improved after breathing training. Moreover, "breathe with touch" brought users better satisfaction during the exercise. However, there was no significant reduction of stress level during a post-training mathematics task. This may be due to it being the participant's first time use of the assistance system; the unfamiliarity with the system brings about new stresses. There were also reservations about the acute effect of 10-minute breathing exercises on stress reduction. These studies suggests that technology using tactile interfaces has the potential to reduce stress, but further study is needed.

While technology has the potential to decrease stress, it has also proved to have adverse effects in the case of internet and social media access (Sagioglou & Greitemeyer, 2014; Fox & Moreland, 2015). Sagioglou and Greitemeyer (2014) found that the longer people are active on Facebook, the more negative is their mood afterwards, and it was demonstrated that this effect is mediated by a feeling of not having done anything meaningful. Contrastingly, Choi and Lim's (2016) study found that social and information technology overload did not exert a direct impact on psychological well-being. However, well-being may not be an accurate indicator of reduced stress and anxiety. Graham and Nikolova's (2013) study found that technology access is positive for well-being in general, but with diminishing marginal returns for those who already have much access. Moreover, signs of increased stress and anger were found among cohorts for whom access to the technologies is new. For example, well-being levels are higher in the countries with higher levels of access to mobile banking, but so are stress and anger. While technology raises aggregate levels of well-being in the long run, high levels of frustration often accompany the process.

A case study: the Aerie (a proof of concept)

Ways to change the approach to open-plan office design have been recently explored, especially in creative enlivenments. When first published, images of the new Google or Miramax offices were considered revolutionary in terms of their colourful and playful approach (Zhang & Guo, 2012). These experimentations still suggest an approach where all workers have to conform to the same environment, although sometimes providing them with a choice of setting. Personal space is still considered a pricey commodity in current work environments and especially the possibility to fully customise one's own experience in the workplace.

The Aerie aims to provide a personal and portable space for mental restoration, which can be situated seamlessly in an open-plan environment (Sawang et al., 2016, see Figure 9.1). The Aerie can be seen as a personal sanctuary, a place to gather thoughts and rejuvenate one's mind; it is meant to be a customisable setting for office workers to unwind and recharge. Kaplan posits "that the sense of being away does not require that the setting be distant and that alternative solutions can be achieved in localized natural environments" (Kaplan, 1995, p.174). Meditation can be seen as a form of "being away", but generally it is not possible to remove oneself from a busy work environment to refocus. The settings of regenerative environments are really important and the most effective regenerative experiences happen when a number of senses are engaged. In order to develop a preliminary concept for the Aerie, different sensory experiences have been selected on the basis of current literature as well as on how practical and realistic developing an intervention affecting specific sensory experiences would be. Different senses are engaged through specific tactics discussed in the literature and provide a positive impact on one's well-being. The approach to each sense in the Aerie is limited in its discussion and focused on the actual production of a working prototype.

Human senses and cognitive experiences: design frameworks for the Aerie

There are five human senses traditionally recognised: sight (ophthalmoception), hearing (audioception), taste (gustaoception), smell (olfacoception or olfacception) and touch (tactioception). Individuals' everyday experience is also influenced by other senses commonly not directly considered; there is debate on the actual number of human senses and their characteristics, but generally researchers also recognise balance (equilibrioception), temperature (thermoception), kinaesthetic sense (proprioception), pain (nociception) and time (chronoception).

When individuals experience these sensory modalities, they treat these stimuli at affective and cognitive levels. At cognitive level, individuals interpret a situation/object based on its semantic and aesthetic qualities (Hassenzahl, 2004). At the affect level, individuals associate stimuli with core affect – neurophysiological state consciously accessible as the simplest raw (non-reflective) feelings evident in moods and emotions (Russell, 2003). How can we integrate sensory modalities to design a compact space within an open-plan environment? Current devices to improve well-being are generally based on stimulating a limited number of human senses; engaging all senses to provide a comprehensive experience is technically quite complicated, but our study aims to develop a prototype catering for the majority of the senses, just excluding taste and pain. In addition to sensory experience, the Aerie also aims to add a psychological experience providing supports for psychological development.

Ophthalmoception through the use of colour and lighting

Colour is a stimulus for our vision which can influence our emotion and feelings (Terwogt & Hoeksma, 1995). Positive emotions, such as happiness, can be associated with light colours (e.g. yellow or blue), and negative emotions, such as anger, can be associated with darker colours (e.g. black or grey) (Boyatzis & Varghese, 1994; Hemphill, 1996). Some specific emotions can also be associated with specific colours, for example, red is associated with excitement, orange is linked to distressing and upsetting, purple has been perceived as dignified and stately and yellow is referred to as cheerful (Ballast, 2002; Stone & English, 1998). Colour can also be associated with temperature based on it wavelength, for example, blue, green and purple are perceived as cool colours, while red, yellow and orange are seen as warm colours (Ballast, 2002). Research also indicates how there is a sensory difference in experiencing a colour as a finish for a surface or in terms of light. For example, blue and purple finishes generally foster relaxation, but blue and purple lights work as stimulating triggers.

Colour in the Aerie can be achieved directly with the use of finishes and materials, this would provide a static environment, but also a neutral setting that can then be customised with different light settings. The latter option is easily achievable with the use of LED lights for example and would provide a more flexible environment tailored for different users.

Audioception through the use of sound

Sound stimulation can generate unpleasant feelings (e.g. noise from an open space). A recent experimental study found that nature-based sound, a mixture of sounds from a fountain and tweeting birds at 50 dB facilitates recovery from sympathetic activation after a psychological stressor (Alvarsson, Wiens & Nilsson, 2010). Soundproofing a space to provide privacy and relaxation can be challenging; the design of the Aerie has to balance the performance of the interior space with a compact design deployable in a variety of settings. Total soundproofing might not be achievable in a limited compact space, so in order to provide a suitable sensory experience to users, the use of headphones would seem a practical solution, but this then opens issues of hygiene. Speakers incorporated in the design of sitting arrangement could provide a similar performance directing sound in a specific area and isolating the user from the broader context. A selection of background natural sounds like rain or the sound of a stream can be provided and customised as a preferred, background, natural white noise.

Olfacoception through the use of aroma therapy

Aromatherapy is the use of essential oils extracted from plants for the treatment of physical and psychological health (Herz, 2009). Drawing from pharmacological literature, inhaling essential oils can interact with and affect the autonomic nervous system/central nervous system and/or endocrine systems. Therefore, the smell can influence individuals' mood, which then can affect one's behaviour. For example, people who worked in the presence of a pleasant ambient odour reported higher self-efficacy, set higher goals and were more likely to employ efficient work strategies than participants who worked in a no-odour condition (Baron, 1997; Herz, 2009).

The essential oil of lavender (*Lavendula angustifolia*) consists of linalyl acetate, β-linalool and β-caryophyllene (Motomura, Sakurai & Yotsuya, 2001; Sayorwan et al., 2012). Lavender oil is known as antibacterial, antifungal, carminative (smooth muscle relaxant), sedative, antidepressant, promoting wound healing (and increasing the detoxification of enzymes associated with insecticide resistance), (Sayorwan et al., 2012). Recent studies confirm the sedative and relaxation effects (Diego et al., 1998). For example, Motomura, Sakurai & Yotsuya (2001) found that exposure to lavender oil decreases stress scores, increases Theta 1 (3.5–5.5Hz) brain wave activity and decreases Beta1 (13.5–20 Hz) which is associated with relaxation. Tongnit et al. (2004) found a significantly decreased blood pressure, heart rate and respiratory rate caused by 3 minutes inhalation of lavender essential oils. A recent study also shows that individuals who inhaled lavender oil reported feeling more active, fresher and relaxed than those who just inhaled base oil (Sayorwan et al., 2012). Our study thus proposes the use of lavender oil inside the Aerie to promote the positive mood for users.

Tactioception through the use of sitting materials

Tactile experience is really important in addressing the materiality of the Aerie. Different finishes can also affect perception in terms of visual experience; natural materials and finishes are generally perceived as more warm and inviting, while smooth finishes and synthetic materials are more often associated with more corporate, formal or clinical environments. Sitting arrangements for the Aerie will have to consider questions of ergonomics, but the actual finishes and materiality of sitting arrangements are important. Materials that allow a certain level of customisation, like foam mattresses or bean bags, can provide a more cosy experience to users that would feel cocooned and protected by soft adaptable surfaces (Siriphorn, Chamonchant & Boonyong, 2016).

Thermoception through the use of room temperature

Thermal comfort mainly depends on two variables: temperature and humidity (Peters et al., 2010). A sophisticated control of these two parameters can be challenging because, although there are ranges recognised as ideal for the majority of people, personal preferences and physiological conditions would impact what is perceived as ideal by different users. Substantial changes between the temperature inside the Aerie and the general surroundings might also have an impact on the body and produce unpleasant experiences while entering or leaving the structure (Shephard & Aoyagi, 2009). Slight changes in temperature while experiencing the Aerie could improve the effectiveness of the installation in providing a rejuvenating environment. Rather than adopting a fixed temperature, the Aerie would need to link the ambient temperature to the actual relaxation exercises users are engaging with (Weinert & Waterhouse, 2007).

Proprioception through progressive muscle relaxation

The word kinesthesia is defined by a dictionary as the sense that detects bodily position, weight, or movement of the muscles, tendons and joints. Kinesthetic sense can be developed through the movement of muscles such as stretching. The stretch-based relaxation approach provides a reasonable alternative to traditional progressive relaxation training procedures, including a 15-second period of muscle stretching followed by a 60-second period of relaxation (Carlson & Curran, 1994). Our study proposes an audio-guided stretching exercise for users to restore their mental and well-being as well as sitting arrangements that foster awareness in body posture.

Psychological components

An intervention with a strong evidence base that has been used extensively to reduce psychological distress is mindfulness-based stress reduction (MBSR). Drawing from Buddhist meditation practices, MBSR is designed for personal development in teaching oneself to be mindful and appreciative of the current moments through mindfulness meditation (Kabat-Zinn, 1982). MBSR can facilitate reduced stress reactivity and resilience in "at-risk stressed workplaces" (e.g. long-term exposure to open-plan environmental stressors). Traditional MBSR training consists of 26 hours of session time including 8 classes of 2.5 hours and an all-day class (Carmody & Baer, 2009). However, recent studies show that a brief pre-recorded audio mindfulness intervention, such as 10-min audio track that contained a guided, mindfulness meditation, can be efficacious (see, for example, Cavanagh et al., 2013, Morledge et al., 2013). Our study proposes to include the brief audio-guided mindfulness mediation in the Aerie as an option for users for mental restoration and well-being recovery.

Drawing from the literature, we propose that that for individuals to recover from daily stressors, especially from an open-plan workspace, a sense of being away, both physically and psychologically will stimulate mental restoration. The restorative environment can be small or vast, but the large spaces are often too overwhelming for humans to comprehend and small spaces of intimacy are preferred (Aben & de Wit, 1999). Office spaces are usually limited in size and therefore the design of Aerie should be compact but comfortable with a sense of being away (Figures 9.1 & 9.2).

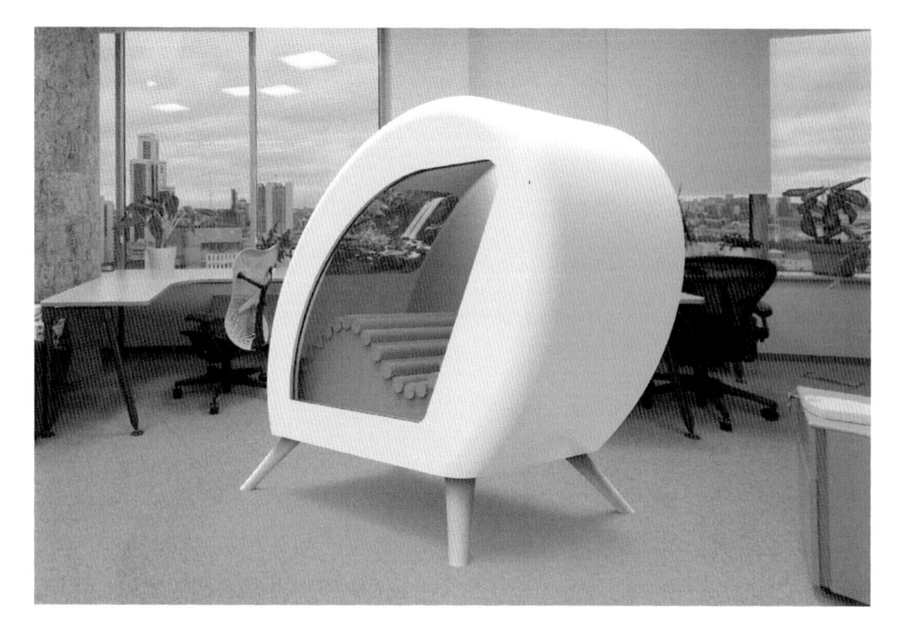

FIGURE 9.1 The Aerie – a concept (© Sukanlaya Sawang)

Conclusion

While the intention of open-plan offices was to encourage more interactive and collaborative work efforts, the design is seen to cause workplace stress resulting from distraction and lack of privacy. However, a complete redesign of office space is not necessarily a feasible or desirable option, some workers are not necessarily opposed to the working environment, and see the negative effects as a reasonable trade-off. More research is needed regarding the best means of offsetting these negative effects while maintaining the open-plan design. In developing the concept for a personal sanctuary that users can customise, it was evident that only some senses could be affected and controlled from a practical point of view. Some experiential variables are in fact easier to manipulate, for example light and sound. Other variables can only be set in the production phase of a personal environment, such as finishes and ergonomics of seating, but also choice of odours to include. Temperature can be hard to effectively customise outside a fully enclosed environment. Technology can aid in the creation of a personal sanctuary, but it can also be distractive as discussed by Graham and Nikolova's study (2013). More research is needed, not only in terms of the potential physical design of a personal customisable sanctuary, but also in the psychological engagement of its potential participants and how active meditation could enhance or make more effective the sensorial experience provided.

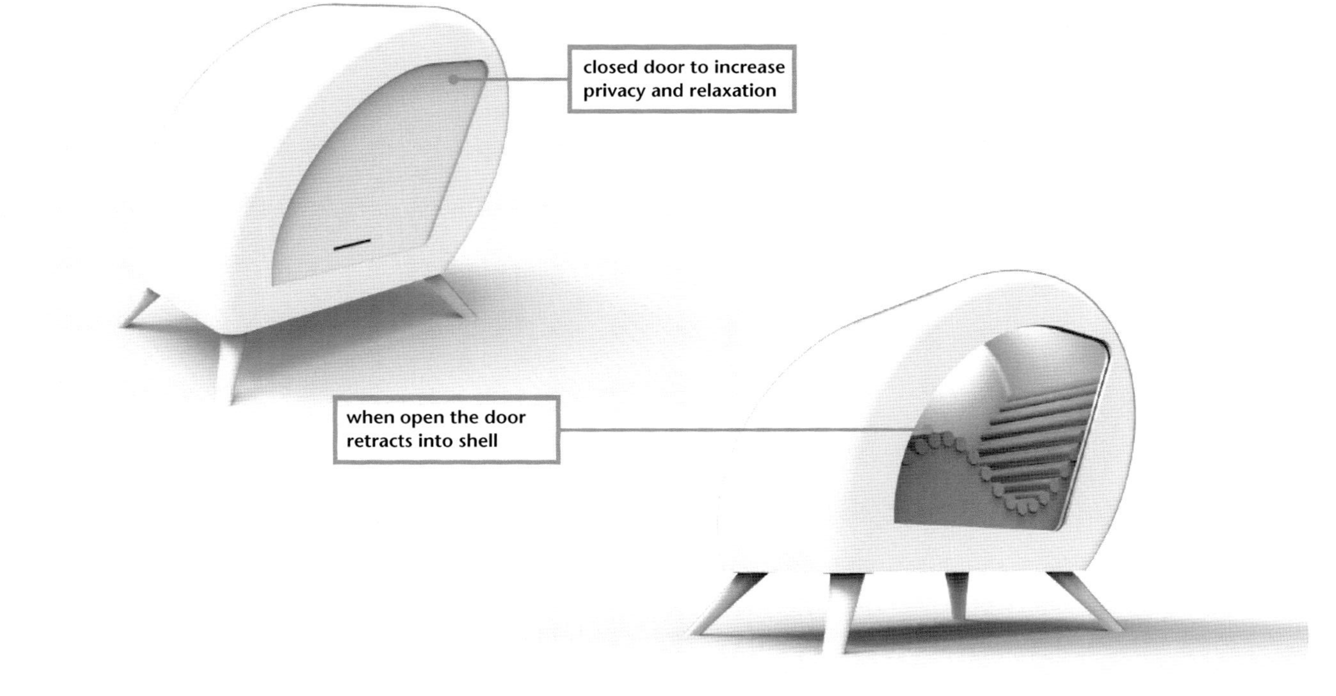

FIGURE 9.2 The Aerie proposed features (© Sukanlaya Sawang)

Acknowledgements

The project is funded by the QUT Engagement and Innovation Grant, led by the first author. The multidisciplinary team members are Dr Mirko Guaralda, Dr Marianella Chamorro-Koc, Dr Veronica Garcia Hansen, Dr Richard Medland and Dr Nigar Khawaja.

References

Aben, R, & Wit, S. D. (1999) *The Enclosed Garden: History and Development of the Hortus Conclusus and its Reintroduction into the Present Day Urban Landscape*, Rotterdam: 010 Publishers.

Alvarsson, J. J., Wiens, S. & Nilsson, M. E. (2010) Stress recovery during exposure to nature sound and environmental noise, *International Journal of Environmental Research and Public Health* 7 (3): 1036–1046.

Ballast, D. K. (2002) *Interior Design Reference Manual*, Belmont, CA: Professional Publisher Inc.

Baron, R. A. (1997) The sweet smell of . . . helping: effects of pleasant ambient fragrance on prosocial behavior in shopping malls, *Personality and Social Psychology Bulletin* 23: 498–503.

Batt-Rawden, K. B. (2010) The benefits of self-selected music on health and well-being, *The Arts in Psychotherapy* 37 (4): 301–310.

Beck, B. D., Hansen, Å. M. & Gold, C. (2015) Coping with work-related stress through guided imagery and music (GIM): Randomized controlled trial, *Journal of Music Therapy* 52 (3): 323–352.

Bergström, J., Miller, M. & Horneij, E. (2015) Work environment perceptions following relocation to open-plan offices: a twelve-month longitudinal study, *Work* 50 (2): 221–228.

Berto, R. (2005) Exposure to restorative environments helps restore attentional capacity, *Journal of Environmental Psychology* 25 (3): 249–259.

Boyatzis, C. J. & Varghese, R. (1994) Children's emotional associations with colors, *The Journal of Genetic Psychology* 155 (1): 77–85.

Carlson, C. R. & Curran, S. L. (1994) Stretch-based relaxation training, *Patient Education and Counseling* 23 (4): 5–12.

Carmody, J. & Baer, R. A. (2009) How long does a mindfulness-based stress reduction program need to be? A review of class contact hours and effect sizes for psychological distress, *Journal of Clinical Psychology* 65 (6): 627–638. Available at doi: 10.1002/jclp.20555.

Cavanagh, K., Strauss, C., Cicconi, F., Griffiths, N., Wyper, A. & Jones, F. (2013) A randomized controlled trial of a brief online mindfulness-based intervention, *Behaviour Research and Therapy* 51 (9): 573–578.

Choi, S. B., & Lim, M. S. (2016) Effects of social and technology overload on psychological well-being in young South Korean adults: the mediatory role of social network service addiction, *Computers in Human Behavior* 61 (August): 245–254.

Dalke, H., Little, J., Niemann, E., Camgoz, N., Steadman, G., Hill, S. & Stott, L. (2006) Colour and lighting in hospital design, *Optics & Laser Technology* 38 (4): 343–365.

Diego, M. A., Jones, N. A., Field, T., Hernandez-Reif, M., Schanberg, S., Kuhn, C. & Galamaga, R. (1998) Aromatherapy positively affects mood, EEG patterns of alertness and math computations, *International Journal of Neuroscience* 96 (3–4): 217–224.

Fox, J. & Moreland, J. J. (2015) The dark side of social networking sites: An exploration of the relational and psychological stressors associated with Facebook use and affordances, *Computers in Human Behavior* 45 (April): 168–176.

Graham, C. & Nikolova, M. (2013) Does access to information technology make people happier? Insights from well-being surveys from around the world, *The Journal of Socio-Economics* 44 (June): 126–139.

Hartig, T., Evans, G. W., Jamner, L. D., Davis, D. S. & Gärling, T. (2003) Tracking restoration in natural and urban field settings, *Journal of Environmental Psychology* 23 (2): 109–123.

Hassenzahl, M. (2004) The interplay of beauty, goodness, and usability in interactive products, *Human-Computer Interaction* 19 (4): 319–349.

Hedge, A. (1982) The open-plan office: A systematic investigation of employee reactions to their work environment, *Environment and Behavior* 14 (5): 519–542.

Hemphill, M. (1996) A note on adults' color – emotion associations, *The Journal of Genetic Psychology* 157 (3): 275–280.

Herz, R. S. (2009) Aromatherapy facts and fictions: a scientific analysis of olfactory effects on mood, physiology and behaviour, *International Journal of Neuroscience* 119 (2): 263–290.

Jahncke, H., Hygge, S., Halin, N., Green, A. M. & Dimberg, K. (2011) Open-plan office noise: cognitive performance and restoration, *Journal of Environmental Psychology* 31 (4): 373–382.

Jiang, J., Rickson, D. & Jiang, C. (2016) The mechanism of music for reducing psychological stress: Music preference as a mediator, *The Arts in Psychotherapy* 48: 62–68.

Kabat-Zinn, J. (1982) An outpatient program in behavioral medicine for chronic pain patients based on the practice of mindfulness meditation: theoretical considerations and preliminary results, *General Hospital Psychiatry* 4 (1): 33–47.

Kaplan, S. (2001) Meditation, restoration, and the management of mental fatigue, *Environment and Behavior* 33 (4): 480–506.

Kaufmann-Buhler, J. (2016) Progressive partitions: the promises and problems of the American open plan office, *Design and Culture* 8 (2): 205–233.

Kim, J. & de Dear, R. (2013) Workspace satisfaction: The privacy-communication trade-off in open-plan offices, *Journal of Environmental Psychology* 36 (December): 18–26.

Klotsche, C. (1993) *Color Medicine: The Secrets of Color Vibrational Healing*, Flagstaff, AZ: Light Technology Publishing.

Krout, R. E. (2007) Music listening to facilitate relaxation and promote wellness: integrated aspects of our neurophysiological responses to music, *The Arts in Psychotherapy* 34 (2): 134–141.

Lesiuk, T., Polak, P., Stutz, J. & Hummer, M. (2012) The effect of music listening, personality, and prior knowledge on mood and work performance of systems analysts, in R. Colomo-Palacios (ed.), *Enhancing the Modern Organization through Information Technology Professionals: Research, Studies, and Techniques: Research, Studies, and Techniques*, Hershey, PA: IGI Global, pp.266–283.

Linnemann, A., Ditzen, B., Strahler, J., Doerr, J. M. & Nater, U. M. (2015) Music listening as a means of stress reduction in daily life, *Psychoneuroendocrinology*, 60 (October): 82–90.

Manzoni, G. M., Gorini, A., Preziosa, A., Pagnini, F., Castelnuovo, G., Molinari, E. & Riva, G. (2008) New technologies and relaxation: An explorative study on obese patients with emotional eating, *Journal of Cybertherapy and Rehabilitation* 1 (2): 182–193.

Millegan, J., Manschot, B., Dispenzieri, M., Marks, B., Edwards, A., Raulston, V., Khatiwoda, I. & Narro, M. (2015) Leveraging iPads to introduce meditation and reduce distress among cancer patients undergoing chemotherapy: a promising approach, *Supportive Care in Cancer* 23 (12): 3393–3394.

Mortledge, T. J., Allexandre, D., Reese, P. (2013) Feasibility of an online mindfulness program for stress management – a randomized, controlled trial, *Annals of Behavioral Medicine* 46 (2): 137–148.

Motomura, N., Sakurai, A. & Yotsuya, Y. (2001) Reduction of mental stress with lavender odorant, *Perceptual and Motor Skills* 93 (3): 713–718.

Nikunen, H., Puolakka, M., Rantakallio, A., Korpela, K. & Halonen, L. (2014) Perceived restorativeness and walkway lighting in near-home environments, *Lighting Research & Technology* 46 (3): 308–328.

Nourse, J. C. & Welch, R. B. (1971) Emotional attributes of color: a comparison of violet and green, *Perceptual and Motor Skills* 32 (2): 403–406.

Oxford Economics (2016) *When the Walls Come Down: How Smart Companies Are Rewriting the Rules of the Open Workplace*, Oxford: Oxford Economics.

Peters, R., Zerwas, M., Krempen, T. & Krause, H. J. (2010) Optimisation of thermal comfort in existing buildings, *BAUPHYSIK* 32 (5): 303–307. Available at doi: 10.1002/bapi.201010034.

Rasila, H. & Rothe, P. (2012) A problem is a problem is a benefit? Generation Y perceptions of open-plan offices, *Property Management* 30 (4): 362–375.

Rodrigues, N. & Deuskar, M. (2016) A Study of the Effect of Color Meditation on Relaxation States, *Journal of Psychosocial Research* 11 (1): 13–20.

Russell, J. A. (2003) Core affect and the psychological construction of emotion, *Psychological Review* 110 (1): 145–172.

Sagioglou, C. & Greitemeyer, T. (2014) Facebook's emotional consequences: why Facebook causes a decrease in mood and why people still use it, *Computers in Human Behavior* 35 (June): 359–363.

Sawang, S., Guaralda, M., Chamorro-Koc, M., Garcia Hansen, V., Caldwell, G. A., Medland, R. & Petty, M. (2016) The Aerie: an innovative way for wellbeing restoration in an open-plan workplace, *Paper presented at the Well-Being 2016 – Co-Creating Pathways to Well-being: Book of Proceedings*, Birmingham, UK. Available at https://eprints.qut.edu.au/101178/.

Sayorwan, W., Siripornpanich, V., Piriyapunyaporn, T., Hongratanaworakit, T., Kotchabhakdi, N. & Ruangrungsi, N. (2012) The effects of lavender oil inhalation on emotional states, autonomic nervous system, and brain electrical activity, *Journal of the Medical Association of Thailand* 95 (4): 598–606.

Sembian, N. & Aathi, M. K. (2015) Chromo therapy: healing power of colors, *i-Manager's Journal on Nursing* 5 (4): 6–12.

Shephard, R. J. & Aoyagi, Y. (2009) Seasonal variations in physical activity and implications for human health, *European Journal of Applied Physiology* 107 (3): 251–271. Available at doi: 10.1007/s00421-009-1127-1.

Siriphorn, A., Chamonchant, D. & Boonyong, S. (2016) Comparisons of the effects of a foam pad, mung bean bag, and plastic bead bag on postural stability disturbance in healthy young adults, *Journal of Physical Therapy Science* 28 (2): 530–534.

Sitzer, V. A. (2013) The effect of a rejuvenation room on reducing subjective workplace stress reported by clinical staff, Paper presented at the Share Inspire Transform Conference at Sharp Memorial Hospital, San Diego, CA.

Small, C. (1999) Musicking – the meanings of performing and listening. A lecture, *Music Education Research* 1 (1): 9–22.

Smith, M. (2008) The effects of a single music relaxation session on state anxiety levels of adults in a workplace environment, *The Australian Journal of Music Therapy* 19: 45–66.

Staats, H. & Hartig, T. (2004) Alone or with a friend: a social context for psychological restoration and environmental preferences, *Journal of Environmental Psychology* 24 (2): 199–211.

Stetz, M. C., Kaloi-Chen, J. Y., Turner, D. D., Bouchard, S., Riva, G. & Wiederhold, B. K. (2011) The effectiveness of technology-enhanced relaxation techniques for military medical warriors, *Military Medicine* 176 (9): 1065–10670.

Stone, N. J. & English, A. J. (1998) Task type, posters, and workspace color on mood, satisfaction, and performance, *Journal of Environmental Psychology* 18 (2): 175–185.

Terwogt, M. M. & Hoeksma, J. B. (1995) Colors and emotions: preferences and combinations, *The Journal of General Psychology* 122 (1): 5–17.

Tongnit, K., Paungmalai, N. & Sukarnjanaset, W. (2004) *Investigation of Physiological Response to Aroma, Special Project in Pharmacy*, Bangkok: Chulalongkorn University.

Ulrich, R. S., Simons, R. F., Losito, B. D., Fiorito, E., Miles, M. A. & Zelson, M. (1991) Stress recovery during exposure to natural and urban environments, *Journal of Environmental Psychology* 11 (3): 201–230.

Villani, D., Riva, F. & Riva, G. (2007) New technologies for relaxation: the role of presence, *International Journal of Stress Management* 14 (3): 260–274.

Waber, B., Magnolfi, J. & Lindsay, G. (2014) Workspaces that move people, *Harvard Business Review* 92 (10): 68–77, 121.

Weinert, D. & Waterhouse, J. (2007) The circadian rhythm of core temperature: effects of physical activity and aging, *Physiology & Behavior* 90 (2): 246–256. Available at doi: 10.1016/j.physbeh.2006.09.003.

Yu, B., Feijs, L., Funk, M. & Hu, J. (2015) Designing auditory display of heart rate variability in biofeedback context, *Paper presented at the 21st International Conference on Auditory Display*, Graz, Austria.

Zhang, L., & Guo, H. (2012) *Tracing the Elephants: Office Designs of The Creative Leaders*. Tortola, British Virgin Islands: Chois Publishing.

10

DESIGNING FOR WELL-BEING IN LATE STAGE DEMENTIA

Cathy Treadaway, Jac Fennell, David Prytherch, Gail Kenning and Andy Walters

Introduction

A different perspective is necessary when considering well-being in the context of dementia as so many aspects of life are affected by the disease. Dementia impacts on memory, perception, behaviour and cognition, leading to anxiety, confusion and difficulties with communication as the disease progresses (Alzheimer's Research UK, 2016). In the advanced stages, people living with dementia frequently become withdrawn, lose mobility and have high dependency needs. The resulting lack of autonomy, perceptual changes and decline in cognitive function means that the accepted "ways to well-being" must be reframed (Aked et al., 2008).

In this context, how do we understand what constitutes well-being for someone with severe communication difficulties, memory impairment and altered perceptions? How can designers address the challenge of designing to support well-being in dementia care and create new appropriate products and services, particularly for people living with the later stages of the disease? These are questions addressed in this chapter exploring the process of participatory research, focusing on how Compassionate Design Approaches are being used to support those with dementia.

The term dementia describes a range of incurable diseases of the brain that affect 1 in 20 people over the age of 65 and 1 in 5 people over the age of 80. Despite significant scientific breakthroughs in understanding the pathology of the disease, an imminent cure seems unlikely. Consequently, understanding how to support people to live well with the disease until the end of life is vital not only for individual families affected, but also for society as a whole (Kane & Terry, 2015).

Understanding the problem

Many of us will experience the impact of dementia at some stage in our lives either through the media, personally through experiencing the disease, or caring for a family member or friend. Dementia is recognised as being one of the major health challenges of the twenty-first century (WHO, 2012) The number of people diagnosed with the disease is estimated to be 46 million globally and this is projected to rise to 131.5 million by 2050 (Prince et al., 2015). This increase will place significant economic pressures on health care and social services (Department of Health, 2013). Many people with the advanced stages of the disease require care in specialist dementia units in residential care or nursing homes. Their needs are complex and specific, depending on the type of dementia and what stage of the disease they are living with. Currently there are very few products designed explicitly to help with advanced dementia care or to enable people to live well, feel pleasure, or experience enjoyment as they transition through the disease to the end of life (Ógáin & Mountain, 2015).

People living with advanced dementia are often some of the most marginalised and vulnerable people in society. Their care requires approaches that affirm their sense of identity, even when they themselves can no longer recall who they are. Highly personalised designs can help people living with dementia to retain their dignity as valued members of society (Hughes, 2014). Universal designs are often not suited to people living with advanced dementia – colours, shapes tonal relationships are perceived differently. Lines, shape and colours "misbehave" by normal design rules. For individuals living with dementia, design can be over stimulating or under-stimulating and furthermore, perception changes as the disease progresses. There are no fixed points; a person living with the disease can experience a spectrum of constant variation from hour to hour.

The complexity of the design problem and sensitivity required to address it, demands expert knowledge that is best informed by those with experience of living with or being in close proximity to someone with the disease. Participatory research approaches that bring together practitioners from a range of disciplines, including health and social care as well as informal carers and people living with dementia, can provide invaluable insights to shape ideas and contribute to the design process (Jakob et al., 2017). The research described in this chapter has been finding ways to unlock this wisdom, in order to co-create designs for playful objects to support the well-being of people living with advanced dementia.

The LAUGH research project (www.laughproject.info) has sought to better understand how people with dementia experience positive emotions and to create designs specifically to stimulate and support subjective well-being (Treadaway et al., 2016). It is partnered by leading charities in the field and guided by an expert group of advisors working in health and social care with relevant dementia experience. People living with dementia, their relatives and carers are also participants in the research via project partner Gwalia Cyf and SE Wales Alzheimer's Society Service Users Review Panel (SURP) members. The acronym LAUGH (Ludic Artefacts Using Gesture and Haptics) reveals the focus of the project on understanding playfulness, positive emotion and hand-use in the context of dementia. These three particular themes have been identified as being pertinent in understanding how to support well-being in advanced dementia.

LAUGH research has involved experts in creative participatory workshops, which have been used to collect qualitative insights, practical knowledge and narratives concerning their experience of being in daily contact with people with advanced dementia. The study has been informed by a series of one to one case study interviews and participatory creative workshops. Data has been captured using audio-visual technology, still photography and materials created during the workshops, including participant completed question cards and flipchart diagrams. The intention was to gain in-depth personal knowledge to help shape design ideas. Empathy, role play and self-reflection through participation in practical creative activities are techniques that have been used extensively to encourage participants to sharpen their focus on the key themes in each workshop and help to reflect upon their experiences of working with people with dementia.

Compassionate Design

Compassionate Design methodology underpins the research (Figure 10.1). This approach has evolved and been tested through design practice and previous research by the authors. Compassionate Design puts love at the heart of the design process and proposes three key components to be considered and prioritised when addressing the requirements of those in the advanced stages of dementia. It advocates that: designs should be personalised (to retain a sense of self and maintain dignity), be stimulating to the senses (to keep in the moment and not rely on past or future) and help the person living with dementia to engage in moments of high quality connection with others. By taking this approach it is possible to create appropriate personalised designs that help craft a more caring world for people living with advanced dementia.

The research involves exploration of the foundational elements that are essential for all human beings to thrive. These "core needs" shape our ability to flourish

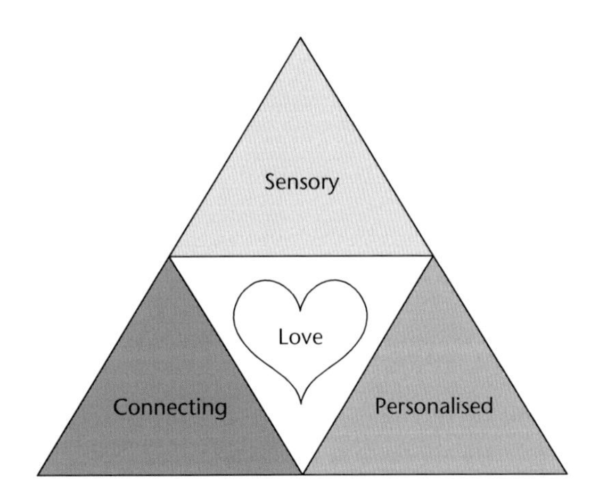

FIGURE 10.1 Compassionate Design diagram

and live well; they are universal and include connection with others, the desire to nurture and be nurtured and the deep emotional responses that arise (often beyond conscious thought) as a result of sensory stimulation. Lived experience shapes our sense of self, builds personhood; it is sedimented through memory, both explicit (cognitive) and procedural (tacitly through bodily knowledge or muscle memory) to build a person's identity (Hughes, 2014). To develop appropriate designs for people living with advanced dementia, new insights are needed to reveal how to connect with these fundamental aspects of an individual's humanity. This is what the first stage of the LAUGH research aimed to examine.

Playfulness and positive emotion

The first two LAUGH participatory workshops focused on playfulness, positive emotion and memory. A group of 25 participants were encouraged to share their personal experiences through a series of playful creative activities and then use these to reflect on the potential differences and similarities for those living with advanced dementia. By contributing their expert knowledge of the disease to the group, insights and observations could be validated and shared with the research team.

The key findings that arose from these workshops included the importance of promoting "in the moment" experience that is playful and engages the senses (Treadaway et al., 2016). Ludic or playful play, fun and humour can be experienced in the present with little cognitive load or reliance on explicit memory. Playfulness is a social activity and laughter and smiles contribute to social bonding and sense of connection with others (Killick, 2013). These positive emotions have proven health benefits and have been found to correlate with a reduction in prescribed medication and hospital admission (Huppert, Baylis & Keverne, 2005). Nevertheless, activities that are ludic, intrinsically playful and without goals are often undervalued by society, despite research evidence of their potential benefits to health and well-being (Tonkin & Whitaker, 2016). The major fear is that playfulness can be perceived as infantilising and playful objects, detrimental to a person's dignity. Overcoming this stigma is not just a challenge within the care and medical professions but to society as a whole. In Western culture, greater value and importance is placed on work compared with playful leisure activities (Kane, 2005). Playful or ludic play is often considered childish and those who engage in it stigmatised (Killick, 2013). In dementia care this is a particular concern when playful objects are used to comfort and soothe, or engage them in stimulating activities. Family members and health and care professionals may feel that the use of "toys" challenges the dignity of the person living with dementia and is ethically unsound (Mitchel, 2016). Although there have been significant changes to attitudes to the use of playful objects in dementia care over recent years (Mitchell & O'Donnell, 2013; Tonkin & Whitaker, 2016), finding ways to design appropriately and sensitively so that ethical issues are not contested has been crucial to LAUGH research.

One of the key ways of addressing these concerns in the research has been through "personalisation". By taking a person-centred approach (Kitwood, 1997), informed by individual life histories and personal preferences, it is possible to design and develop objects that are not only highly appropriate for the person living with dementia, but also of relevance to family and carers (Treadaway & Kenning, 2015). Personalisation enables information about the previous life of the person living with dementia to be integrated and embedded in the design, acting as a prompt to elicit emotional memories or a catalyst for conversation. Visiting a person with advanced dementia can be a challenge even for loved ones and family members who know the person well. Altered perceptions, loss of explicit memory, withdrawal and resulting difficulties with verbal communication make meaningful conversation problematic. Personalised playful objects can help bridge these issues by providing an alternative focus of attention that is 'in the moment' and without cognitive demands on the person living with dementia.

Emotional memory is retained into the later stages of dementia (Zeisel, 2011). The implications of this for personalised design is that "feel good" memories can be triggered through embedded music and other sensory prompts that relate to a person's lived experience. Although it is impossible to know exactly what a person who is unable to communicate verbally is remembering, observations of facial expressions and body language can reveal when pleasure and enjoyment is experienced. Stimulating these kinds of positive emotions is vital for enhancing well-being (Fredrickson, 2004) particularly as many people living with dementia also experience depression (Rahman, 2017).

Procedural memory and craft

Recent research has identified the therapeutic benefits of hand-use on emotional well-being (Lambert, 2008). Lambert identifies a particular brain circuit, which she calls the "effort-driven reward circuit", as crucial in maintaining emotional resilience and avoiding depression. She contends that "engaging the effort driven rewards circuit appears to be the equivalent of taking a preventive dose of the most powerful anti depressants" (Lambert, 2008, p.90). Her theory identifies and implicates a neural network comprising three particular regions of the brain – the accumbens-striatal-cortical regions, which are intimately connected and located in close proximity. The accumbens is identified as "a critical interface between our emotions and actions" and is positioned between the area of the brain that controls movement (striatum) and the prefrontal cortex that controls thought processes, problem-solving, decision-making and planning. The hands dominate the activity of the motor cortex and "moving them activates larger areas of the brain's complex cortex than moving much larger parts of our bodies" (Lambert, 2008, p.33). Activating the effort-driven rewards circuit results in the secretion of neurochemicals, such as dopamine and serotonin, which contribute to the stimulation of positive emotions. This theory is supported by the everyday experience of emotional satisfaction and well-being that most people gain from activities requiring physical effort, hand movement and coordination - with a degree of cognitive challenge. This pleasure is often derived from activities such as crafts and hobbies (e.g. knitting, woodwork, drawing) and even simple day-to-day chores such as folding and ironing clothes or cooking.

Most people living with advanced dementia are passive recipients of care and have little opportunity to engage in the routine activities likely to stimulate the effort-driven reward brain circuitry. They are often relocated from their personal home environment into residential care, usually when they require more intensive attention than can be provided at home. Once in care, they lose the necessity to engage in many of the activities that have punctuated their daily experience – such as cooking, cleaning and personal care. As the essentials of daily living are provided for them, the effort needed to engage with life diminishes (Brooker, 2008). Research has highlighted how meaningful occupation – especially with the hands, can boost well-being. According to Rahman (2017, p.175) occupation can be meaningful, in the context of advanced dementia, when it provides a sense of "pleasure, connection" and "autonomy"; the activity need not be complicated or structured. The connection between meaningful occupation and well-being in dementia through creativity and the arts has been the focus of a number of recent research studies and government reports. These have evidenced the benefits of arts practice to health and well-being for people living with dementia (Windle et al., 2014; Kenning, 2016; All-Party UK Parliamentary Group on Arts, 2017). Creative activities with people living with dementia in residential care and day centres are often heavily directed and take place during specified art or craft sessions led by an Artist or Activity Co-Ordinator (Coleman et al., 2016). For the majority of the day, however, there may be limited opportunity for meaningful or creative occupation. Hands that have experienced a lifetime of skilled work or domestic activities rest in the lap with nothing purposeful to do for long periods of time (Brooker & Duce, 2000).

Hand skills and craft practices, acquired throughout life, become sedimented in the body through lived experience. Hand eye coordination, tactile and haptic perception essential in craft making, becomes automatic and is stored as muscle or procedural memory (Sennett, 2008). Recall of these embodied actions requires little conscious thought and is not reliant on cognitive processing. Hand skills, that involve haptic sensation and manipulation acquired over a number of years, gradually become "tacit knowledge" (Dormer, 1994). People who engage in tacit hand-crafting activities are able to enter a "flow state" involving total immersion or absorption in the activity (Csikszentmihalyi, 1996). This has been found to be both deeply satisfying and beneficial to a person's sense of well-being (Haworth, 2016). Despite explicit memory being significantly impaired by dementia, some people living with the advanced stages of the disease continue to be able to access a range of procedural memories involving skills such as playing the piano, knitting, bread making etc. They may however, be unable to follow instructions, patterns, sequences or recipes, which require cognitive processing. Access to procedural memory implies the potential for people living with dementia to also retain some capacity to experience the flow states that are beneficial to well-being, through activities using the hands.

In order to explore this further, the third LAUGH participatory workshop examined how people living with advanced dementia routinely engage in activities involving hand-use. The aim was to understand how to design for purposeful hand-use and consider how this might enhance well-being. Those attending the participatory workshop included occupational therapists based in hospital dementia units and residential care, art therapists, representatives from the charity sector, carers, designers and researchers. The event was divided into four stages: two practical activity sessions each followed by a group discussion session. The aim was to enable participants to engage in and then reflect on their own experiences of handcraft activities and tool use. These practical exercises were designed to sharpen and focus the later discussion sessions concerning hand-use, craft and procedural memory in relation to people living with advanced dementia.

Developing designs for well-being

As a result of the participatory workshops six key themes were identified that have been used to inform the subsequent development of LAUGH playful objects. The following section briefly describes the themes that emerged and presents examples of some of the objects that have been designed. In each case, designs were highly personalised. "Portrait information", including personal preferences and life histories from individuals living with advanced dementia, was gathered from care staff and family members. Design concepts were developed into prototypes using this information following two further participatory co-design workshops guided by the six themes outlined below.

1. Nurturing (Hug; Figure 10.2)

One of the fundamental aspects of being human is the desire to nurture others. This is evident in self-grooming, cuddling, cradling and caring for others, animals, plants and things. The desire to nurture is instinctive, low level and subconscious and frequently involves touch and hand-use. Participants at the workshop identified activities that involved people living with dementia in nurturing activities they had observed that had been seen to be beneficial to their well-being. Their examples included: stroking pets, visitors bringing animals, children and babies into care homes, dolls and soft toys. Textile and animal fur was highlighted as being comforting and one occupational therapist noted that "fur is always appealing". Textile blankets, towels and clothing were described as nurturing and comforting – wrapping and enfolding the body. Participants also included caring for plants; activities involving simple hand-based gardening tasks such as potting plants were observed to bring pleasure to people living with dementia.

In response to this theme a soft textile object was designed for a lady with advanced dementia. Her carers explained that they considered what she needed most was a hug. The object that was designed for her is cushion-like but also reminiscent of a soft toy or doll. The arms and legs are long and weighted in order to

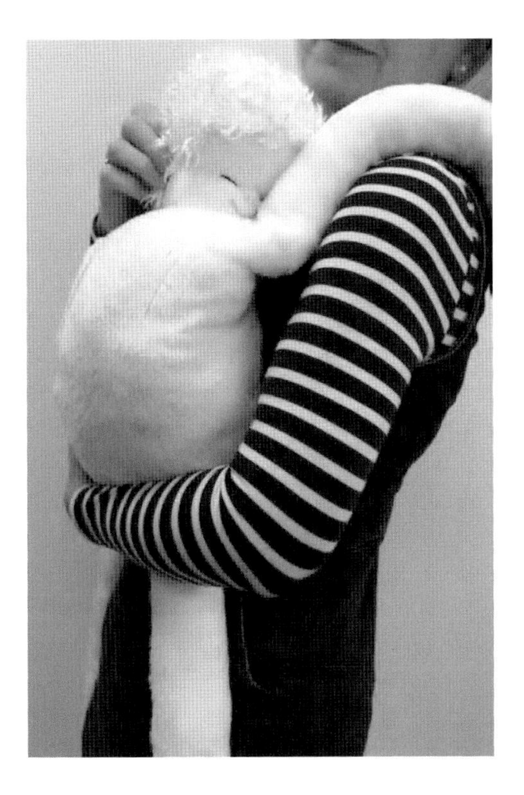

FIGURE 10.2 Hug

wrap around the body and provide the physical sensation of a hug. It has a "beating heart" that is activated through movement via a small electronic sensor inside the body cavity. The object is highly personalised and plays her favourite music, which is stored on and played via a small microcontroller with speakers inside the body.

2. Security (Fidget jewellery box; Figure 10.3)

Aspects of security and objects that represent home, personal identity or "keeping things safe" were noted as being vitally important to people living with dementia. These included items such as handbags, wallets, purses, pens, key rings and money. Pockets were considered particularly important for men and handbags for women. The idea of being able to grasp, hold, finger or fiddle with the item seems to provide a sense of security and therefore offer comfort.

A jewellery box was designed in response to this theme. The box was made for a lady who was fond of beads and particularly pearls. Inside, the box contained a series of fiddle jewellery pieces designed to fit on her hand. Her personal preferences and interests informed the designs and included, for example, a seaside themed piece containing pearls, shells and driftwood; another referenced textile crafts she had once practised as hobbies, with buttons, lace and embroidery.

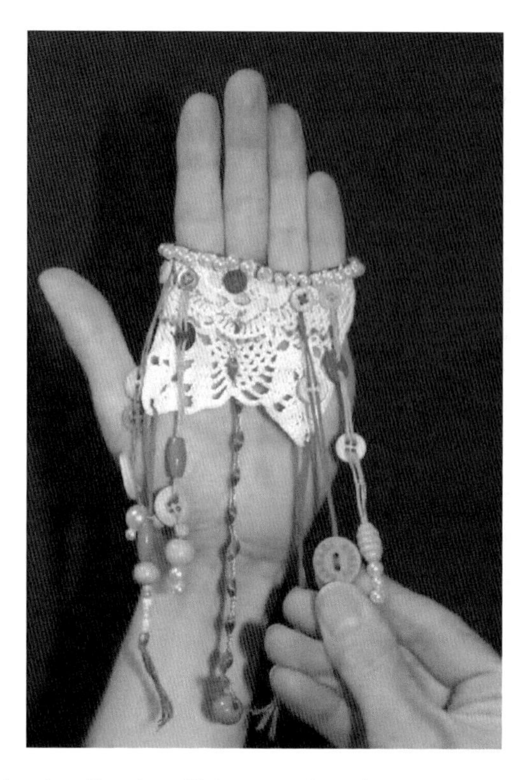

FIGURE 10.3 Fidget jewellery box (© image and product courtesy of Cathy Treadaway (Principal Investigator), Project LAUGH)

The pieces were designed to rest gently over the fingers and dangle into the palm of the non-dominant hand where they could be manipulated by the fingers of the dominant hand.

3. Movement (Steering wheel; Figure 10.4)

Although movement maybe increasingly restricted through the progression of the disease, the desire to move, particularly to music and rhythm, is fundamental and intuitive. Dance and larger body movements are encouraged in residential care using simple activities and props such as balls, balloons and computer gaming consoles. Drumming and rhythmic responses in group situations can involve people living with dementia in both hand and foot movement. One participant described music as "a lubricant to move". Many of those in the more advanced stages of the disease however, are chair or bed bound with limited ability to move and often require greater assistance or motivation to participate in activities. Occupational therapists working in a hospital environment noted that, on admission to hospital, people often exhibit "pyjama paralysis" and become increasingly sedentary and immobile.

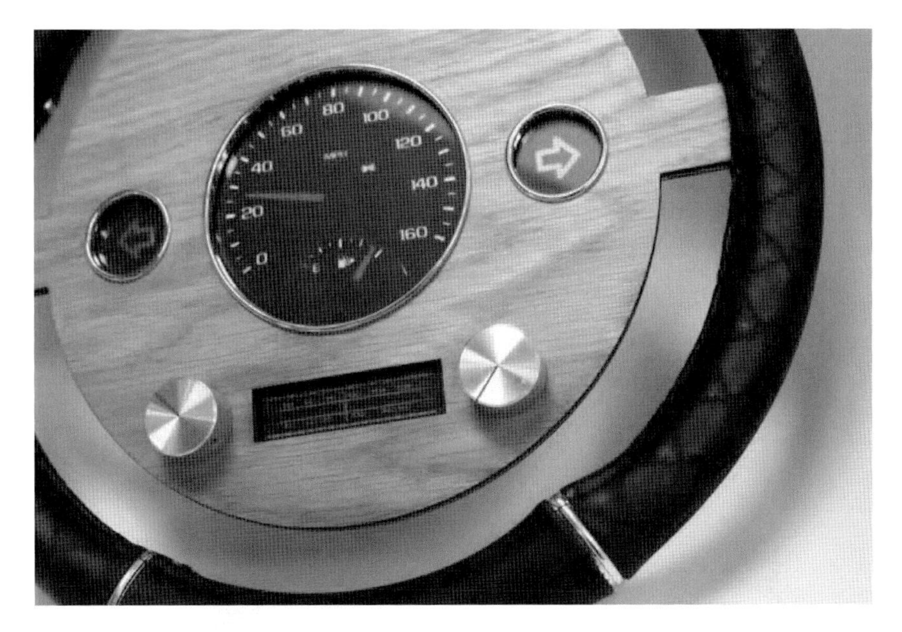

FIGURE 10.4 Steering wheel (© image and product courtesy of Cathy Treadaway (Principal Investigator), Project LAUGH)

A steering wheel was designed in response to this theme, for a man who loved driving and had worked as a motor mechanic. The steering wheel is hand held and contains electronics that provide vibration to imitate the engine running, working indicators with light and sound and an old-fashioned tune-in radio, complete with favourite music, to provide personalisation and an incentive to move. The steering wheel uses haptic sensation to provide emotional memory prompts and encourages conversation.

4. Purposeful (Wooden nuts and bolts; Figure 10.5)

A dominant theme that emerged from the data was the importance of purposefulness and meaningful activities. One of the participants commented on the ways in which people who are capable of domestic activities find themselves without a sense of purpose and without opportunity to contribute to their care:

> "People moving into care homes suddenly have everything taken away from them (purposeful activities), even if they're able. You then see a sudden decline."

Activities that replicate baking and cooking become more like entertainment rather than integral components of daily life and lack the rewards of social appreciation and sense of achievement. Purposeful tasks, such as folding napkins and clothing, dusting, laying the table and washing up, are examples of activities that some people living with dementia are able to do with assistance. There was a consensus that craft activities were seen as being imposed on residents in care, often directed by external facilitators and viewed as entertainment. Hobbies and craft activities that were intrinsically motivated by people with dementia were considered more beneficial and examples given by participants included knitting and collage. A need was highlighted for gender-neutral activities and participants noted there are currently more activities available for women than men. There was some discussion around observations that men like to take things apart whereas women enjoy repetitive tasks.

One Care Home Manager noted that simple one step activities were observed to be pleasurable and over complicated tasks were demotivating for a person living with dementia. This is especially so for someone who is aware that they are no longer capable of performing the activity, as a result of the progression of the disease or for other health reasons, such as arthritis in the fingers. Building on this theme, a series of large turned wooden nuts and bolts were crafted for a man who had worked as an engineer.

5. Attention (Giggle balls; Figure 10.6)

Participants commented on the need for activities to help with everyday tasks that people living with dementia find stressful, such as washing and dressing, and to "turn around some of that anxiety and turn it into something fun". As the disease

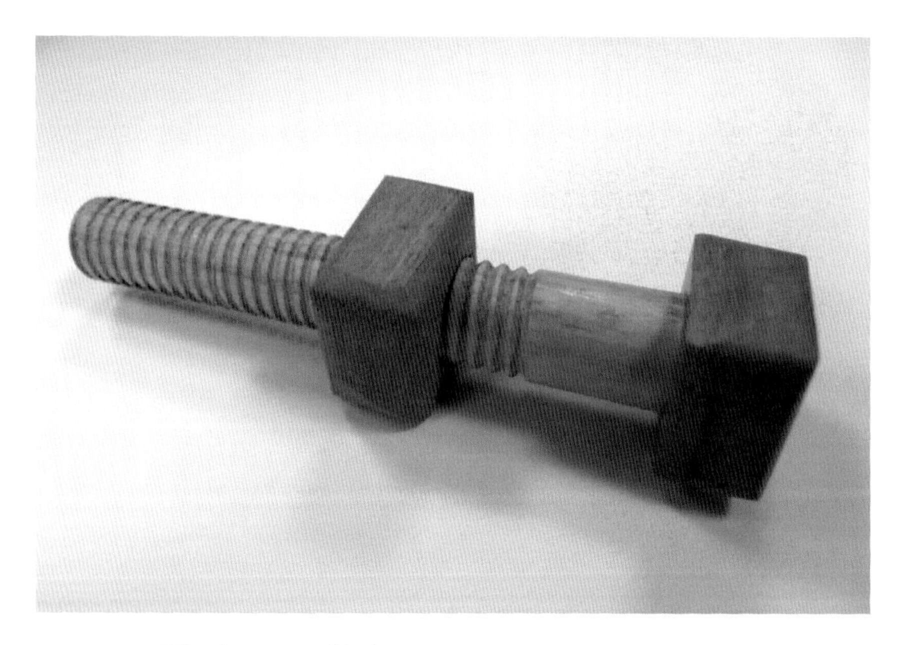

FIGURE 10.5 Wooden nuts and bolts

progresses and mobility decreases "there is a need for distractions – something to focus on". Suggestions included: "something at the window" and mobile kinetic devices. Twiddle muffs and textiles that are personalised can be used to refocus attention and soothe, but it was noted that people with advanced dementia often needed help or encouragement to use them.

Using humour to defuse a potentially stressful situation with a person living with dementia is a ploy well known to care professionals. Laughter and a sense of fun are contagious and keeping care staff positive and happy enables them to emotionally support the person being cared for. A set of small hand held felt "giggle balls" were developed in response to this theme. Each ball has a simple laughing face and contains embedded electronics with a sound file of a giggling child. The balls are soft, warm to touch and rest easily in the palm of the hand.

6. Re-play (Telephone; Figure 10.7)

The final theme brings together a number of sub themes including music and rhythm, reminiscence and playfulness. Rummage boxes and memorabilia are frequently used in dementia care to stimulate interest. In the later stages of the disease these may arouse emotional memories and fingering and touching objects can evoke new thoughts and feelings. Music in particular was noted as being important as a prompt for procedural memory, such as the use of musical jingles; for example, the Fairy liquid washing up commercial song, to help in hand washing.

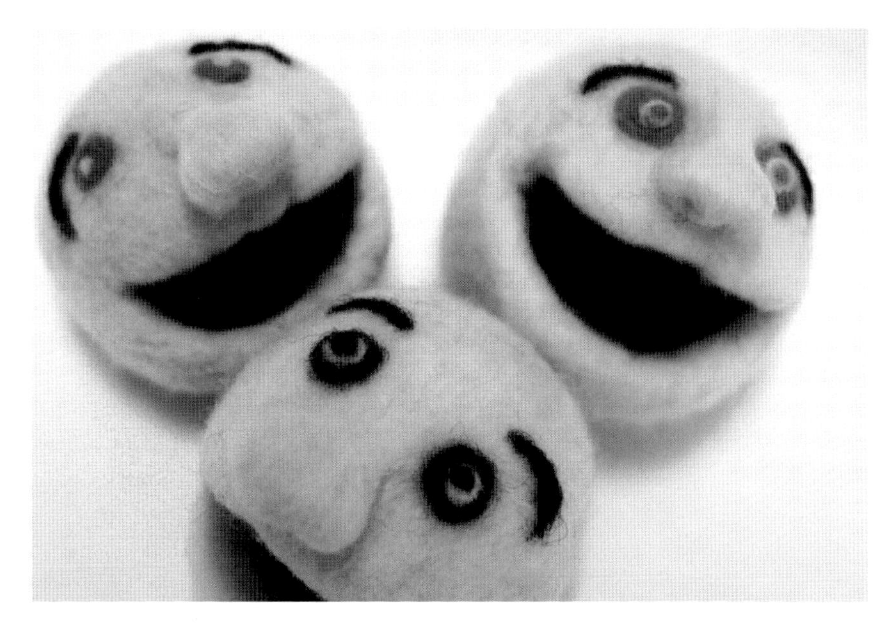

FIGURE 10.6 Giggle balls (© image and product courtesy of Cathy Treadaway (Principal Investigator), Project LAUGH)

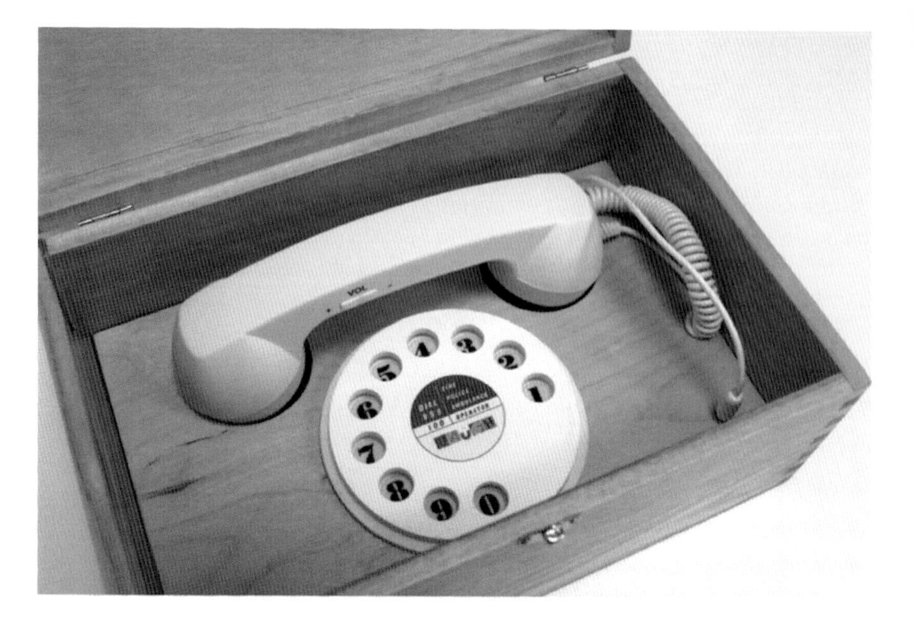

FIGURE 10.7 Telephone (© image and product courtesy of Cathy Treadaway (Principal Investigator), Project LAUGH)

In response to this theme a wooden box containing a retro telephone was developed for a lady who had grown up in Spain and whose first language was Spanish. The sprung dial mechanism, operated by inserting a finger, is designed to prompt procedural memories through haptic sensation and is reminiscent of telephones that existed prior to the advent of press or touch button devices. Dialling any series of numbers selects sounds files containing a selection of pre-recorded Spanish conversation and music.

Music and well-being

Music has been found to be vitally important in the care of people with dementia and is an overarching theme that can be linked with each of the above. It can be used to soothe, calm and relax, initiate waking or sleeping, be individual or social, participatory, performative or passive and can stimulate deep emotion. When combined with hand activities it can assist movement, speed up or slow down action and provide a regular rhythm. There are a number of studies to show that an individual's preferred music can reduce agitation and depression in people living with dementia and improve their well-being (Rahman, 2017).

Music can stimulate emotional memories very quickly and transport a person to a particular time and place; it can kindle associations with people and relationships such as parents, partners or children. Memory of popular songs, rhymes and hymns learned in childhood or adolescence is often retained even when short-term memory is compromised (Capstick, 2012). It is important to find the right musical triggers to benefit a person emotionally. Information from family friends or caregivers about a person's life history can help to pin point particularly meaningful genres of music or specific songs or melodies. When the music is right for the person it can bring enormous pleasure, lift mood and stimulate connection with others. It can create a moment of 'magic' that can reconnect a person living with dementia with the world around them.

Designing for well-being to the end of life

A person living with advanced dementia is in a state of decline and withdrawal from the world. The reality they experience, depending on their dementia diagnosis, maybe very different from that experienced by carers and loved ones. As they transition through the disease, physiological changes in the brain lead to them to experience an alternative reality that can be both frustrating and frightening. Finding ways to keep the person living with dementia connected in a "shared" reality with those around them demands empathy, imagination and acceptance of the changes from carers and loved ones. The creative arts can help create a magical shared reality through music, poetry, visual art making etc. (Capstick, 2012; Killick, 2013). For a person with advanced dementia, shared realities can be prompted by sensory stimulation, especially via music or touch. Hand held objects can play a vital role in helping to stimulate in the moment sensory pleasure and also bring carers and loved ones into a shared reality with the person living with dementia. Laughter, smiles and singing are examples of reciprocal expressions of positive emotion that can ensue.

When a person's mobility and speech are challenged through the disease, the hands become the primary means of interacting with the world beyond the body. Hands act as a conduit, exploring and translating experience of the world through touch and then responding to it outwardly from the body through gesture and finger movement (Wilson, 1998; Treadaway, 2009). Touch can trigger deep emotional and procedural memories and touching objects can stimulate conversation and non-verbal sharing when visiting is difficult for loved ones (Tanner, 2017). Personalised objects are particularly valuable since they can reinforce a person's identity and express the accumulated experience of their "lived life" that they may no longer remember for themselves. This helps both carers and visitors to see the whole person, not just the disease and so retains the dignity of the person living with dementia.

In advanced dementia people gain attachment to objects from which they derive sensory pleasure; they may also provide them with a sense of security in much the same way as a comforter does for a child (Kenning & Treadaway, 2017). Touching sensory textiles and objects can provide a variety of visual and tactual experiences that can comfort, engage and soothe a person in the later stages of the disease (Treadaway & Kenning, 2016). Transitional objects of this kind encourage emotional engagement, stimulation via the hands and opportunities for connection with others.

The pathology of dementia is that it is a degenerative terminal disease for which there is currently no cure. However, finding ways to help people live well through their dementia journey to the end of life should be an imperative in a humane and caring society. Compassionate Design offers an approach that can guide designers to create products, environments and services that can support the well-being of people living with advanced dementia and assist in their care. Compassionate Design focuses attention on three key themes: *personalisation, sensory stimulation* and *connection* in order to embed love (moments of high quality connection between people) into the design process. According to Fredrickson (2014), moments of love, high quality connection or *positivity resonance* between people can have both physiological and psychological benefit to well-being (Fredrickson, 2014). This approach builds on person-centred and relational care perspectives, valuing the caregiver and loved ones of the individual living with dementia as being co-supporters in promoting a person's well-being (Rahman, 2017).

LAUGH research has successfully trialled Compassionate Design Approaches in the development of the playful objects that are described in this chapter. Informed by an interdisciplinary group of dementia experts and working in collaboration with people living with dementia and their families, it has been possible to co-create highly personalised designs for playful objects to help people live well with the disease until the end of life.

Acknowledgements

LAUGH research is supported by an AHRC Standard Grant Ref: AH/M005607/1; we would like to acknowledge our project partner Pobl Gwalia Care and are grateful for the support and participation of Alzheimer's Society Service Users Review Panel, Dementia Positive, Age Cymru, My Home Life and participants who attended LAUGH project workshops throughout the research.

References

Aked, J., Marks, N., Cordon, C. & Thompson, S. (2008) *Five Ways to Well-being: A Report Presented to the Foresight Project on Communicating the Evidence Base for Improving People's Well-being*, London: New Economics Foundation.

All-Party UK Parliamentary Group on Arts, Health and Wellbeing (2017) *Creative Health: The Arts for Health and Wellbeing*, London: UK Government.

Alzheimer's Research UK (2016) *All About Dementia*, Cambridge: Alzheimer's Research UK.

Brooker, D. (2008) What makes life worth living, *Aging & Mental Health* 12: 525–527.

Brooker, D. & Duce, L. (2000) Wellbeing and activity in dementia: a comparison of group reminiscence therapy, structured goal-directed group activity and unstructured time, *Ageing and Mental Health* 4: 354–358.

Capstick, A. (2012) Dancing to the music of time: an experiential learning exercise in dementia care, *Journal of Applied Arts and Health* 3: 117–131.

Coleman, S., Treadaway, C. & Loudon, G. (2016) Avenues, values, and the muse: an ethnographic study of creative activity to support the wellbeing of residents living with

dementia in residential care, *10th Design and Emotion Conference*, Amsterdam: Design and Emotion Society.
Csikszentmihalyi, M. (1996) *Creativity: Flow and the Psychology of Discovery and Invention*, New York: HarperCollins.
Department of Health (2013) *Dementia: A State of the Nation Report on Dementia Care and Support in England*, London: UK Government.
Dormer, P. (1994) *The Art of the Maker: [Skill and its Meaning in Art, Craft and Design]*, London: Thames & Hudson.
Fredrickson, B. L. (2004) The broaden and build theory of positive emotions, *The Philosophical Transactions of the Royal Society* 359: 1367–1377.
Fredrickson, B. L. (2014) *Love 2.0: Creating Happiness and Health in Moments of Connection*, New York: Penguin Group.
Haworth, J. (2016) Enjoyment and wellbeing, in I. Bache, A. Martinez-Perez & A. Tsuchiya (eds.), *CWiPP Working Paper Series*, Sheffield: Centre for Wellbeing in Public Policy, University of Sheffield.
Hughes, J. C. (2014) *How We Think About Dementia: Personhood, Rights, Ethics, the Arts and What They Mean for Care*, London: Jessica Kingsley.
Huppert, F., Baylis, N. & Keverne, B. (2005) (eds.) *The Science of Well-being*, New York: Oxford University Press.
Jakob, A., Manchester, H. & Treadaway, C. (2017) Design for dementia care: making a difference, *Nordes 2017, 7th Nordic Design Research Conference*, Oslo, Norway.
Kane, M. & Terry, G. (2015) *Dementia 2015: Aiming Higher to Transform Lives*, London: Alzheimer's Society.
Kane, P. (2005) *The Play Ethic: A Manifesto for a Different Way of Living*, London: Pan.
Kenning, G. (2016) *Art Engagement for People with Dementia: Independent Evaluation of the Art Access Program Art Gallery of New South Wales, Sydney*, Australia: Art Gallery New South Wales.
Kenning, G. & Treadaway, C. (2017) Designing for dementia: iterative grief and transitional objects. *Design Issues* 34.
Killick, J. (2013) *Playfulness and Dementia: A Practice Guide*, London: Jessica Kingsley Publishers.
Kitwood, T. M. (1997) *Dementia Reconsidered: The Person Comes First*, Buckingham: Open University Press.
Lambert, K. (2008) *Lifting Depression: A Neuroscientist's Hands-On Approach to Activating Your Brain's Healing Power*, New York: Basic Books.
Mitchell, G. (2016) *Doll Therapy in Dementia Care*, London: Jessica Kingsley.
Mitchell, G. & O'Donnell, H. (2013) The therapeutic use of doll therapy in dementia, *British Journal of Nursing* 22: 329–334.
Ógáin, E. N. & Mountain, K. (2015) *Remember Me: Improving Quality of Life for People with Dementia and their Carers Through Impact Investment*, London: NESTA.
Prince, M., Wimo, A., Guerchet, M., Ali, G., Wu, Y. & Prina, M. (2015) *World Alzheimer Report 2015: The Global Impact of Dementia – An Analysis of Prevalence, Incidence, Cost and Trend*, London: Alzheimer's Disease International.
Rahman, S. (2017) *Enhancing Health and Wellbeing in Dementia*, London: Jessica Kingsley.
Sennett, R. (2008) *The Craftsman*, London: Allen Lane.
Tanner, L. (2017) *Embracing Touch in Dementia Care*, London: Jessica Kingsley.
Tonkin, A. E. & Whitaker, J. E. (2016) *Play in Healthcare for Adults: Using Play to Promote Health and Wellbeing Across the Adult Lifespan*, Abingdon, Oxon: Routledge.
Treadaway, C. (2009) Hand and mind – shaping experience, *Australasian Journal of Arts Health* 1: 1–15.

Treadaway, C. & Kenning, G. (2015) Designing sensory e-textiles for dementia, in A. Chakrabarti, T. Toshiharu & Y. Nagai (eds.), *The Third International Conference on Design Creativity (3rd ICDC), 2015 Indian Institute of Science*, Bangalore, India, pp.235–232.
Treadaway, C. & Kenning, G. (2016) Sensor e-textiles: person centered co-design for people with late stage dementia, *Working with Older People* 20: 76–85.
Treadaway, C., Prytherch, D., Kenning, G. & Fennell, J. (2016) In the moment: designing for late stage dementia, in P. Lloyd & E. Bohemia (eds.), *DRS2016, 27–30th June 2016 Brighton*, Brighton, UK: Design Research Society, pp.1442–1457.
WHO (2012) *Dementia: A Public Health Priority*, Geneva: World Health Organisation Alzheimer's Disease International.
Wilson, F. R. (1998) *The Hand*, New York: Pantheon Books.
Windle, G., Gregory, S., Newman, A., Goulding, A., O'Brien, D. & Parkinson, C. (2014) Understanding the impact of visual arts interventions for people living with dementia: a realist review protocol, *Systematic Reviews* 3: 91.
Zeisel, J. (2011) *I'm Still Here: Creating a Better Life for a Loved One Living with Alzheimer's*, London: Piatkus.

11

ALONE TOGETHER – DOCUMENTARY FILMMAKING AND STORIES OF WELL-BEING IN OUTDOOR SPACES

Esther Johnson

Introduction

Alone Together: The Social Life of Benches is an 18-minute poetic documentary made by Esther Johnson, created as part of the collaborative research initiative the Bench Project, exploring how individuals and groups use public space. One of the aims for this research was to test how making a film can help tell stories about encounters, exclusion and well-being in outdoor spaces. Revolving around the micro-space of the humble bench, *Alone Together* includes a series of oral testimonies which identify and illuminate the thoughts of frequent users of two public spaces in London.

> "On a day such as this, while roaming around this park,
> If you see a thousand faces then it is good for you.
> My ancestors used to say that."
>
> – *Chila Kumari, General Gordon Square, Woolwich*

The filmmaking approach relates to the historiographical tradition that addresses "history from below" (Thompson, 1966; Lynd, 1993) with a focus on "people's history" of everyday life. Of particular interest to social historians are narratives that explore the stories of people who have eluded historical records (Thompson, 1991), rather than from the perspective of well-documented leaders and officials. The emphasis for *Alone Together* was to illuminate "people's experience" and the stories and thoughts of users of each location, voiced in contributors' personal oral testimonies. The film acts like a stranger who joins you to "watch the world go by", and to break the ice by starting a conversation with their fellow bench user.

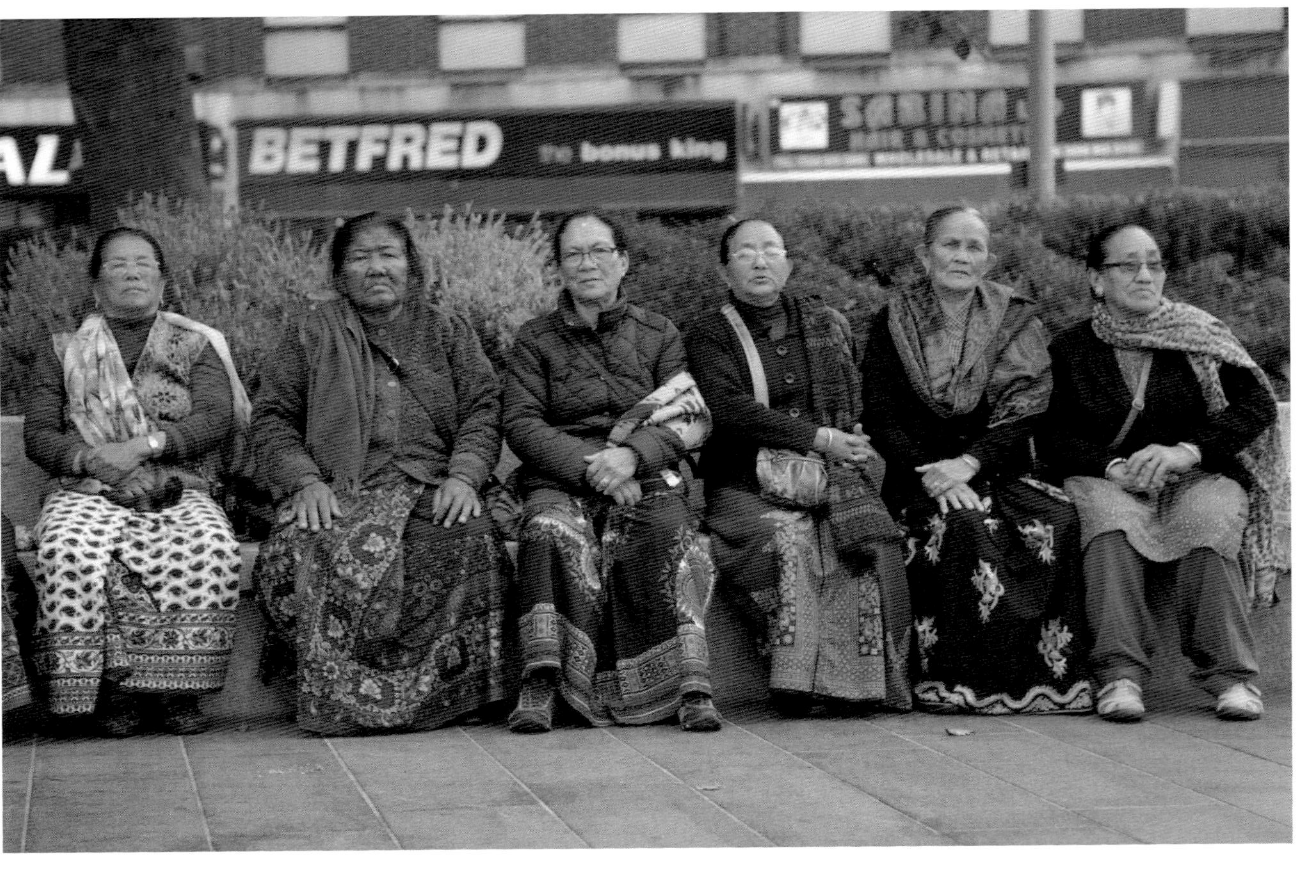

FIGURE 11.1 Nepalese ladies in General Gordon Square, Woolwich

In the historian Lynd's "Oral history from below", he discusses the notion of "accompanying" interviewees, and how an interviewer and interviewee can meet as equals:

> To accompany another person is to walk beside that person; to become a companion; to be present . . . we are implicitly saying: your life is important. It's worth my time to talk to you. It may be worth your time to talk to me. People like me need to know what people like you have learned.
>
> *(Lynd, 1993)*

The project sought to experiment with a mixed approach, including the social and natural sciences, in order to gain a personal and fully rounded point of view from the perspective of the inhabitants of the locations. This mixed perspective aims to develop a reflexivity to articulate "feeling and being" that is beyond the written word, and situate the film viewer within the fabric of filmed existence. This attentive approach of combining aesthetics and ethnography is exemplified in the works made in the Sensory Ethnographic Lab (SEL), an "experimental laboratory" at Harvard University, that "opposes the traditions of art that are not deeply infused with the real, those of documentary that are derived from broadcast journalism, and those of visual anthropology that mimic the discursive inclinations of their mother discipline" (https://sel.fas.harvard.edu).

Urban micro-territories of encounter and intimidation

Discussion draws on a wider collaborative research project, The Unsociable Bench, and Other Urban Micro-Territories of Encounter and Intimidation (http://the-bench-project.weebly.com) developed as an Arts and Humanities Research Council bid in response to a call to address the challenges of disconnection, division and exclusion. This bid was developed alongside a group of researchers (following a Connected Communities event, https://connected-communities.org/index.php/project/the-bench-project), the research coming from a collective interest in how individuals and groups use public and liminal spaces, and in particular the micro-space of the bench.

The project team was characterised by cross-disciplinary collaboration in which research was co-designed by the group from the conception stage, allowing for a close consideration of a creative approach and filmmaking methods from the start. The group consisted of three academics: Dr Clare Rishbeth, Lecturer in Landscape Architecture at the University of Sheffield; Ben Rogaly, Professor of Human Geography at the University of Sussex and Esther Johnson, Professor in Film and Media Arts at Sheffield Hallam University. Individuals from community groups were fully embedded in the research and included: Radhika Bynon, Programme Lead at The Young Foundation (https://youngfoundation.org); and Dr Jasber Singh, former Co-ordinator of Greenwich Inclusion Project (https://griproject.org.uk).

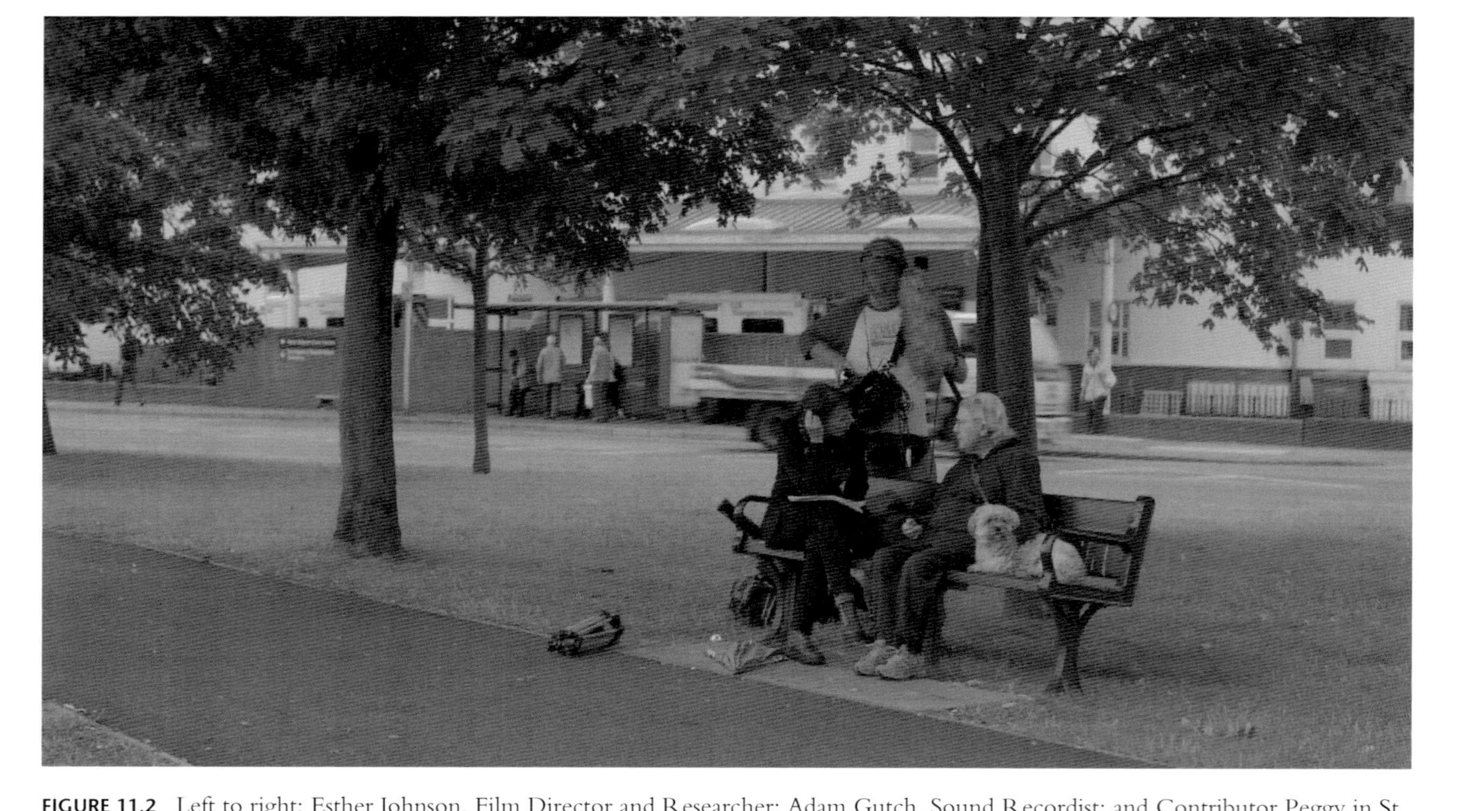

FIGURE 11.2 Left to right: Esther Johnson, Film Director and Researcher; Adam Gutch, Sound Recordist; and Contributor Peggy in St Helier Open Space, Sutton

The micro-space of the humble bench

As an artist and filmmaker, my overarching aim for the development of the film was to test how making a film can help to tell detailed and nuanced stories about encounters, exclusion and well-being in outdoor spaces, including:

- How the media of moving image and audio, can elicit the stories and memories of visitors to the chosen research locations.
- Explore the micro-histories and memories of visitors to the chosen locations.
- How each place could provide a space for social interaction, well-being and respite from everyday concerns.

The film revolves around the micro-space of the bench as a means to access stories and opinions of frequent users of two public spaces in London, chosen for their contrasting features, and for their closeness to sites of work undertaken by the two community groups involved in the project. The locations of focus were General Gordon Square, Woolwich and St Helier Open Space, Sutton.

The characteristics of the two squares are identifiable in the images (Figures 11.1–11.6). General Gordon Square, situated in South London, is a busy public urban square located next to Woolwich Arsenal train station and a large supermarket. The architectural characteristics include: integrated granite benching, grass terraces and landscaped areas, a water feature and a big screen. Regeneration of the area, by Gustafson Porter and Bowman (www.gp-b.com/woolwich-squares), took place in 2011, in time for the London Olympics the following year.

St Helier Open Space, also in South London, is a green outer-urban area. The space incorporates sports activity areas including a skateboard park, a playground, an outdoor gym and a ball court. The area is dotted with traditional wooden benches and has a meadow, a field with football pitches and is situated near a busy hospital and sports centre.

Project development was facilitated by five group workshops undertaken over the eleven-month research period, including an outward-facing website, a group only blog, and an online project folder to track the project progress and share research materials. Fieldworkers Samprada Mukhia and Diana Coman, each connected to one of the community groups, were employed to assist in collecting data from the locations as integral components of the methodology. This data took several forms:

- Written observations of the use of the space, generally taken on different days and times to the film project.
- Interviews with users of the spaces, also at different times to filming. Each fieldworker had meetings with user groups in the local area, such as Age Concern and youth groups, in order to gain a deeper insight into the use of the locations.

- Rogaly and Rishbeth conducted additional observational fieldwork, including interviews with the wardens for General Gordon Square and the designer of the square, Gustafson Porter.
- Preliminary extensive film fieldwork for each space, involving interviews with potential film participants, and stills photography to allow reflection on each location and envisage possibilities and restrictions for filming each space.

Alone Together – the filmmaking process

The filmmaking process is not only a technical and creative process, but is a social and embodied act. Film has the capacity to capture and personify the psychological and lived experience of people, and can democratise the telling of sensitive personal histories. Rather than take a didactic approach, in which an authoritative voiceover would tell the viewer about the design and use of the spaces, the direction of filmmaking was to approach the work in a way that the viewer would gain a heightened perceptual sense of place, becoming a stranger who joins one of the contributors on their bench. In order to achieve this, in the making of the film, emphasis is placed on capturing the specific sensorial characteristics of filmmaking, in tandem with individuals' reflections. Observational filmmaking allowed for a general overview of the rhythm and flow of visitors throughout the day and early evening, surveying the different uses to which these spaces are put. By mixing observational filmmaking of the spaces with portraits and oral testimonies by individual users of the places, it was possible to gain both a macro and micro view of the use of space and the themes that arose from interviewing and observing.

The hidden dimensions of the use of the urban realm, and opinions on the space, are revealed through the filmmaking, for example – the Nepali community bringing along cardboard to sit on instead of sitting directly on the cold granite benches; skateboarders using the ramp as a bench; visitors sitting on the back of granite benches rather than the intended seat section; and pavement slab demarcations indicating out-of-bounds skateboarding areas.

The film foregrounds the rich pool of first-hand audio testimonies as voiceover, so contributors could speak for themselves. Reading transcribed interviews is very different to listening to/hearing the words being said, the voice being a means of expressing memory and experience through nuances of intonation, accent, timbre and pause. How the stories are told, and how they sound, is as important as the words being said.

To avoid a "parachute" approach, by which a filmmaker spends little time in the location or with the interviewees, it was imperative to undertake an integrated process whereby the Researcher visited each location multiple times during the project period in order to meet and get to know the users of these spaces. In the spirit of "accompanying" contributors for the film (Lynd, 1993), a lot of preparation time was involved talking with users at the locations and experiencing what it was like to spend lengthy periods there.

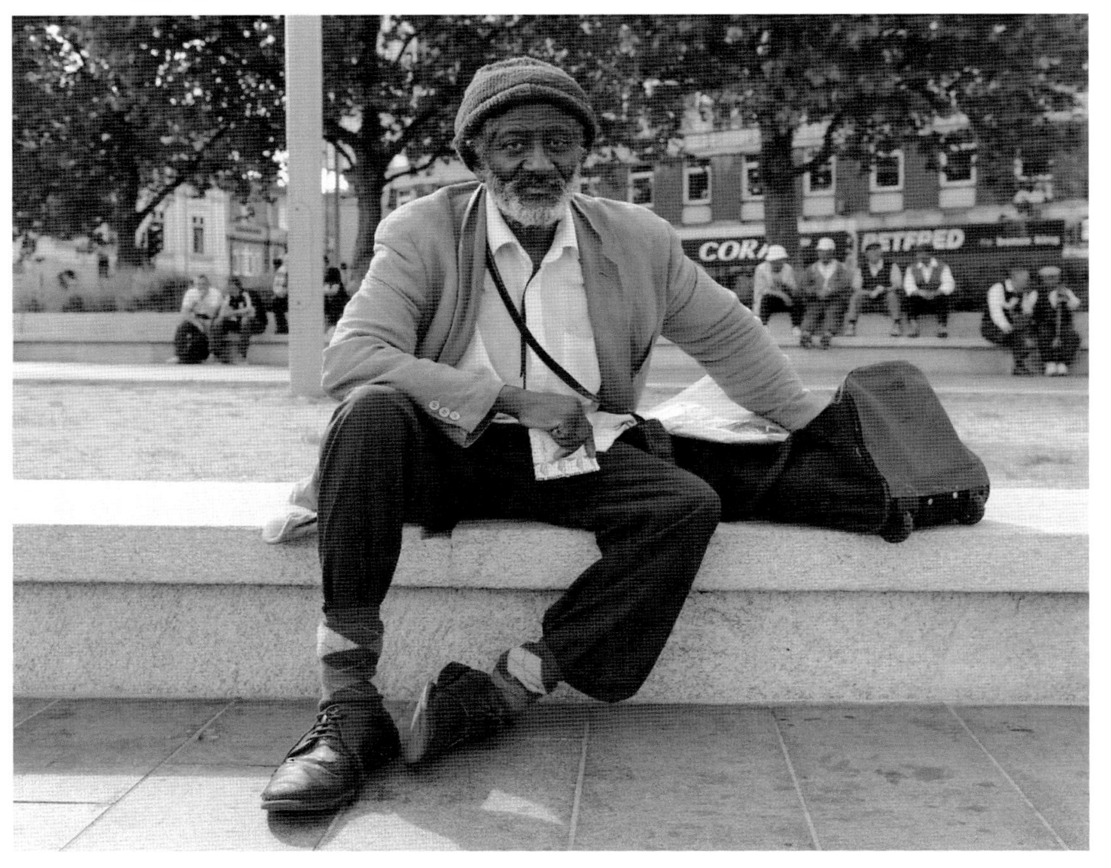

FIGURE 11.3 Michael, General Gordon Square, Woolwich

Repeated field trips were made to both locations on different days and times to meet potential film participants and observe life in each space. Audio recording can be less intrusive than a camera when a contributor is invited to tell their story. This is especially the case when meeting for the first time. Approaching potential contributors by chatting and audio recording, without a camera in sight, is generally less threatening, allowing a dialogue to be formed, and creating space in which the project can be explained in full. Conducting interviews on each field visit, sometimes talking with the same person, helped to earn the trust of potential contributors and to gain a deeper understanding of their stories, experiences, and use of the specific spaces. Some interviews were undertaken with individuals, while others, such as a group of young men, were collectively interviewed, group members correcting, embellishing, or modifying each other's statements, thus creating a shared, cooperative, and often infectious camaraderie.

Incorporated are several filmmaking methods – from traditional observational, ethnographic documentary of personhood and place, to a poetic approach through interstitial "observational scenes" between "interview scenes", slow-motion footage and careful attention to sound design and recorded anthropological soundscapes. Accordingly, filming captures a series of intimate portraits in which contributors are given space to tell us, in their own words, about their specific relationship to place. These are interspersed with sequences that observe the ebb and flow of each location. The voiceover is akin to poetic radio documentary and the filming of people and place, with static long takes, borrows from portraiture stills photography.

To echo broadcaster and oral historian Studs Terkel (Prial, 1992) reflections on oral history interviewing, "it's like prospecting. The transcripts are the ore. I've got to get to the gold dust. It's got to be the person's truth, highlighted. It's not just putting down what people say".

Over the course of the project, approximately 50 individuals were interviewed. In the final film there are 15 contributors, the majority were interviewed more than once. There was an attempt to get a diverse range of experience for the film and the interviewing process garnered a large number of connected but varied viewpoints and memories relating to the questions and fieldwork discussions.

TABLE 11.1 Manifesto for the good bench

1	Benches are valued as public, egalitarian and free.
2	Bench-space allows people to loosely belong within the flow of city life, to see and be seen.
3	Sitting on benches supports healthy everyday routines by enabling people to spend longer outside.
4	Benches function as a social resource – they are flexible places to spend time at no cost.
5	Design of benches is important. Comfort and accessibility are basic requirements.
6	People need to feel safe. Frequently used, visible spaces with a choice of seating can support this.

Interviews were undertaken in the knowledge that the raw recordings would be used both for the film and as social data, the resulting transcriptions aiding the research project in multiple ways, with the interview questioning being extended to address all the project research aims.

Insights gained from the interviews were utilised in a report written by Rishbeth and Bynon (2015), *Benches for Everyone: Solitude in Public, Sociability for Free* and in the creation of a "Manifesto for the good bench" (Table 11.1), which was printed as a postcard, presenting some of our findings in the form of a very concise list. In addition, further research articles have been written in response to the research (Rishbeth & Rogaly, 2017).

Interview material was organised into themes, which included: why and how contributors use the spaces; how frequently they visited; the length of time they spent there; how the space made them feel; specific memories of the place; whether they felt safe or threatened in the space; and thoughts on design of the environment and everyday street furniture; recommendations for possible changes; and what they thought about while sitting in the respective spaces.

Asynchronicity and film editing

Carl Jung described his concept of synchronicity as an, "acausal connecting principle" and "temporally coincident occurrences of acausal events" (Jung, 1960), in which cause and effect occurring at the same time, reveal a collective unconscious. In many films there is an attempt to create a synchronous replication of daily life. *Alone Together* was edited so that audio interviews are "out-of-synch" with the picture, in opposition to an in-synch approach. This out-of-synch audio promotes closer attention to, and understanding and empathy with what is being said by the contributors. In other words, we do not see contributors speaking directly in-synch to camera/interviewer, as might be seen in a traditional news item. We hear and see the contributors, but these are never in-synch. What the film does show, are portrait vignettes of the contributors using the spaces, and in the film soundscape we hear them talking about their thoughts and experiences. By discouraging a totalising approach to synchronous representation, there is an uncoupling of spatial-temporal links between eye and ear. An audience is encouraged to observe a person within a space, and hear intimate stories and thoughts at the same time – the non-synch technique being an attempt to create a gap in which viewers are able to place themselves in the contributors' world. This approach aims to elicit a deeper sensory engagement, to emotionally connect and empathise with contributors' stories.

Sound design and edit

As previously mentioned, a journalistic "news item" approach was not taken for this film, in which an interviewer interviews a contributor on camera. The idea of the film was to gain a deeper insight and to help a viewer to experience and "feel" a specific environment. The intermediary interviewer thus became invisible. Both environments were noisy and a journalistic approach would have necessitated a different production technique. By using interviews as voiceover, a longer segment of interview material could be mined without worrying about visual "jump-cutting".

In addition to the oral testimonies, there is a focus on sound design, using location recordings to articulate the sonic world of each space – water, birds, traffic, barking dogs, whistling, shouting and chattering. This sound design is enriched with a musical track composed by oberphones and based upon the singing of the Nepali elders who were interviewed for the film. This tri-layered use of sound – interviews, atmospheres and music – heightens the sensory capacity of the film image, promoting an audience "sensation" of being in "place".

The editing framework for the film begins at dawn, fluctuating through a 24-hour period and then on to the following morning. This approach allowed for a change in light, weather, viewpoint, and shifting denseness of visitors to each location.

Production

Due to the nature of filming in public outdoor spaces, the film necessitated a small crew consisting of Sound Recordist, Camera Operator, Community Fieldworker and the Researcher (Figure 11.2). In Woolwich, the Fieldworker Mukhia also spoke Nepalese so acted as an intermediary and translator for the Nepalese community that feature in the film (Figure 11.1). This small crew size impacted on the practicalities of kit, which as a result needed to be transportable by the small crew. The shoot in each location for the final film was around four days, from early morning to early evening. As we were very present and embedded in a busy public environment, there needed to be a thorough consideration of public liability protection, risk assessments, consideration of the impact of weather on filming/recording, and the care and well-being of the contributors and crew.

Obstacles – filming in public space

With the concentrated filming in outside public places permission was sought to film in each location from the respective council's film office. This proved difficult for Woolwich with filming permission being granted a few weeks later than the dates originally planned. This meant that some of the contributors where no longer available for the filming dates. Their interviews were, however, not wasted as these where utilised in the various reports and articles that have been written by other members of the team.

Unlike a film in which you make an appointment to meet someone and interview them usually indoors, an outdoor environment has the obstacle of contributors potentially not turning up due to, for instance, weather. Some of the contributors had a relatively unstable home environment that necessitated them spending a long time in public locations such as those used in the film. The chaotic living conditions that many endured also meant that being available for scheduled filming days was hit-and-miss. On the scheduled filming days a few contributors who had agreed to be available did not turn up. As a result, the final film includes a mix of contributors who were interviewed multiple times, with other one-off contributors, being people who the film team met on the filming days.

Other interviews could not be audio recorded, whether by request from the interviewee or, for example children who were with a youth worker rather than their parents/guardian and thereby not able to readily give permission. It was not possible to interview or film the Woolwich Wardens for the film, however this was outside the scope of the film as the focus was visitors to the square rather than those that worked in the square. Wardens were later interviewed by other members of the team for inclusion in the written research reports and articles.

All interviewees that feature in the film were requested to sign a release form, or in the case of children, have the permission of their parents or guardians. The release form allowed contributors to depart from the project at any time, or request anonymity. As the Nepali contributors did not read or speak English, the release forms for them were translated by Mukhia.

Although *Alone Together* did not employ a full range of participatory filmmaking methods, as seen in projects such as the National Film Board of Canada Challenge for Change: The Fogo Island Film Project (www.nfb.ca/playlist/fogo-island) there was a consideration of involving participants in the "making". Contributors were invited to view the film mid-edit and thereby allow them the opportunity to engage in the filmmaking process. There were options of how to access the edit at this stage, with a physical review session in each location, in addition to an online link for feedback. As previously mentioned this review session also allowed contributors to voice any concerns they may have had as to whether they felt the edited material was a true and fair representation of what they said and felt.

The bench and well-being

Through the interviews conducted, it was clear that sitting outdoors on public benches was a vital part of many contributors' routines, affording them space to rest, think and spend time.

For example, the booklet that accompanies the DVD (Johnson, 2015) of the film states that:

> Sitting on benches supports healthy everyday routines by enabling people to spend longer outside. These opportunities to rest can be restorative for mental health and support local walking when personal mobility is limited. Benches function as a social resource, and are flexible and affordable places to spend time. This is appreciated by many, and especially vital for many people who are largely marginalised from other collective environments such as work, cafes, and educational or leisure facilities. They are contrasted positively with crowded, lonely or boring home situations.

Sentiments which are best expressed in the words of the users themselves.

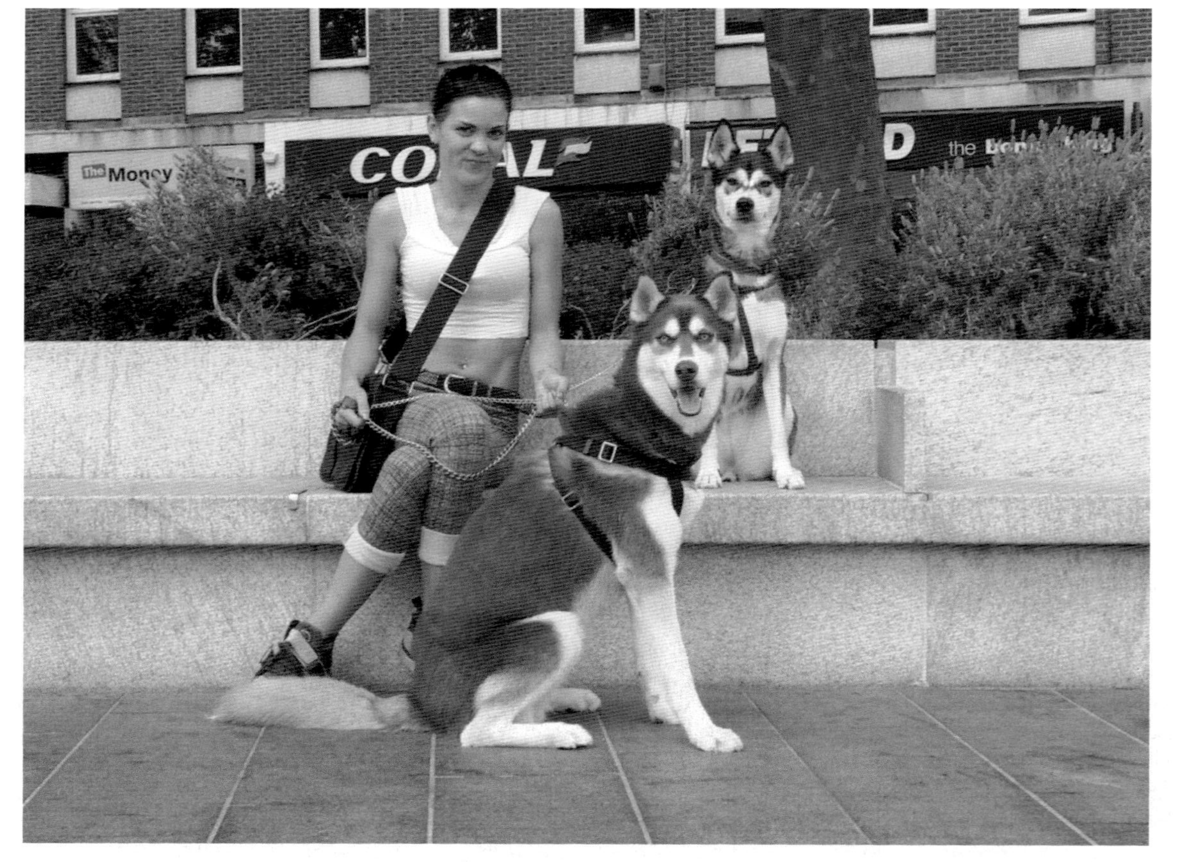

FIGURE 11.4 Lauren, General Gordon Square, Woolwich

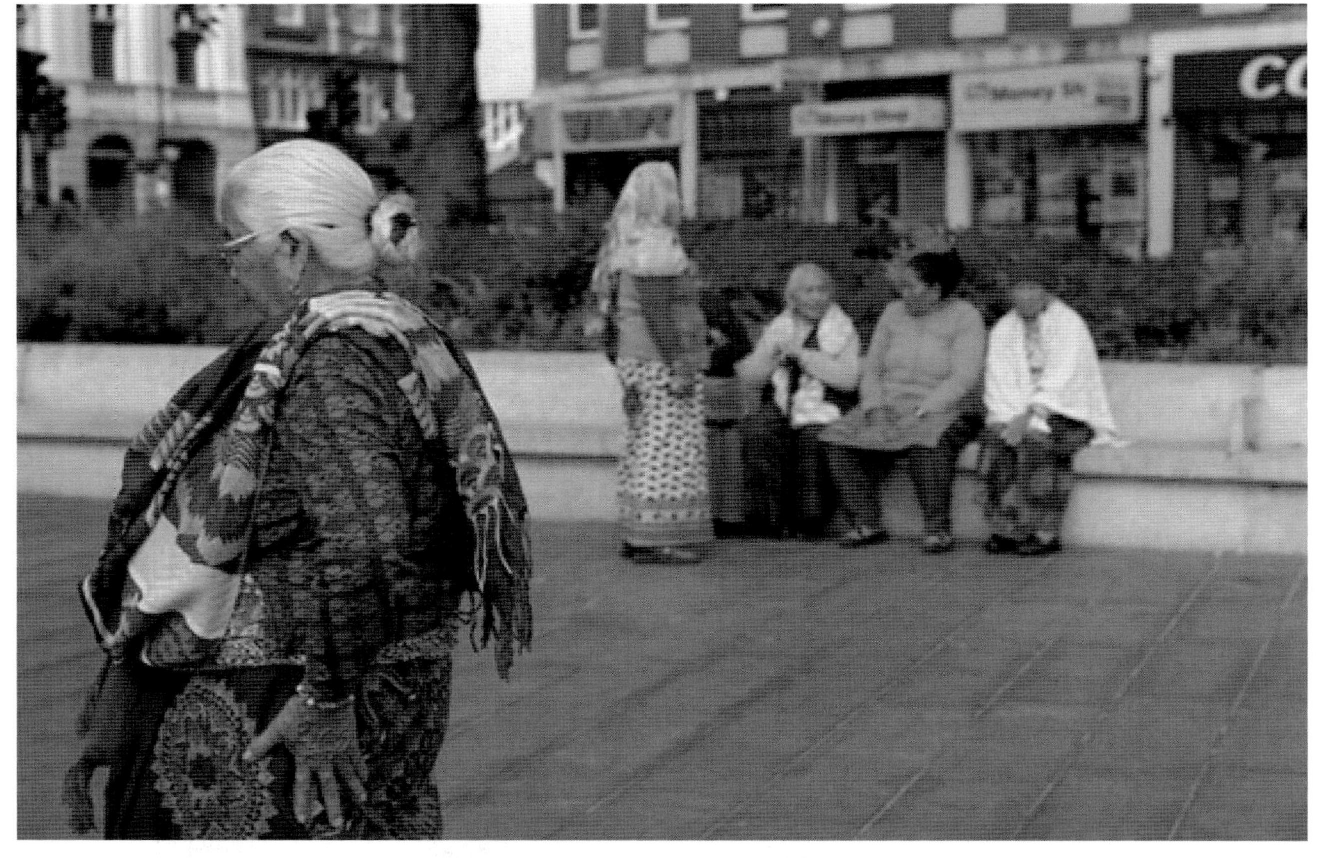

FIGURE 11.5 Nepalese ladies, General Gordon Square, Woolwich

General Gordon Square, Woolwich

"When I sit at home, it's lonely.
There are worries I think of.
But when I come here I watch the TV,
Or cars passing by, or people walking,
And I forget about issues at home.
It feels peaceful here."

– *Till Sana*

"It's a good place to like,
Get away from things and sit and think."

– *Lauren*

"Being out here in the park,
You can actually feel a little bit more
. . . free.
. . . I'm here most days . . .
The atmosphere is a lot better than what it was,
A few years ago"

– *Roy*

"I'm from Nepal.
Some people are nice
They say 'Morning' when they pass us
So we say 'Morning' as well.
If we knew how to speak English,
We could be friends with others.
We would have really liked to socialize with others,
But can't.
We have cried because of the language."

– *Till Sana*

"People come here to shop,
People come here to have coffee,
People come here to go t'pubs,
People come here and watch telly
. . . or like us,
You just come here to chill.
And we come here hanging with friends,
Chill out, and that's it really, init,
That's it really.
. . . if you spent longer than a week in Woolwich, yeah

You would see so much stuff,
You'd just see everything"

– Fitz and Ali

"A while ago, while we were here just looking,
Somebody was stabbed just there.
The police immediately came and took the perpetrators away.
It's good here.
Help comes fast."

– Till Sana

St Helier Open Space, Sutton

"It makes me feel happy,
Because I'm out with my friends.
I'm not indoors, like,
Stuck playing with my X-Box and stuff"

– Owen

"People will go and use benches all the time,
And it is, I think it is a social meeting point . . .
And it can sort your day out.
You think, right, this is what you've got to do . . .
Without benches everyone would be a bit more,
Lost.
They wouldn't talk as much.
It's good, old-fashioned face-to-face chat."

– Philip

"We just live nearby.
So whenever we pass by here.
She go's on here.
Actually it's good for her.
Because she's got autism, so,
For us,
It's really beneficial.
She loves, because of the sense issue.
She takes off her shoes, she likes to be on the grass."

– Margaret, talking about her daughter Khusi

"Does you good to get out, don't it?
Better that staying in sitting indoors, init?
Watching the television all day."

– Peggy

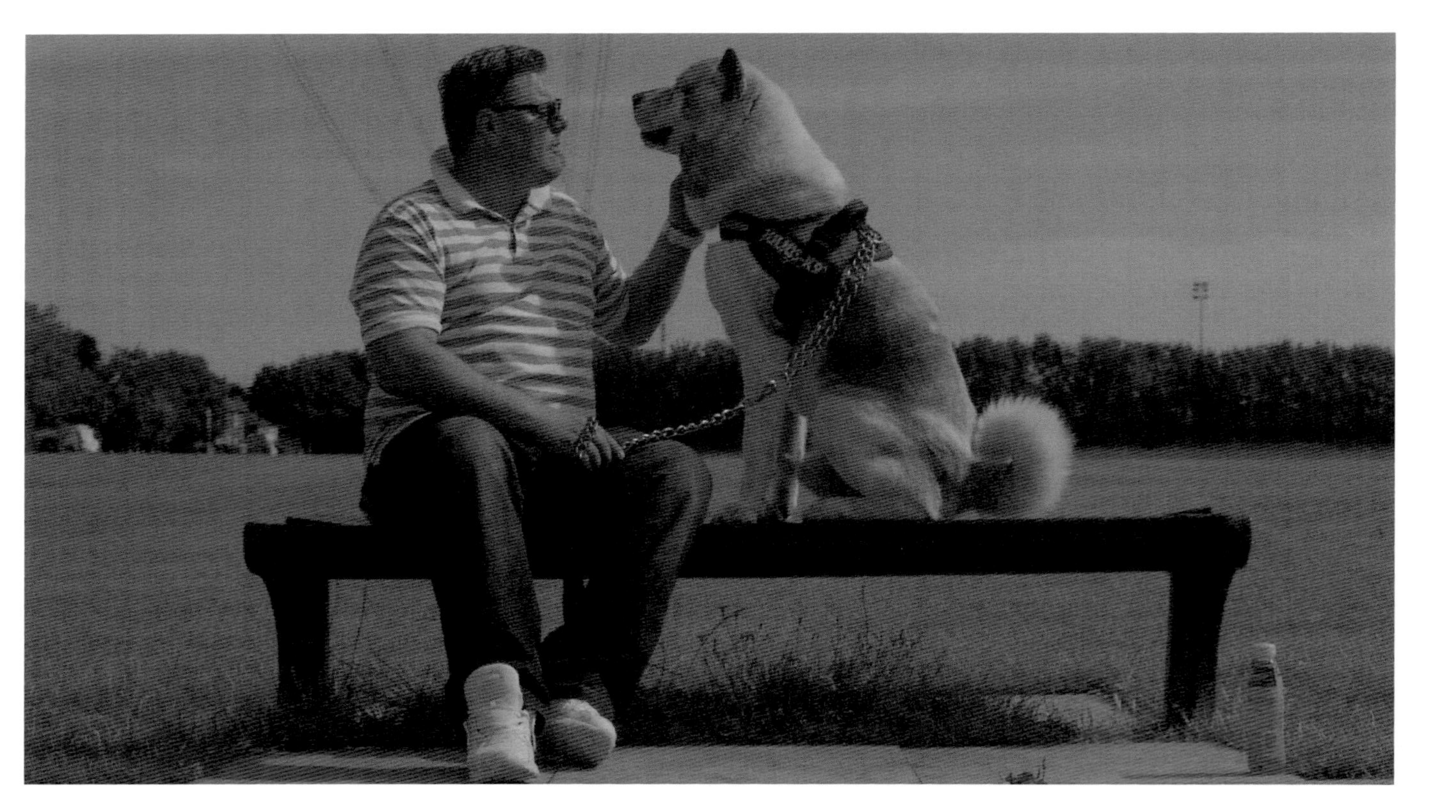

FIGURE 11.6 Philip, St Helier Open Space, Sutton

"She sits sometimes for . . .
On this bench for some time.
I think outdoors is better for her.
That makes them calm.
So they like to be in a place like this."

– Margaret, talking about her daughter Khusi

"Well I must have been four,
And my brother was coming up for a year,
And we moved in round the corner there
But nothing of this was here.
The field was here,
And that was a field.
It was very nice
I thought it was heaven living out here after living in the middle of London,
You know."

– Joy

Conclusion

Creating the film *Alone Together: The Social Life of Benches* for this research allowed for a different layer of engagement and understanding of research data traditionally written as a report. Film allows social data to be brought to life in an immediate way that permits an emotional reaction. The film gives life to the voices of those that used the research locations daily – voices that may otherwise have gone unheard. The work shows, in both visual and aural form, the need for such places of public respite for all sections of society.

On completion of the film there was an end-of-project screening and party held in each community location to which contributors were invited, in addition to local residents, support groups, including Age Concern, Sutton Vision, mental health organisations and local MPs, councillors and policy makers. These forums provided a space for contributors, and the research team to engage in further dialogue about the research aims, discuss how the film revealed new insight into and understanding of the importance of outdoor spaces for people, on multiple levels. Verbal feedback at these events stated that the use of film was an evocative and immediate method of really showing and experiencing the locations, and allowed one to be closer to people's concerns and points and view – film embodying an emotive and personal response. There were audience members who expressed how they were physically moved by the portraits in the film and made them think about public space in a new light.

Each contributor received a copy of the final film on DVD within a designed slipcase (Figure 11.7). The booklet articulated the filmmaking and research process. The *Benches for Everyone* research report, available as a hard or electronic

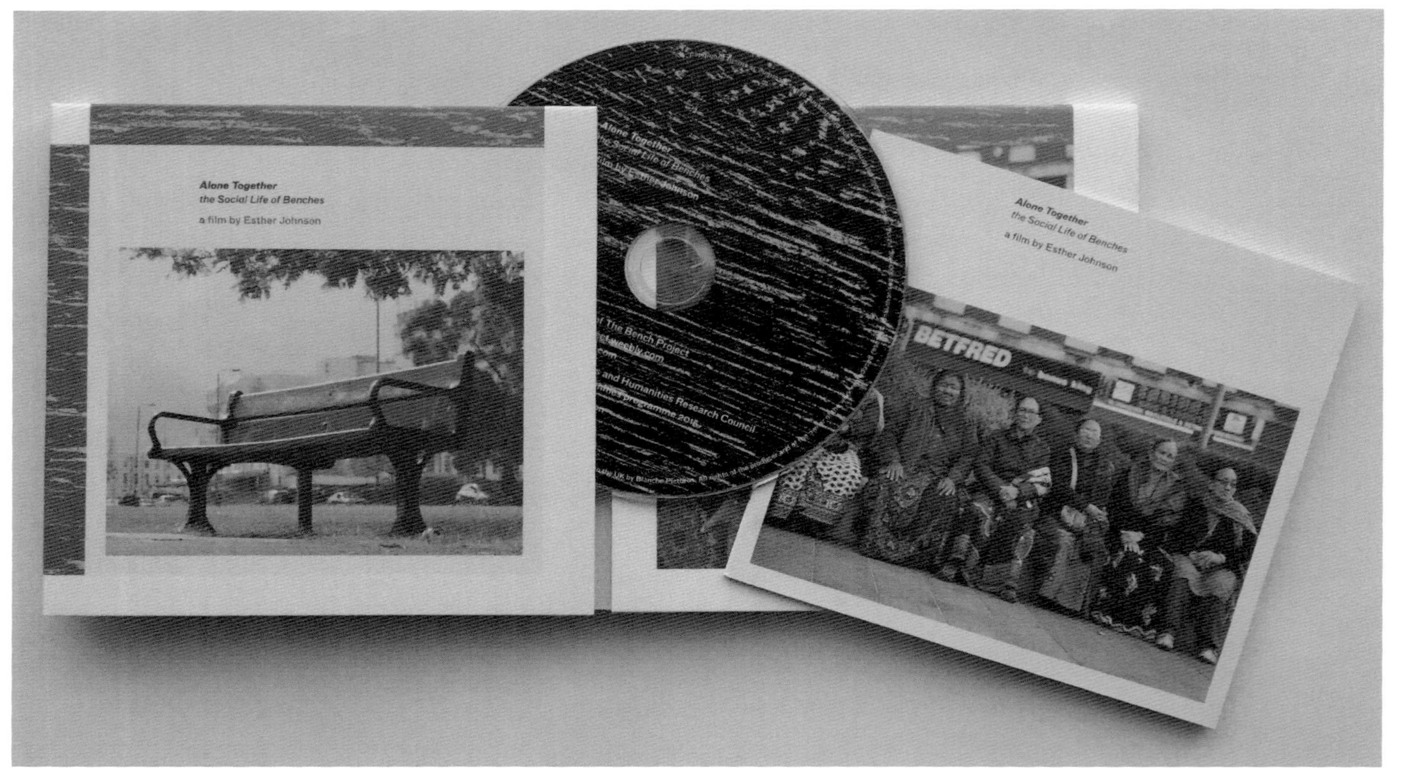

FIGURE 11.7 Souvenir DVD and booklet

copy, was also handed-out at these screenings. The report includes production film stills and interview quotes, and social, geographic, and design research undertaken for the project.

The film has since been screened in multiple contexts, including: academic institutions, art galleries, community groups, conferences, film festivals, museums and research groups. The research findings have continued to be promoted with professionals involved in policy development for: well-being; mental health; community engagement and safety; landscaping and planning.

After the completion of the eighteen-minute film and the initial screenings, a short, four-minute, version of the film focusing on the Nepali community was produced (www.nowness.com/story/alone-together-the-social-life-of-park-benches-esther-johnson). This edit allowed for a short introduction to the project, and as the Nepali community had expressed how sorry they felt at not being able to communicate with others in the square due to the language barrier, it felt appropriate that wider access to their story and experience was made available online. This edit also extended on the intensive work that the Greenwich Inclusion Project had undertaken with them, through photography workshops, language lessons, well-being and social care support.

Acknowledgements

The author would like to thank the Arts and Humanities Research Council; the Art and Design Research Centre, Sheffield Hallam University for supporting this research; her research colleagues; and all the contributors to this project.

References

Johnson, E. (2015) *Alone Together: The Social Life of Benches (documentary film)*, BP028, DVD and booklet. Available at www.nowness.com/story/alone-together-the-social-life-of-park-benches-esther-johnson.

Jung, C. (1960) *Synchronicity: An Acausal Connecting Principle*, Princeton, NJ: Princeton University Press.

Lynd, S. (1993) Oral history from below, *Oral History Review* 21 (1) (Spring): 1–8.

Prial, F. J. (1992) At lunch with: Studs Terkel; "Everyone Around Here Knows Me", *New York Times*, 6 May 1992. Available at www.nytimes.com/books/99/09/26/specials/terkel-lunch.html.

Rishbeth, C. & Bynon, R. (2015) *Benches for Everyone: Solitude in Public, Sociability for Free*. Available at http://the-bench-project.weebly.com/research.html

Rishbeth, C. & Rogaly, B. (2017) Sitting outside: conviviality, self-care and the design of benches in urban public space. *Transactions of the Institute of British Geographers, ISSN 0020-2754*. Available at http://onlinelibrary.wiley.com/doi/10.1111/tran.12212/full.

Thompson, E. P. (1966) History from below, *The Times Literary Supplement*, 7 April 1966, pp.279–280.

Thompson, E. P. (1991) *The Making of the English Working Class*, Toronto: Penguin Books.

Additional internet sources

http://the-bench-project.weebly.com.
https://connected-communities.org/index.php/project/the-bench-project.
https://griproject.org.uk, last accessed 4th February 2018.
www.gp-b.com/woolwich-squares, last accessed 4th February 2018.
www.nfb.ca/playlist/fogo-island, last accessed 4th February 2018.
https://sel.fas.harvard.edu, last accessed 4th February 2018.
https://youngfoundation.org, last accessed 4th February 2018.

12

PATHWAYS TO WELL-BEING

Richard Coles, Sandra Costa and Sharon Watson

Frameworks of disciplinary practice and academic enquiry

We start this discussion by considering the frameworks surrounding well-being investigation evident within each chapter. These frameworks are defined by the context of the investigation, the disciplinary or academic focus behind each and the professional practices implicated. The academic/practitioner dialogue inherent in each chapter is unique in presenting strong frameworks which can be considered in terms of existing practice or developing good practice. The frameworks are further defined by the methodologies involved and the user group targeted, plus the underpinning theory or the niche of theoretical development to which the studies contribute.

Taking account of the complexity of each framework and how each is underpinned by supporting literature, the reader will be aware that several chapters cite the same material in exploring theory, but within different disciplinary contexts. We consider this an advantage since it allows the reader to make connections between different strands of literature and different areas of practice. The practical circumstances surrounding each exploration make this task particularly valuable. Frameworks are also identified by the remit of the organisation (or discipline) involved. The reader is thus able to identify, with some confidence, the framework behind each chapter the disciplines involved, the context of exploration, the nature of the professional interface with well-being and the stance being taken. This also allows the reader to interrogate the material in relation to their own identity or circumstances.

These frameworks are also defined by the user group or participants in the study and the environment in which they are undertaken, outside, inside, leisure, work, health care, the internet and e-interface, to give a good representation of the diverse circumstances and niches that are being explored by researchers and practitioners. This also shows the variety of disciplines who are considering or applying their professional and organisational experience within the specifics of well-being and thus evaluating and defining their area of practice; supporting case studies and examples are evident in the chapters. As identified, these circumstances represent real-life situations, i.e. lived experiences. The combination of material and the context of each chapter thus presents a spectrum of experience which spans a range of life situations and circumstances although related primarily to urban based activities. It also demonstrates how the move to an alternative paradigm of supporting well-being is being driven by bottom up approaches and increasingly reflected in national policy.

The work of The Children's Society

An investigation of children's well-being seems a fairly critical consideration in understanding how well-being is defined and experienced by children (McGoldrick, 1991), and as identified by Pople et al. (Chapter 1), there is a need to qualify general assumptions about well-being which have mainly focused on adults. As such, Chapter 1 introduces *the Five Ways to Well-being* developed by the New Economics Foundation (Aked et al., 2008) and collaboration between the two organisations demonstrates the high profile that well-being is now assuming.

By necessity the *Five Ways to Well-being* is broad but does form a well-researched and valuable framework in which to consider other initiatives and how the *Five Ways* are manifest in specific activities; thus it is likely that studies on well-being will, increasingly, be analysed in relation to the *Five Ways*, for example, Steemers discusses the *Five Ways to Well-being* in considering the professional remit of architects (Steemers, 2015). This is the approach taken by The Children's Society and the parameters identified further validate the *Five Ways* in relation to children's lived experiences.

The approach taken is child-centric (Ergler & Kearns, 2014) and the focus is on everyday activities, where initial enquiry adopts an open questioning methodology to allow the children to raise aspects concerning "what contributes to making life good for them". The extent of the responses demonstrates that children have little difficulty in identifying the specific experiences and relationships which relate to their personal well-being with the later analysis by The Children's Society qualifying the specifics of these relationships and as indicated, how they cross reference the *Five Ways*.

The authors highlight "playing for fun" as outside the *Five Ways*. Play is of course a complex activity but one that engenders positivity and might be related to physical activity, learning and social engagement, aspects which are identified within the *Five Ways*. Play is not an activity much discussed outside child related contexts, it is often considered trivial in an adult context, although this stance is criticised (Spencer et al., 2014) and is discussed later by Treadaway et al. (Chapter 10) in relation to dementia and Compassionate Design.

Comment is also made regarding mindfulness (Keng et al., 2011; Davis & Hayes, 2011) another term which is increasingly being aired in relation to well-being, but which in Western contexts has an association with alternative lifestyles (Sun, 2014). Quotes from the children, included by the authors, affirm that being aware and taking notice are linked to feeling good, i.e. "noticing surroundings", however the chapter also points out that the relationship is one of "diminishing returns". Clearly children are very aware of their progress through the environment as a positive aspect of feeling good, but that over awareness might be indicated as a qualifying factor and it is interesting to speculate if this could be associated with aspects such as anxiety, e.g. feeling unsafe, findings which are indicated in other studies regarding childhood use of their local environments (Ergler & Kearns 2014; Carroll et al., 2014).

The authors conclude that: "Association between everyday activities and children's well-being does not in itself provide evidence of a causal link, although it is plausible that they do . . . encouraging children to engage in these activities may lead to improvements in their well-being." The findings in this chapter thus guide others in opportunities to embed well-being potential through the design of places and cities which takes account of children's lived experiences and the user interface.

Designing for well-being

Taking the lead from this initial chapter it is clear that all chapters consider the user and user interface in respect of supporting or understanding well-being, but two chapters (2 & 6) consider in more detail the actual design process or education of professionals, both showing innovation in approach and in responding to the well-being agenda.

As a guide, Table 12.1 summarises several design concepts discussed in different chapters, but it is co-design and empathic design approaches which are considered in this section. Biophilic Design, explored by Calabrese and Dommert, takes its theory from the concept of biophilia and is considered after reviewing the therapeutic impact of nature; Compassionate Design is an approach developed by Treadaway regarding her work on supporting dementia sufferers so properly belongs to this chapter and is discussed later.

From these examples, in the context of developing pathways to well-being, it is possible to identify some principles regarding engaging with users or supporting the user to access a service, be it a designed service based on e-assisted technology (Chapter 2), an Ecosystem Service based on access to nature (Chapter 3), or the education of built environment design professionals (Chapter 6).

The examples given help clarify what constitutes a pathway to well-being and different processes to facilitate alignment with users. While these are developed/applied in very different circumstances, they have the common remit of supporting the well-being of the individual, paying close attention to the lived experience. In this respect, in exploring how individual well-being might be

TABLE 12.1 Design processes and the user interface discussed within chapters

- **Participatory Design:** A design process involving engaging with user groups, but where design decisions are largely taken by the professional (see Chapter 2).
- **Co-Design:** The design process is characterised by all stakeholders equally contributing to the process through a range of engagement procedures to develop effective solutions founded upon user experience and knowledge of the user interface (see Chapter 2, Holliday et al.).
- **Empathic Design:** Characterised by the engagement with wider society or groups where the designers or the design team undergo the same experience as the potential end users and thus become aligned and sensitised to their experiences and emotional state (see Chapter 6, Amrit Phull).
- **Biophilic Design:** An approach which draws its inspiration from the positive effect of nature on the human being and thus the natural affinity of human beings to align themselves or seek out contact with nature, the process thus seeks to reinforce these connections (see Chapter 5, Calabrese & Dommert).
- **Compassionate Design:** A design process that places loving and kindness at the centre of the process, especially regarding vulnerable people and which is personalised, draws on sensory experience, emphasising the moment and encouraging high quality connections (see Chapter 10, Treadaway et al. & compassionatedesign.org.uk).

supported, i.e. establishing a pathway, there are principles that can be applied or translated to wider situations. For example, from our own research in considering the restorative effect of nature, there are critical pathways concerning perceptions of safety, physical and visual access, where and how nature is presented and in what form (Coles & Bussey, 2000; Coles & Caserio, 2015). Accordingly, effective pathways are grounded by an informed approach regarding the user interface and access to that provision.

Chapter 2 explores in detail the Co-Design process regarding the creation of tools and methodologies to generate support services leading to product development, specifically in terms of the elderly, where Assistive Living Technology (ALT) is to be delivered through an "e-interface". The examples presented purposely show both failures and successes and that technological excellence alone, i.e. reflecting state of the art, needs to be assessed in terms of the user interface.

The broader context of Chapter 2 is health care provision and the move towards services and technology that can be accessed by the individual to suit their specific needs when required, in a way that suits the user requirements and understanding the opportunities that may be present. The future of health care and the provision of support services and tools in supporting well-being is in itself most interesting, but specific aspects of the design process identified by Holliday et al. and thus pathway creation are worth highlighting:

- Identifying stakeholders or the wider stakeholder community which is implicated, i.e. the intended recipients of the technology, and those that interface with the target group, e.g. the family.

- Customer Journey Mapping and the development of a persona, in this case a fictitious persona which visualises or models the life characteristics of the target user group.
- The identification of touchpoints where users are identified as likely to interface with the provision, or which represent a potential interface.

Holliday et al. construct the fictitious persona of "Ada". Using this persona the design team is able to visualise "what aspects were most important in future service possibilities"; a process illustrated by Customer Journey Maps. The Journey Maps "focus primarily on the customers' perspectives", but leads onto the identification of "touchpoints" where users are likely to interface with the service provision. As discussed earlier, while the idea of Customer Journey Mapping and touchpoints are considered in relation to the Service Design, their translation to other situation would seem appropriate in critically assessing the potential to establish an effective accessible well-being pathway.

Developing empathy

Holliday et al. demonstrate a set of design approaches which involves the modelling of a customer persona, a process which ensures alignment with the end user and reflects lived experience, but Phull (Chapter 6), considers more specifically the wider responsibilities and ethical principles of professionals, in this case architects, and a programme of training that ensures sensitisation to such.

Central to the approach is "how people conduct their lives learning about each other as humans". The process is additionally described as "co-mentorship", "entering into another's being and coming to know what they feel and think" (see also Chapter 2). Empathic Design thus "presents a pathway of practice through experiential transition and prompts connection". The process enables both participants and designers to widen their comfort zones, engage in open discussion and access related emotional states, i.e. those inherent when discussing well-being. The location of events is significant involving real everyday places, coffee shops, parks, a range of activities and the variety of locations and modes of engagement clearly involves different bodily senses, sensations and emotional states. As such, the professional enters the world of the potential end user and through a series of tasks or events shares a common experience developing a mutual understanding of each other and in particular experiences the world through the eyes of the users. Thus the designer actually adopts or empathises with the personae of the wider user community with consequent impact on the design process.

An empathic response and a shift to Empathic Design, would seem to indicate "a natural synergy with well-being" involving a re-centring of professional approaches towards society in general, accountability, sustainability and the consequences of their actions. Through this approach, Phull discusses how diverse student cohorts with disparate philosophies and approaches are able to interface with publics that may have equally diverse profiles and their lived experiences.

As Phull states: "The simple design of the group has allowed for an open discussion of well-being at the university and for each individual to feel as if they can have agency within creating it."

Nature related pathways – therapeutic interaction with nature

The impact of accessing nature on mental and physical health has received considerable attention with a range of health indicators employed to validate findings and which are discussed in Chapters 3, 4 and 5. Accordingly, access to natural environments is fast becoming a recognised part of health prescribing with the adage The Natural Health Service adopted in the UK as an alternative for the acronym NHS (the National Health Service).

Access to nature as a pathway to good health is underpinned by a range of theories, explored in these chapters, foremost of which is ART (Attention Restoration Theory). The term refers to restoration to a calm mental state from the stressed state caused by modern urban living which is relieved by access to nature. However, while physical access to nature invokes ART, views of nature, i.e. from a window, also impact positively and features in Biophilic Design criteria (Chapter 5). Nature can be defined quite widely, e.g. to include urban greenspaces typified by extensive vegetation rather than just wild places (Coles et al., 2013). Designed systems are perfectly capable of providing a positive link to well-being (Coles et al., 2013; Coles & Costa, 2018; Costa & Coles, 2018).

Nature thus presents a key pathway in supporting well-being and can be defined by different modes of engagement (Chapter 5) and accepted as a legitimate health intervention, e.g. in Green Prescribing and the NHS Forest (Chapter 4). However there are qualification regarding how we interface with nature especially safety. Unsafe environments are avoided and for the therapeutic impact to be realised the location must be perceived as safe (Coles & Bussey, 2000; Coles & Caserio, 2015). Also included is the theory of "prospect and refuge" developed by Appleton (1975) which indicates viewing the landscape from a situation of safety, or refuge, as a survival strategy (see also Chapter 5). Purposely the idea of a refuge is introduced here as it is examined further when reviewing later chapters.

Greenspace as infrastructure in the built environment

The extent to which nature is acknowledged as a pathway to good mental and physical health is now recognised in the concept of Ecosystem Services, discussed in detail by Douglas et al. These authors take a critical stance based upon "life-course appraisal" and the different green and blue space requirements pertinent to each life stage, how the ecosystems inherent in green and blue (water-based) spaces are a key urban component critical to city infrastructure. There are similarities here regarding the user interface and touchpoints highlighted from Holliday et al. (Chapter 2), i.e. user identities, how spaces might be accessed, their location, distribution and related factors to introduce a critical design, user focused approach, to the planning of green infrastructure which has health as its goal.

In the context of greenspace planning, Douglas et al. (Chapter 3) identify that it is the buffering effect of greenspaces, their direct impact on air quality and other urban "bads" plus the emotional positivity and role in promoting healthy active health styles in situations that can be accessed by populations as and when desired, which is a recognised pathway in urban development. Urban development might thus be considered as removing the "bads", recognising the "goods" plus retro-fitting the latter to present an effective greenspace interface as a strategy towards sustainable cities where well-being is a key driver and measure of progress. Douglas et al., however, are critical of the different policy silos regarding health, amenity, landscape and planning which currently inhibit integrated development.

Accordingly, from these chapters it is possible to identify "different modes" of nature interaction' related to, how nature is accessed and thus how it is experienced, i.e. the interface (see Calabrese & Dommert, Figure 5.6). Contact with nature is not restricted to physical access. Indirect contact and surrogate representations of nature expand the definition of nature in the context of its potential for mental restoration.

The importance of pathways to health through accessing nature is now well-established and is reflected in a range of health-related terminology including "Green" or "Social" prescribing (Natural England, 2017), the Green Gym® (Betz, 2012) and the NHS Forest, a national programme in the UK to increase the use and quality of greenspace on or near healthcare estates for staff, patients and the local community to use for exercise, rest and relaxation (https://sustainablehealth-care.org.uk; https://nhsforest.org).

The case study of the Queen Elizabeth Hospital (Birmingham, UK) presented by Barry and Blythe (Chapter 4) is one example of the NHS Forest and demonstrates how far nature as a pathway to well-being has become recognised as an integral part of a package of clinical referral, the hospital dealing with acute care and its associated green estate dealing with patient and staff needs for recuperation, and mental restoration.

The second case study presented by Barry and Blythe offers further insights into practice, aptly termed growing pathways, where the processes of food growing, contact with the soil, producing food, seasonal change, indicate a strong biophilic interaction with complex social engagement. These require participants to be aware of conditions, the soil and weather, as well as aspects of sharing of produce and contact with nature. Community urban food growing thus presents a specific mode of interaction. However, despite its potential, it remains isolated from formal urban planning activities, but is now beginning to move more to the centre of policy debate (Coles & Costa, 2018).

Biophilia

The idea of biophilia and Biophilic Design explored by Calabrese and Dommert in Chapter 5 have already been briefly discussed. Biophilia and Biophilic Design are gaining ground as a potentially attractive approach at both local and city scales; several international cities have adopted Biophilic Principles to guide their planning approach signing up as "Biophilic Cities". A Biophilic City thus demonstrates a political will to embrace biophilic ideals and associations, as well as recognising existing biophilic resources (Figure 12.2). The example of Singapore can be highlighted as exceptional in this respect as "A City in a Garden" (biophiliccities.org) where re-naturing is ubiquitous and extends extensively to roof gardens and vertical building surfaces, sometimes referred to as vertical forests (Thorns, 2018). It is interesting to compare Figure 12.2 with Calabrese and Dommert's Biophilic Design Principles (Figure 5.5) and also the *Five Ways to Well-being* regarding the extent to which they are complementary.

At building scale these principles can be translated into a design language to ensure appropriate contact with nature, making explicit where this contact is built in, but also extending ideas to the nature of materials and processes to provide designs which endorse a positive biophilic response. The five Principles of Biophilic Design (Figure 5.5) present a strong context at all scales. At city scale, authorities can undertake an audit to identify the biophilic profile, but also to identify the interface between different aspects of the profile, how they are accessed or might be accessed. There seems no reason why biophilic profiling cannot be taken down to an individual-level to audit a person's lived experience, or could be undertaken on a district level by community groups where there exists much potential for retrofitting greenspace, as the examples described by Barry and Blythe, explore.

Emotional transition

Several chapters explore or include ideas of emotional transition including Sparrow (Chapter 7), Sawang and Guaralda (Chapter 9) and Treadaway et al. (Chapter 10), although each of these chapters is very different in their contexts and of course relate primarily to the individual chapter focus. Emotional transition is indicated in Attention Restoration Theory but the ideas discussed in these three chapters enable us to further interrogate the processes that underpin the formation of a pathway to well-being. Sparrow identifies well-being as "the experience of life going well" (compare to the terminology used by The Children's Society) and his work is considered first.

Sparrow examines well-being in relation to the internet and internet use on emotional well-being and e-coaching. Purposeful engagement with the internet can lead to positivity, i.e. positive well-being outcomes, in that it "enhances personal assessments of social capital" regarding the identity of self (related to the individual's persona). Emphasised is the importance of a positive self-identity, which needs to be and can be reinforced via e-coaching. Sparrow thus introduces us to a range of underpinning theory gleaned from his disciplinary perspective and the dynamics of "self-talk" in the context of e-coaching. E-coaching concentrates on cognition, personal belief, helping the coachee to appraise them in the form of "Positive Emotional Attributes", e-coaching thus consists of a series of planned

TABLE 12.2 Example Biophilic City profiles

City	*Biophilic profile*
Austin Texas (USA)	Nature integrated into the legal and planning process, development that prioritises vegetation, ecosystem function and the human experience, access to a daily dose of nature, connecting children with nature, Neighbourhoods Free Tree Project, 20,000 acres of parkland, 30 miles of urban trails, 38,361 acres of water quality protection, 13,610 acres of habitat preservation, City Code emphasising vegetation and ecosystem management, Imagine Austin Plan.
Birmingham (UK)	Green Living Spaces Plan, linking health and greenspace, mapping Health Improvement Zones, 570 parks, 73,000ha of greenspace; extensive network of accessible canals, Multiple Challenge Ecosystem Services Maps, Natural Capital Planning Tool, Birmingham Green Commission; Nature Improvement Areas; Birmingham Open Spaces Forum; community gardens and allotments.
Singapore	Singapore city motto "Singapore Garden City", changed to "City in a Garden", networks of trails and paths, integration of nature in vertical, spaces, vertical forests, roof gardens, indoor hanging gardens, increase in city greenspace from 36% to 47% over 21 years, National Parks Board, Garden City Fund, internationally famous botanic gardens, Center for Urban Greening and Ecology providing skills training, repository of best practice, Gardens by the Bay leisure destinations, foster pride of ownership of the City's gardens.
Vitoria-Gasteiz (Spain)	High biodiversity index, over 25sq metres greenspace per capita, named as European Green Capital, restoration of greenbelt surrounding the city, Environment Studies Centre, urban ecological gardens promoting urban horticulture, Local food production and consumption, promoting healthy eating and leisure.

Note: the cities are defined by their biophilic attributes or credential plus a commitment to the natural environment through policy or action (for full details see Biophiliccities.org)

computer-generated components that engage proactively. The coachee thus moves to a positive place where positive identity, self, is understood and reinforced. Ideas are explored in detail through the case study.

Self and self-talk

A widening of the discussion surrounding the notion of self and self-talk is useful as self, involving self-talk are attributes shown in other well-being pathways, i.e. indicated in other studies. In this case, these involve both real and virtual biophilic environments, situations involving immersion in real settings or viewing biophilic saturated images. Both images of nature or actual access to nature, have been shown to move individuals to positivity and form a strong context in which to explore self-identity especially when it was accompanied by verbalisation in the form of associated narratives (Costa et al., 2014; Costa & Coles, 2018). In these examples the narration (which participants were asked to include as they accessed nature) demonstrated emotional change and to paraphrase Sparrow's terminology, "enhanced personal assessments of natural capital in relation to self-identity". On the other hand situations associated with negative anti-biophilic features, principally urban generated noise and views, were also assessed but did not lead to any positive emotional change.

These findings and the theory of biophilia suggests that a "biophilic-self" is also indicated, refined by the individual in the experience of places, particularly in childhood (Sobel, 1990; Sebba 1991; Ward Thompson et al., 2008) and is reinforced in appropriate nature associations. The biophilic-self aligns itself to environments which accord with this identity. Biophilic-self and positive self-identity would seem to be components of a strong pathway to well-being with huge potential for developing self-coaching systems based on real environments or e-environments. One can integrate the ideas of eALT (Holliday et al.), Sparrow and Calabrese and Dommert to realise the potential offered.

Restoration in the workplace

Sawang and Guaralda in Chapter 9, explore the positives and negatives of working in modern, typically open-plan office situations regarding the design of an installation that is capable of restoring one from a stressed condition to a restful positive state. The approach has some similarities to other aspects discussed regarding the stress induced by modern environments where the underpinning principles leading to its development as a restorative installation are based on sophisticated interactive technology offering bespoke multisensory experience embodied in nature-based and other situations. The "Aerie" would thus seem to offer access to surrogate biophilic elements via a computer screen as interface, but also with control over different sensations, through touch, light, smell and sound. The Aerie concept is thus designed to offer a personal (tailored) sanctuary facilitating rapid recharge to positive valence (Barrett, 2006), particularly where the individual cannot remove themselves from the work location.

The concept of the Aerie is described in detail with images of the installation, i.e. its size and appearance. While one might think of access to real environment as a restorative force the Aerie concept offers isolation from a stressful situation, immediacy and a bespoke multisensory experience which can be aligned to self, to offer a fine-tuned restorative experience. Additionally, it would seem that the parameters behind its development and the experience of users would substantially advance understanding of technological solutions, the nature of mental restoration, restoration therapy and the parameters which are contextual to personal well-being. It is interesting to speculate on the therapeutic potential of such designs and the potential role of such beyond workplace situations, although this is the niche in which the concept was designed.

Well-being dimensions and dementia

Discussion above has emphasised aspects of cognition, identity, and self, but Chapter 10, by Treadaway et al., takes ideas to a new dimension. Treadaway et al. discuss the situation surrounding well-being and dementia. With dementia, the condition impacts on cognitive ability, perception, memory, behaviour, thus it involves substantial difficulties with communication and seriously impacts on an individual's well-being. In this situation, as Treadaway et al. identify, "well-being must be reframed".

Treadaway et al. emphasise the need for a personal approach that establishes connections and flows related to identity and positivity. The identity of the individual cannot be accessed directly so is uncovered through an understanding of a person's life revealed by those that know them. Connections are re-established by targeting the inherent memory developed by the body through skills and practices stored through the body, especially the hands as "muscle or procedural memory". As explained, procedural memory can be stimulated through tacit hand-crafting activities where recall requires little conscious thought and cause a flow state involving total immersion or absorption in that activity.

Stimulating bodily knowledge requires little reliance on explicit memory, but can target emotional memory to create in the moment experiences needing very little cognitive load, including accessing emotional memory through practical playful activities. Thus feel good moments, identified through body language and facial expressions, are initiated. Treadaway et al. discuss the process in relation to theory and the development of Compassionate Design which emphasises, humour and play, giving examples of interventions which exploit this pathway. The approaches discussed illustrate the innovation being applied within clinical and support situations, the thinking that goes towards the support of dementia sufferers and in particular, the alternative approaches or frameworks that are being developed. Compassionate Design places emphasis on play and being in the moment, the pathways thus developed are both innovative and extremely elegant.

Bodily, procedural memory is also indicated in relation to biophilia. The concept of biophilia (as an innate affinity with nature) would suggest the presence of a basic instinct inherent in body actions, thus to engage with the natural environment needs little cognitive load. Accessing natural environments involves total bodily immersion and the stimulation of multi-senses (Ingold, 2000; Pallasma, 2005; Howes & Pink, 2010) and requires the body to orientate itself to facilitate engagement, touch, smell etc. Biophilia would suggest that the body is programmed to interpret the natural environment, with little load on cognitive memory and, as described by Treadaway et al., causes a flow situation and thus the establishment of a positive flow state. Such appears to be indicated in ART which is experienced as being "in the moment". Access to nature-based environments also has positive impacts on dementia sufferers which suggests that this is the case (Detweiler et al., 2012; Kershaw et al., 2017).

Chilling out

Sawang and Guaralda identify their workplace installation, the Aerie, as a refuge, a place to undergo mental restoration, or chill out. Other aspects associated with mental restoration, discussed above, also indicate the need to get away from the stress of urban life and seek out restorative experiences. In this context we can consider the approach taken by Johnson (Chapter 11) in collecting narratives surrounding the use of benches, what the author calls "the social life of benches".

The humble bench is, of course, a common feature of urban places, but is an invitation to stop, sit down and rest, a place where social engagement takes place and the individual observes the world from a favoured location. There is good evidence from the film, i.e. the quotes given, that these locations and activities do represent a refuge and offer places in which to undertake mental restoration, while it is also possible to consider their locations and the process of observing the scene as conforming to prospect and refuge theory in the way that the individual is positioned in the landscape (see Chapter 5). Johnson identifies filming as an appropriate approach which invites local users to talk about their bench related experiences, to verbalise them, i.e. self-talk, but also, emotional response, empathy and movement into another's world.

The approach of film making thus has features associated with movement to well-being, elicits voice, involves a narrative and explores identity and self, but the bench also has tactile properties which may be enhanced by the orientation of the user. Of course, the provision of benches is specifically undertaken to allow users to enjoy the view, but Johnson's film demonstrates the well-being related activities taking place, i.e. similar to those taking place in other restorative locations or installations. Emphasised by Johnson's approach is the need to examine all aspects of the built environment as a potential well-being resource in that they (as is the case with the bench) actually represent "well-being capital" and that these properties need to be made explicit. In addition, Johnson's approach as a filmmaker, further identifies the importance of considering or adopting diverse methodologies when exploring the well-being interface.

The future, embedding well-being as a common goal

The ideas offered by chapter authors demonstrate our understanding of well-being in different situations and that there are good indications that supporting well-being is becoming more mainstream in relation to different aspects of built environment design and related practice. Well-being is now featured as a measure of human social progress and realised as an appropriate goal featured in policy. However, there is some way to go before it stands equally alongside typical urban development parameters which prioritises economic development as the driver, but here we can consider the discussion by Davies (Chapter 8).

The *Well-being of Future Generations (Wales) Act 2015* establishes a right for future generations that is capable of being reinforced through the courts. Davies discusses the implications of the Act and how it is enforced exploring the duties placed upon public bodies; importantly, it recognises well-being and the rights of future generations, plus policing through the appointment of a "Future Generations Commissioner, the guardian of the interests of future generations".

Davies critically explores the powers of the Future Generations Commissioner but also identifies some of the weaknesses. For example, he lists the public bodies in Wales to which the Act applies. They include local authority, health, education, national parks, arts and sports councils as well as museums and libraries. The majority of these sectors are already exploring and supporting aspects of well-being, although the critical aspect of safeguarding the interests of future generations is not usually explicit. However, it does seem that the shift is gaining momentum fuelled by the reality of practice. For example Phull's discussion of training architects clearly impacts upon future generations, while The Children's Society exploration of childhood experiences related to well-being indicates obvious interest in investing in children's well-being futures.

Thus the Act adds to the consideration of duty, responsibility, obligations and the collective nature of this obligation. The Act would seem to demand a more unified approach to considering future generations and the actions of the public bodies identified should lead to greater coordinated approaches and invites these bodies to look for synergies between their approaches, as Davies identifies to make well-being "a central organising principle". Increasingly, these synergies are becoming identified forming a raft of activities, approaches and provision that cross different sectors.

Concluding remarks

A good starting point is to quote Davies once more where well-being is becoming "a central organising principle" crossing professional divides and there is substantial evidence that this is becoming so with professions and authorities aligning themselves to the well-being agenda and through their activities, exploring what supporting well-being actually means. In the UK, for example, the ways that interaction with greenspace has become recognised as part of health care provision within the National Health Service in supporting physical and mental health, is moving towards the norm. In other areas, including design, there are practice related pathways, substantiated by theories, which are advocated as best practice (Calabrese & Dommert, Chapter 5; Phull, Chapter 6).

Accordingly we see the development of pathways which, when analysed, show some consistency in the way that they operate, but originate from quite diverse perspectives. Pathways are represented across professional divides but also operate within policy levels. For well-being to become embedded as an organising principle needs political will and as Davies discusses, a supporting legislative framework.

However, what is significant is that, internationally, cities are beginning to express a pride in their green infrastructure and its relationship to well-being in supporting citizens and in initiatives that serve to ensure salutogenic environments, subscribing to the notion of a Biophilic City (Table 12.2).

In collating the chapters, we purposely identified approaches ranging from identifying well-being related activities, therapeutic impact of greenspace, principles of Biophilic Design through to restorative interventions and installations that provide a refuge away from stress. It appears that these might be as simple as the humble bench, with the pathway indicated clearly linking to existing concepts of landscape perception which were explored earlier. The importance of the natural world in the design of and access to salutogenic environments is clearly identified and in reality does not present any problems in their design as they are an extension of existing practice; they can be designed into urban environments including retrofitting. What needs more consideration is how such are made available and accessed in order to maximise therapeutic potential. There are implications of life stages (Douglas et al., Chapter 3) but also how associated activities, such as urban gardening (Barry & Blythe, Chapter 4) further define a well-being pathway. Yet, in many locations it has been found that these types of green related activities are still not recognised in conventional planning models (Coles & Costa, 2018). The importance of understanding the interface, the stakeholder community, developing empathic approaches to design are well demonstrated in the various chapters.

Discussion concerning self, identity and emotional transition help to explain the processes that occur, including measures that assist the individual process the information by accentuating the positive impact of the experience. For example, in the context of everyday environments, we have undertaken self-narrated walks in local parks where volunteers from the local community verbalised their walking experience (Costa & Coles, 2018). These resulted in clear emotional transition, endorsement of a positive self and reinforcement of identity. This is only one such supportive intervention, filming is clearly another (Johnson, Chapter 11); community made films and local walking initiatives are well within the scope of current practice. It is in these aspects that the arts, humanities and design professions excel and can help individuals to learn to effectively interface with well-being resources. Neither is the resource restricted to the physical environment. Discussion on eALT (Holliday et al., Chapter 2), e-coaching (Sparrow, Chapter 7) demonstrate pathways that can be developed via an internet interface and the principles inherent in their design.

The authors of the chapters contained within this book have taken the step to align their work and investigate their professional roles in the context of well-being, encouraging others to do the same, with highly significant results. This has resulted in a realisation that their professional activities impact upon well-being outcomes, leading them to become immersed in the new paradigm of well-being futures and thence act as advocates. This is a situation that we are happy to endorse and encourage others to take the same pathway as well-being becomes a central organising principle for future city development.

References

Aked, J., Marks, N., Cordon, C. & Thompson, S. (2008) *Five Ways to Well-being: A Report Presented to the Foresight Project on Communicating the Evidence Base for Improving People's Well-being*, London: New Economics Foundation.

Appleton, J. (1975) *The Experience of Landscape*, London: John Wiley & Sons.

Barrett, L. F. (2006) Valence is a basic building block of emotional life, *Journal of Research in Personality* 40 (2006): 35–55.

Betz, A. (2012) People-powered health – co-creating a new story of health, *BHMA Journal of Holistic Health* 9 (3), December.

Carroll, P., Asiaiga, L., Tava'e, N. & Witton, K. (2014) Kids in the city: Differing perceptions of one neighbourhood in Aotearoa/New Zealand, in R. W. Coles & Z. Millman (eds.), *Landscape, Well-being and Environment*, London: Routledge, pp.129–146.

Coles, R. W. & Bussey, S. C. (2000) Urban forest landscapes in the UK, progressing the social agenda, *Landscape and Urban Planning* 52 (92–93): 181–188.

Coles, R. W. & Caserio, M. (2015) *Social Criteria for the Evaluation and Development of Urban Green Spaces. EU Report Number: D7 EVK4-CT-2000-00022*. Available at www.researchgate.net.

Coles, R. W. & Costa, S. (2018) Food growing in the city: Exploring the productive urban landscape as a new paradigm for inclusive approaches to the design and planning of future urban open spaces, *Landscape and Urban Planning* 170: 1–5.

Coles, R. W., Millman, Z. & Flanningan, J. (2013) Everyday environmental encounters, their meaning and importance for the individual, *Urban Ecosystems* 16: 819–839.

Costa, S. & Coles, R. (2018) The self-narrated walking. A user-led method to research people's experiences in urban landscapes, *Landscape Research*. Available at doi: 10.1080/01426397.2018.1467004.

Costa, S., Coles, R. & Boultwood, A. (2014) Walking narratives: interacting between urban nature and self, in C. Sörensen & K. Liedtke (eds.), *SPECIFICS: Discussing Landscape Architecture*, Berlin: Jovis. pp.40–43.

Davis, D. M. & Hayes, J. A. (2011) What are the benefits of mindfulness? A practice review of psychotherapy related research, *Psychotherapy* 48 (2): 198–208.

Detweiler, M. B., Sharma, T. & Kim, K. Y. (2012) What is the evidence to support the use of therapeutic gardens for the elderly, *Psychiatry Investigation* 9 (2): 100–110.

Ergler, C. & Kearns, R. (2014) Children as explorers: revealing children's views on well-being in intensifying urban environments, in R. W. Coles & Z. Millman (eds.), *Landscape, Well-being and Environment*, London: Routledge, pp.184–199.

Howes, D. & Pink, S. (2010) The future of sensory anthropology/the anthropology of the senses, *Social Anthropology* 18 (3): 331–340

Ingold, T. (2000) *The Perception of the Environment: Essays on Livelihood, Dwelling and Skill*, London: Routledge.

Keng, S. L., Moria, J. & Robins C. J. (2011) Effects of mindfulness on psychological health: a review of empirical studies, *Clinical Psychology Review* 31 (6): 1041–1056.

Kershaw, C., McIntosh, J., Marques, B., Cornwall, J., Stoner, L. & Wood, P. (2017) A potential role for outdoor, interactive spaces as a healthcare intervention for older persons, *Perspectives in Public Health* 137 (4).

McGoldrick, D. (1991) The United Nations convention on the rights of the child, *International Journal of Law, Policy and Family* 5 (2): 132–169.

Natural England (2017) *Good Practice in Social Prescribing for Mental Health, the Role of Nature Based Interventions, Natural England Publications, Report NECR228*. Available at www.naturalengland.org.uk.

Pallasma, J. (2012) *The Eyes of the Skin: Architecture and the Senses*, third edition, New York: John Wiley and Sons.

Sebba, R. (1991) The landscapes of childhood: the reflection of childhood's environment in adult memories and in children's attitudes, *Environment and Behavior* 23 (4): 395–422.

Sobel, D. (1990) A place in the world: adults' memories of childhood's special places, *Children's Environments Quarterly* 7 (4): 5–12. Available at www.jstor.org/stable/41514753?seq=1#page_scan_tab_contents.

Spencer, B., Williams, K., Mahdjoubi, L. & Sara, R. (2014) Third places for the third age: the contribution of playable space to the well-being of older people, in R. W. Coles & Z. Millman (eds.), *Landscape. Well-being and Environment*, London. Routledge, pp.109–128.

Steemers, K. (2015) Architecture for well-being and health, *Daylight and Architecture* 23 (Spring): 6–27. Available at http://thedaylightsite.com/architecture-for-well-being-and-health/.

Sun, J. (2014) Mindfulness in context: a historical discourse analysis, *Contemporary Buddhism* 15 (2): 394–415.

Thorns, E. (2018) Stefano Boeri Architetti's Vertical Forest is the very first to be used in social housing, *Archdaily*, 10 January 2018. Available at www.archdaily.com/886899/stefano-boeri-architettis-vertical-forest-is-the-very-first-to-be-used-in-social-housing/>, last accessed 1 February 2018.

Ward Thompson, C. (2007) Playful nature: what makes the difference between some people going outside and others not? In C. Ward Thompson & P. Travlou, *Open Space, People Space*, London: Taylor & Francis, pp.23–37.

Ward Thompson, C., Aspinall, P. & Montarzino, A. (2008) The childhood factor: adult visits to green places and the significance of childhood experience, *Environment and Behavior* 40: 111–143.

INDEX

Note: page numbers in italics refer to the figure or table on the page.